AI and Digital Health Technology in Animal Health Care and Welfare

NIPA® GENX ELECTRONIC RESOURCES & SOLUTIONS P. LTD.
New Delhi-110 034

About the Editors

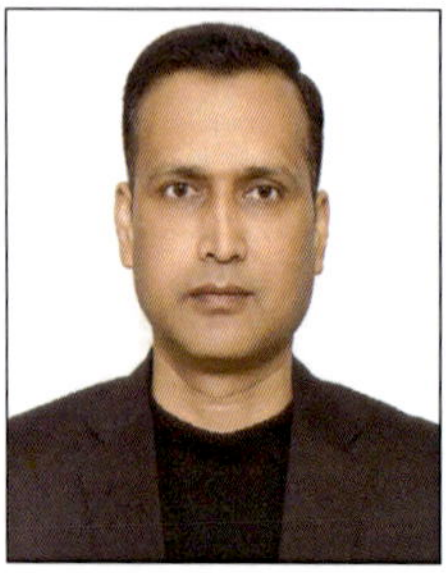

Professor (Dr.) S. R. Upadhyay did his BVSc & AH from Nagpur Veterinary College, Maharashtra, India in the year 2000. MVSc in Veterinary Medicine from Veterinary College Anjora, Durg (under I.G.K.V, Raipur, Chhattisgarh, India) in the year 2003 and subsequently Ph.D. in Veterinary Medicine from Faculty of Veterinary Sciences and Animal Husbandry Sher-E-Kashmir University of Agriculture Sciences Jammu J & K, India in the year 2015. Dr. Upadhyay started his Carrier as Research Associate at prestigious Centre for Animal Disease Research and Diagnosis, Indian Veterinary Research Institute, Izatnagar, Bareilly, Uttar Pradesh, India. At present he is working as Professor of Veterinary Medicine at Faculty of Veterinary Sciences and Animal Husbandry, Sher-E-Kashmir University of Agriculture Sciences, Jammu, J & K, India and Heading Division of Veterinary Animal Husbandry Extension Education.

Dr. Upadhyay has more than 22 years of teaching, research and extension experience. He has more than 80 publications to his credit in various national and international journals of repute. Apart he is also author and co-author of 10 books/ research monographs/manuals and had also written approximately 19 chapters in books. He also presented more than 49 research papers in various national and international conferences and received more than 10 best paper/poster presentation awards. He has guided 04 MVSc and 01 Ph.D. student so far as major advisor and member in advisory committee of 10 PG/PhD students. Dr. Upadhyay is recipient of merit cum mean scholarship in graduation, honours in post graduation and merit scholarship in his Ph.D. Dr Upadhyay has been conferred with Fellow of Academy of Science for Animal Welfare and highly prestigious DC Blood Gold Medal and Professor Sushovan Roy Gold Medal for Best Teacher in Veterinary Medicine by Indian Society for Veterinary Medicine for his outstanding contribution in Veterinary Medicine. Apart, he has also been conferred with Young Scientist Award by Council for Science and Technology, Government of Chhattisgarh, India for his outstanding research in master's degree. He has also been conferred with Young Scientist Award by Indian Society for Veterinary Medicine and Indian Association for Advancement of Veterinary Research. He is recipient of Appreciation award by various professional organisations like ISVM, ISACP, AVDI, VIPM and SBBS. He is life member of various professional and scientific bodies like ISCA, NAVS, IVA, ISVM, ISACP, ISIIP, IAAVR and VCI.

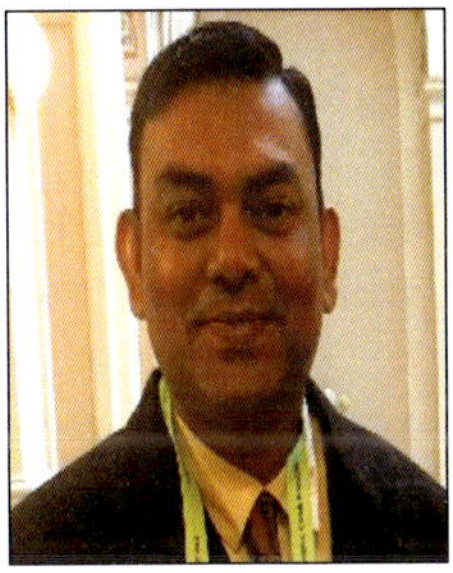

Dr. Hussain's research broadly focused on healthcare aspects of small, large, and exotic animal species. He has a rich experience in veterinary clinical medicine/mineral and vitamin deficiency disease/endocrine disorders/ zoo animal healthcare research. He has worked on techniques of non-invasive endocrine monitoring including sample workup preparation, performance of enzyme immunoassays (EIA) data collection and interpretation at Endocrine Laboratory Department of Reproduction Biology, Leibniz Institute for Zoo and Wildlife Research (IZW), Berlin, Germany. He has guided 9pg students co guided 30 pg students, 1 Ph.D student and co advisor of 3 Ph.D students. In addition to this, he has more than 20 years of experience in teaching research and extension in veterinary medicine. Dr Hussain published more than 100 papers in international, national journals and Conferences/ Seminars/ Symposiums. He is active member of many international society including American Association of Zoo Veterinarian, Florida United States, European Association of Zoo and Wildlife Veterinarians (EAZWV) and International Primatological Society (IPS). Dr Hussain is a recipient of international recognition Award -Murray Fowler International Conference Scholarship Award instituted by American Association of Zoo Veterinarian. He is fellow of Academy of Science for Animal welfare recipient of Young scientist award by Indian Society for Study of Animal Reproduction (ISSAR), Award of Honour from Soc. of Mob. and Indian Society of Veterinary Medicine Appreciation award.

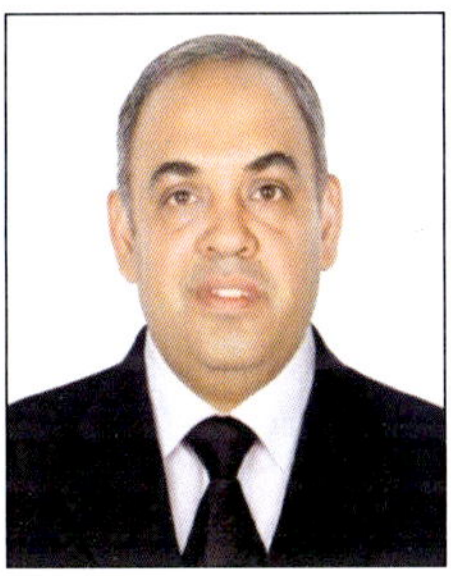

Dr Neelesh Sindhu, Assistant Professor, Veterinary Medicine and working in Department of Veterinary Clinical Complex and also at Haryana Pashu Vigyan Kendra, Jhajjar, Haryana joined the Veterinary Profession in 2000 as Veterinary Student. He completed graduation in 2005 Master's in Veterinary Clinical medicine from CCSHAU Hisar in 2007 and PhD in Veterinary Clinical Medicine in 2010 from COVS, CCSHAU, Hisar. In June, 2010, he joined as Veterinary Surgeon in Govt of Haryana and worked as field Veterinarian for Animal health Care and in December 2013, he joined as Faculty of Veterinary Medicine and is working for welfare of dairy farmers and companion animal owners.

Being associated directly with Farmers and animal owners especially since 2006 (A total experience of more than 18 years) when his Post graduate research started on Staphylococcal mastitis, he has tried his level best to understand the ground reality challenges of farmers and dairy owners and tried level best to solve their issues at their doorsteps. In true spirit of Faculty of Veterinary Medicine his research is associated with practical problems (Lab to Land) so that his students can excel in research, education and animal welfare and care and become inspiration for farmers and animal owners especially dairy farmers. Being having passion to excel in Media along with Veterinary Skills, he is associated with many professional societies as Media Incharge and helped in conduction of webinars and dissemination of knowledge especially during COVID crisis. Being social media Incharge of ISVM, he has been given responsibility to manage Society's Social Media handles to provide information to all members/non-members.

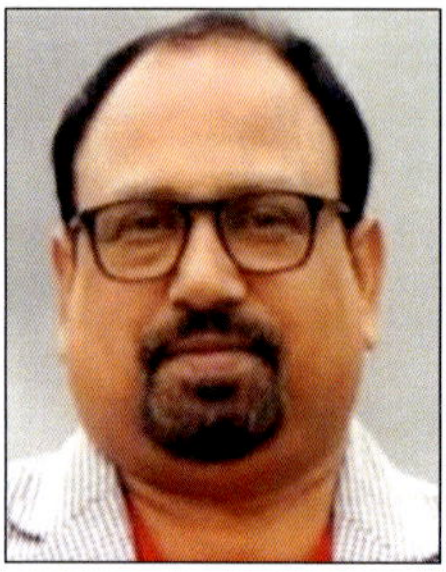

Dr. Pranav Kumar is a Veterinary Extension Education scientist with more than 18 years of experience in government and private sectors. Born in Begusarai, Bihar, he pursued his academic career at prestigious institutions like Sainik School Tilaiya, College of Veterinary Sciences, Hyderabad. He earned his Master Degree in Veterinary Extension Education from Indian Veterinary Research Institute (IVRI) Bareilly and Ph.D. in Veterinary Extension Education from Sher-e-Kashmir University of Agricultural Sciences and Technology (SKUAST), Jammu. Dr. Kumar's professional journey began as a Subject Matter Specialist at PRADAN, an NGO in New Delhi. He later worked in various roles, including Senior Executive at Mother Dairy and Assistant Manager at Hariyali Kisan Bazar. In 2010, he joined Division of Veterinary & Animal Husbandry Extension Education, Faculty of Veterinary Sciences, SKUAST-Jammu as an Assistant Professor and is currently working as Associate Professor.

As an academician, Dr. Kumar has taught various undergraduate and postgraduate courses, guided 11 Masters students, and published 49 research papers. He has developed innovative extension programs, including ICT based web modules on Scientific Dairy Practices, Organic Dairy Farming, Scientific Goat and Broiler Farming. He has also designed and developed several training manuals, extension booklets, and folders on various aspects of animal husbandry for the benefits of farming and scientific community. A prolific writer, Dr. Kumar has authored four books, edited two books, and contributed to 26 book chapters. He has received several awards, including the Best Extension Scientist Award, Fellow Award Young Scientist Award, and Excellence in Extension Award. He is also involved in several externally funded projects as PI and Co-PI. Dr. Kumar is actively involved in extension activities, including training programs, workshops, and Kisan Melas. He is a life member of several professional societies and aims to bridge the gap between the veterinary scientific community and farming community through innovative extension programs. He possesses a never-ending passion for extension outreach and connecting to the people

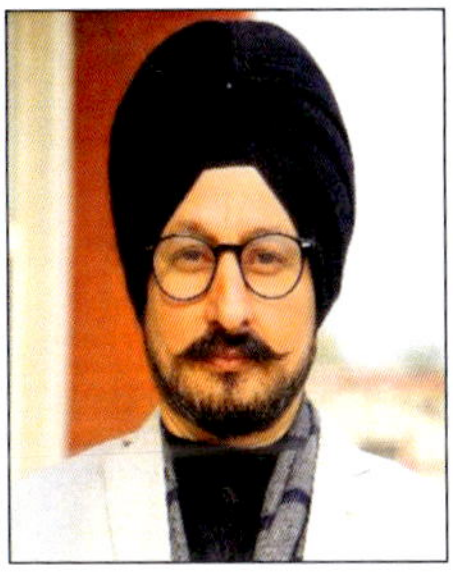

Dr. Mandeep Singh Azad is an animal genetics and breeding scientist with over 13 years of experience in research and innovation in animal sciences. He holds a Ph.D. in Animal Genetics and Breeding from Sher-e-Kashmir University of Agricultural Sciences and Technology of Jammu. His research expertise includes molecular characterization, animal breeding, and genetics. Dr. Azad has received 18 international fellowships and attended 28 fully funded international events. He is currently associated with 10 projects as PI and Co-PI and holds a patent for an IoT-based solar-powered agricultural robot. He has also developed a mobile app with over 10,000 users. With over 100 publications, including research papers, popular articles, and books, Dr. Azad is a prolific writer. He has authored 10 books in English and Hindi and serves as an editor for a scientific periodical. Dr. Azad is a member of 11 international and national scientific organizations and has completed an international project in collaboration with organizations from the UK and Vietnam. As a scientist at SKUAST-Jammu, Dr. Azad has experience running demonstration cum training units, including dairy, poultry, and feed block units. He excels in team-based research, collaborating with national and international researchers, scientists, farmers, and experts.

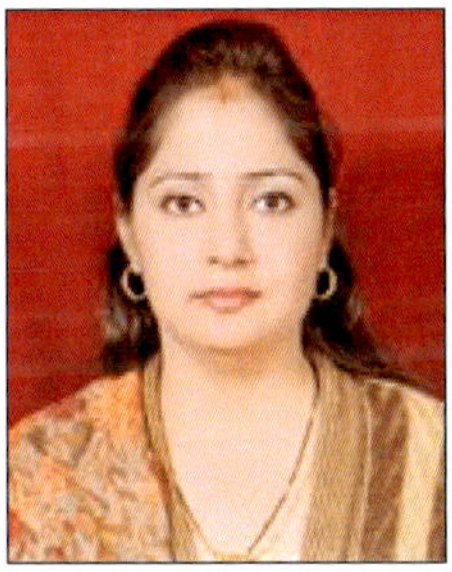

Dr. Shikha Sharma completed her graduation and then master's and PhD in Veterinary Parasitology from SKUAST-Jammu respectively in the year 2009, 2011 and 2016. She is recipient of Young Scientist Award, Merit Scholarship during her doctoral studies & few best paper/poster presentation awards in various national and international conferences. Dr Shikha has more than 10 scientific publications in high impact journals of repute, coauthored two books and presented 10 papers in various conferences. In her brief scientific carrier Dr Shikha has studied zoonotic potential of canine Giardiasis in Jammu district, complexity and pathology of induced hook worm infection in healthy and diabetic murine model and as a junior research fellow she was associated with DBT project to study impact of backyard poultry on socio-economic status of rural population of border area of Jammu. At present she is associated as faculty in private veterinary college in Haryana.

AI and Digital Health Technology in Animal Health Care and Welfare

Editor-in-Chief

S.R. Upadhyay

Professor, Veterinary Medicine
Sher-e-Kashmir University of Agricultural Sciences & Technology-Jammu
Jammu and Kashmir, India

Editors

Kafil Hussain

Professor, Veterinary Medicine
Sher-e-Kashmir University of Agricultural Sciences & Technology-Jammu
Jammu and Kashmir, India

Neelesh Sindhu

Assistant Professor
Lala Lajpat Rai University of Veterinary & Animal Sciences
Hisar, Haryana, India

Pranav Kumar

Associate Professor
Department of Veterinary Extension and Animal Husbandry
Sher-e-Kashmir University of Agricultural Sciences & Technology-Jammu
Jammu and Kashmir, India

Mandeep Singh Azad

Scientist, Directorate of Extension
Sher-e-Kashmir University of Agricultural Sciences-Technology-Jammu
Jammu and Kashmir, India

Shikha Sharma

MR College of Veterinary Sciences and Research Centre
Jhajjar, Haryana, India

NIPA® GENX ELECTRONIC RESOURCES & SOLUTIONS P. LTD.

New Delhi-110 034

NIPA® GENX ELECTRONIC
RESOURCES & SOLUTIONS P. LTD.

101,103, Vikas Surya Plaza, CU Block
L.S.C. Market, Pitam Pura, New Delhi-110 034
Ph : +91-11-43860225, Mob.: +91 9717133558, 9540816132
E-mail: newindiapublishingagency@gmail.com
Website: www.nipaersources.com

Print ISBN: 978-93-58878-47-9

ebook ISBN: 978-93-58871-92-0

Composed and Designed by NIPA®.

Preface

As we stand at the forefront of a new era in animal health care, it is evident that digital health technology and artificial intelligence (AI) are poised to revolutionize the field. The rapid evolution of these technologies has opened up unprecedented opportunities for improving animal health, welfare, and productivity. As editors of this book, we are honored to bring together a diverse group of experts who share our passion for harnessing the potential of digital health technology and AI to transform animal health care.

The book commences with an exploration of digital veterinary medicine and AI, highlighting the potential of these technologies to enhance clinical decision-making and patient outcomes. The authors delve into the realm of digital veterinary medicine, discussing the applications of AI-powered technologies in disease diagnosis, treatment, and prevention. The chapter on reaching the unreached emphasizes the potential of digital health technology and AI to improve animal health care in resource-poor settings, where access to veterinary care is limited.

Clinical decision support systems are a crucial aspect of modern veterinary medicine, and the chapter on clinical decision support using animal data: artificial intelligence and tele-veterinary medicine provides valuable insights into the applications of AI-powered technologies in this realm. The authors discuss the potential of AI-powered clinical decision support systems to enhance patient outcomes, reduce healthcare costs, and improve the overall efficiency of veterinary care.

Veterinary nuclear medicine (VNM) and targeted drug delivery systems for infectious diseases are two areas that hold tremendous promise for improving animal health care. The chapter on VNM and targeted drug delivery systems explores the potential of these technologies to revolutionize the treatment of infectious diseases in animals. The authors discuss the applications of VNM in disease diagnosis and treatment, as well as the potential of targeted drug delivery systems to improve treatment outcomes and reduce side effects.

Climate change and animal health and diseases are two topics that are intricately linked. The chapter on climate change and animal health and diseases provides a comprehensive overview of the impact of climate change on animal health, highlighting the need for urgent action to mitigate the effects of climate change on animal health and welfare.

Antimicrobial resistance is a pressing concern in both human and animal health, and the chapter on antimicrobial resistances in food and companion animals provides a timely and insightful analysis of the issue. The authors discuss the temporal, spatial, and genomic aspects of antimicrobial resistance, highlighting the need for a comprehensive and multifaceted approach to addressing this pressing concern.

The application of modern technology in the health and wellbeing of captive and free-range elephants is an area that holds tremendous promise for improving animal welfare. The chapter on the application of modern technology in elephant health and wellbeing explores the potential of digital health technology and AI to enhance the health and wellbeing of elephants, highlighting the need for further research and development in this area.

A comparative study of AI/ML algorithms for modeling chronic canine epilepsy and enhancing homeopathic interventions provides valuable insights into the applications of AI-powered technologies in veterinary medicine. The authors discuss the potential of AI-powered algorithms to enhance the diagnosis and treatment of chronic canine epilepsy, highlighting the need for further research and development in this area.

Fostering antibiotic stewardship in farming communities is an essential aspect of addressing the pressing concern of antimicrobial resistance. The chapter on fostering antibiotic stewardship in farming communities provides a comprehensive overview of the importance of antibiotic stewardship, highlighting the need for a multifaceted approach to addressing this pressing concern.

The final chapter on smart animal health: transforming animal welfare through digital and AI-powered technologies provides a comprehensive overview of the potential of digital health technology and AI to transform animal welfare. The authors discuss the applications of AI-powered technologies in animal health monitoring, disease diagnosis, and treatment, highlighting the need for further research and development in this area.

In conclusion, this book provides a comprehensive overview of the applications of digital health technology and AI in animal health care and welfare. The chapters provide valuable insights into the potential of these technologies to transform animal health care, highlighting the need for further research and development in this area. We hope that this book will serve as a valuable resource for animal health professionals, researchers, and students who are interested in exploring the applications of digital health technology and AI in animal health care.

We would like to express our gratitude to all the contributors who have made this book possible. We would also like to thank our publisher for their support and guidance throughout the publication process.

Editors

Contents

1

Digital Veterinary Medicine© & Artificial Intelligence Reaching The Unreached

P. Selvaraj

BVSc, PGDBM, MVSc, Ph.D (Clin.Med.), Dip.Regen.Med., Fellow.Regen.Med.
Professor of Clinical Medicine, Professor and Head, Veterinary University Peripheral Hospital, Madhavaram, Tamil Nadu Veterinary and Animal Sciences University (TANUVAS), Chennai, Tamil Nadu
&
Lead PI, ICAR-NASF Project on Artificial Intelligence & IoT based Smart Vet Ecosystem, Department of Veterinary Clinical Medicine, ICAR Centre of Advanced Faculty Training in Veterinary Clinical Medicine, Madras Veterinary College, Vepery, TANUVAS, Chennai, Tamil Nadu

Introduction

In the last decade, digitalization has transformed every aspect of life and society, changing almost every area of our day-to-day lives. Not just that; the rate of change that is happening is astonishing and only going to accelerate further. From the way, we work and communicate to how we organize our lives, digital tools and technologies are everywhere including the veterinary sector. Veterinarians are recognizing the need to depart "the analog island" and increasingly willing to embrace digital solutions. Undoubtedly, digitalization is crucial when it comes to boosting efficiency and quality in veterinary medicine and delivery of animal healthcare to masses across various geographies and resource poor setups. Uniquely these digital tools helps vets also to focus on the needs of patients and animal owners.

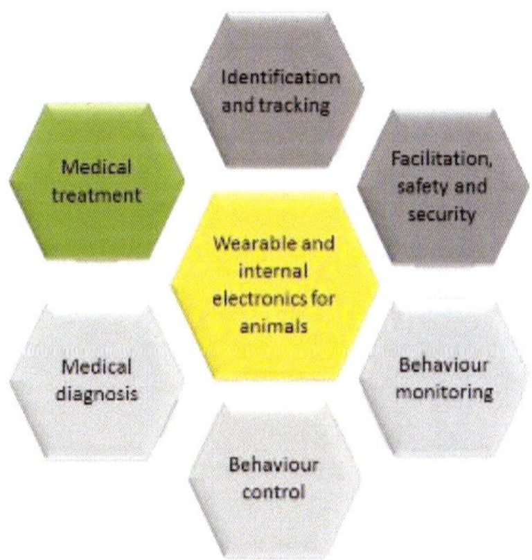

Digital Technologies that Advances Veterinary Medicine

Various digital technologies and their usage are now widespread in veterinary medicine. These were made possible with rapid expansions of cloud computing, whereby users take advantage of resources such as servers, storage, databases, network components, and software available via the web (or cloud). With cloud computing, the user only pay for the services they use, which not only saves money on hardware and software, but also improves the efficiency.

Computing speed and storage capacity can now be precisely tailored to the needs of the veterinary practice or the clinics, and helps to increase the business and growth. Reliable technology service providers guarantee reliability and disaster recovery, which is an added advantage. Today, many interactions and transactions between veterinary practices and service providers are already handled via such digital platforms. Examples includes transferring lab and image data, forwarding invoicing data to settlement agents or insurance companies, sending orders to suppliers for medicines and equipment, and more.

Big Data and Enhanced Disease Prevention through Digital Revolutions

Electronic Medical Records are the key in animal health and disease management interventions; they revolutionized disease monitoring and prevention approaches; they also generates huge volumes of not only valuable but also researchable animal health data. This brings in "Big Data".

The Technology of"Big Data" is that it lets every participant manages and processes the daily flood of data various veterinary practice and institutions generates about animals, like details of examination results, treatments, and prescriptions. This data is then analyzed so that one can can pinpoint the right diagnosis and the course of therapy. The Stakeholders and participants will have access to investigating ways to detect and prevent outbreaks of infectious diseases by combining and analyzing data from various agencies and service providers involved in the whole chain of the sector of veterinary medicine.

Digital Technologies that Transforms Veterinary Medicine

Technologies such as portable sensors, or wearables, are revolutionizing veterinary medicine. A US study reveals that animal owners in the USA spent an estimated 2.3 billion dollars on monitoring the health of their pets via wearables in 2023. Wearables thus provided veterinarians with valuable data and insights regarding the patient's medical history, which would otherwise not be available in meaningful volumes, if at all. New sensors and related technologies also supported therapy by logging various vital parameters.

Rehabilitation Medicine, 3D-Printed Implants and Prostheses

Enabling a good quality of life for animals with ambulation issues are the major expectation by the animal keeping families. 3D printers are used to produce precision prostheses or implants, anatomical models for preparation, and sawing and drilling templates for the intended interventions or surgical procedures. Now 3D printing has made its way into veterinary medicine in recent years. It is already being utilized in veterinary practices, where in implants and prostheses are created using 3D printers.

Digital Technology Enabled Client Interactions

Smartphones had brought in an unimaginable transformation for health care sector. Families and People with Pets want to access information and services anywhere, any time. Animal Health and Veterinary Medical Care is immensely benefitting from digital communication tools. Websites, newsletters, blogs, social networks such as Facebook and Instagram, messenger services like WhatsApp, as well as many other apps such as petsXL are helping to share content and news and interacting with clients, customers and stake holders.

First Point Contacts and Initial Care support through modern social media tools are increasingly being used across small animal practitioners. They also enabled better data management for further referrals and second opinions. Practices benefit operationally from the inventory management tools and such data from the various clinic's in-house software can help to predict the demand status for medications and consumables in such clinics and practices. This also makes it easy to order the required supplies electronically, saving both time and money. Suppliers easily can then transmit the available quantities, prices, batch numbers, and shelf lives via an invoice or delivery note directly to your inventory management system. All this enables better work flows and operational efficiency.

Benefits of day-to-day Digital Tools for Small Practice Setups

- Very efficient workflows
- Clients can book appointments online; they need not stress the minimal staff on conventional phone.
- Practice assistants will be free to devote themselves to the patients already in the practice.
- Digital technologies also hugely boost client loyalty.
- Certain Apps focusses on customer communications and helps staying in contact with the practice easy.
- Any clinic or practice that uses digital tech is more competitive as it saves time, effort, and money.
- Digital tools lets us keep your existing customers happy, attract new ones, and also raise the profile of the clinic or practice.

Artificial Intelligence Revolutions

Artificial intelligence (AI) totally revolutionized all the fields and Veterinary medicine was not an exception. AI refers to the simulation of human intelligence in machines that are programmed to think like humans and mimic their actions. The term may also be applied to any machine that exhibits traits associated with a human mind such as learning and problem-solving. The ideal characteristic of artificial intelligence is its ability to rationalize and take actions that have the best chance of achieving a specific goal.

A subset of artificial intelligence is machine learning (ML), which refers to the concept that computer programs can automatically learn from and adapt to new data without being assisted by humans. Deep learning techniques enable this automatic learning through the absorption of huge amounts of unstructured data such as text, images, or video.

Applications of Artificial Intelligence

Veterinary Hospitals, Standalone clinics and veterinary professionals across the globe are beginning to experiment with artificial intelligence and developing solutions with AI that can help them take better care of their patients while striving to improve efficiency. As the benefits of AI emerge along with multiple products, some risks too are beginning to appear and future research will address them.

The applications for artificial intelligence are endless. It can be applied to many different sectors and industries. AI is being tested and used in the healthcare industry for dosing drugs and doling out different treatments tailored to specific patients, and for aiding in surgical procedures in the operating room.

Other examples of machines with artificial intelligence include computers that play chess and self-driving cars. Each of these machines must weigh the consequences of any action they take, as each action will impact the end result. In chess, the end result is winning the

Artificial Intelligence in Veterinary Medicine

Current Developments in India

The Indian Council for Agricultural Research under its National Agricultural Science Fund has supported an advanced research programme on Developing Artificial Intelligence Tools for Applications in Veterinary Medicine at the Tamil Nadu Veterinary and Animal Sciences University (TANUVAS), Chennai.

This frontier research program is a multi-institutional project involving lead institutions like Indian Institute of Technology, BHU, Varanasi (Cooperating Centre CC-1), ICAR-Indian Veterinary Research Institute, Izatnagar (CC-2), Indian Institute of Information Technology, Design & Manufacturing, Chennai- 600127 (CC-3) and Sri Sivasubramaniya Nadar (SSN) College of Engineering, Chennai – 603110 (CC-4) with TANUVAS, Chennai as the Lead Centre.

This Project titled as "Artificial Intelligence & IoT based Smart Vet Ecosystem for Animal Health, Patient Care & Precision Farming", and led by Dr.P.Selvaraj, a Senior Faculty in the field of Veterinary Medicine. Interested Veterinarians can contribute and collaborate in this programme. (email:smartvet23@gmail.com).

game. For self-driving cars, the computer system must account for all external data and compute it to act in a way that prevents a collision.

AI in Human Medicine

- The future of 'standard' medical practice might be here sooner than anticipated, where a patient could see a computer before seeing a doctor.
- Through advances in artificial intelligence (AI), it appears possible for the days of misdiagnosis and treating disease symptoms rather than their root cause to move behind us.
- Think about how many years of blood pressure measurements you have, or how much storage you would need to delete to fit a full 3D image of an organ on your laptop?

The accumulating data generated in clinics and stored in electronic medical records through common tests and medical imaging allows for more applications of artificial intelligence and high performance data-driven medicine.

- These applications have changed and will continue to change the way both doctors and researchers approach clinical problem-solving.
- Some algorithms can compete with and sometimes outperform clinicians in a variety of tasks, yet they have to be fully integrated into day-to-day medical practice.

Machine Learning has made great advances in health care, pharma and biotech efficiency. The top applications of AI in medicine are discussed herein.

AI to Diagnose Diseases!

- Correctly diagnosing diseases takes years of medical training.
- Even then, diagnostics is often an arduous, time-consuming process.
- In many fields, **the demand for experts far exceeds the available supply**. This puts doctors under strain and often delays life-saving patient diagnostics.

Machine Learning – particularly Deep Learning algorithms – have recently made huge advances in automatically diagnosing diseases, making diagnostics cheaper and more accessible.

How Machines Learn to Diagnose

- Machine Learning algorithms can learn to see patterns similarly to the way doctors see them.
- A key difference is that algorithms need a lot of concrete examples – many thousands – in order to learn.

- And these examples need to be neatly digitized – machines can't read between the lines in textbooks.

Machine Learning (ML) is particularly helpful in areas where the diagnostic information a doctor examines is already digitized. Examples includes, but not limited to:

- Assessing the risk of sudden cardiac death or other heart diseases based on electrocardiograms and cardiac MRI images
- Classifying skin lesions in skin images
- Detecting lung cancer or strokes based on CT scans
- Finding indicators of diabetic retinopathy in eye images

Advantages of ML usage

Since there is plenty of good data available in these cases, algorithms are becoming just as good at diagnostics as the experts. The difference is:

- The algorithm can draw conclusions in a fraction of a second, and it can be reproduced inexpensively all over the world.
- Soon everyone, everywhere could have access to the same quality of top expert, for example in radiology diagnostics, and for a low price.

More Advanced AI diagnostics

The application of Machine Learning in diagnostics is just beginning – more ambitious systems involve the combination of multiple data sources (CT, MRI, genomics and proteomics, patient data, and even handwritten files) in assessing a disease or its progression.

AI Won't Replace Doctors Anytime Soon

It's unlikely that AI will replace doctors outright. Instead, AI systems will be used to highlight potentially malignant lesions or dangerous cardiac patterns for the expert – allowing the doctor to focus on the interpretation of those signals.

AI in Clinical Veterinary Medicine

AI is a tool that should be used in tangent with veterinary professionals completing full clinical exams, and AI will not replace any of it. Over the years, AI will likely diffuse into clinical practice, though it is in small way, it will be in tangible ways that could release the burden of what might be considered mundane tasks. In case of Imaging based diagnostics, AI-based auto-segmentation has been explored in human medicine and can save time (30% or more) while also providing a consistent approach to segmentation (reduce inter- and intra-observer variations). Those time-savings can be re-invested into more patients accessing care or other clinical tasks.

AI in Small Animal Medicine

AI in Veterinary Medical Imaging – Cardio Thoracic Medicine

AI and ML is being increasingly used in the medical imaging field. In practice, the evaluation of medical images is very subjective and complex, and therefore the application of AI tools and methods to automatize the analysis process would be very beneficial to vets. Researchers had already applying these methods to image analysis, and developing software capable of assisting veterinary doctors or radiologists in their daily practice.

ML in veterinary imaging diagnosis has mostly been applied to the thoracic region, with various studies on the identification of pulmonary patterns and cardiomegaly detection. Commercially available softwares, such as "PicoxIA", enable abdominal, thoracic, and hip image analyses, although studies have only been published validating the thoracic analysis. "Vetology" is another clinically certified software, which was created for the analysis of radiographs of the thorax, heart, and lungs in dogs. The nervous system and the abdominal region are the least studied regions for ML in veterinary medicine.

AI Chatbots in Veterinary Medicine

Recent advancements in AI and chatbot technology have opened up new possibilities for streamlining patient care in areas including, but not limited to

- Client-facing triage,
- Diagnostic recommendations,
- Research enhancements,
- Literature review, and
- Hospital workflow
- Write surgery reports,
- Client communications,
- Emails, etc.

AI chatbots are basically computer programs that use natural language processing and machine learning algorithms to interact with users. There has been a significant advances in the development of AI chatbots for use in health care. These chatbots, are known as virtual health assistants or chatbot nurses, and have been used to help patients schedule appointments, manage prescription refill requests, and even monitor health from home.

There have been a growing interest and investment in using AI chatbots to improve workflow and patient care in the field of veterinary medicine. A potential application is in the area of diagnostics, where chatbots could help veterinarians quickly and accurately diagnose a variety of conditions based on inputs of patient history, physical exam findings, laboratory results, and more. It is a potent enhancement, allowing dramatically faster review and diagnosis of patient files.

For example, a chatbot could be programmed to ask a series of questions to a pet owner about their animal's symptoms and behavior. Based on the answers provided, the chatbot could then suggest potential diagnoses or recommend further testing to the veterinarian. Chatbots—including the likes of OpenAI's ChatGPT, Google Bard, Perplexity AI, and Microsoft Bing—can be programmed to triage cases, take histories, and even help to translate a doctor's recommendations to clients. Some have been trained to calculate drug dosing and flag adverse drug interactions.

The potential use for AI chatbots in veterinary medicine is not limited to doctors in streamlining workflow. Chatbots could be used to automate certain tasks, such as scheduling appointments, keeping records, writing surgery reports, producing discharge instructions, and even following up on a patient's wellbeing by prompting communication with the client. While a chatbot may not yet be able to be employed without monitoring and review, the possibility of more autonomous AI is on the horizon.

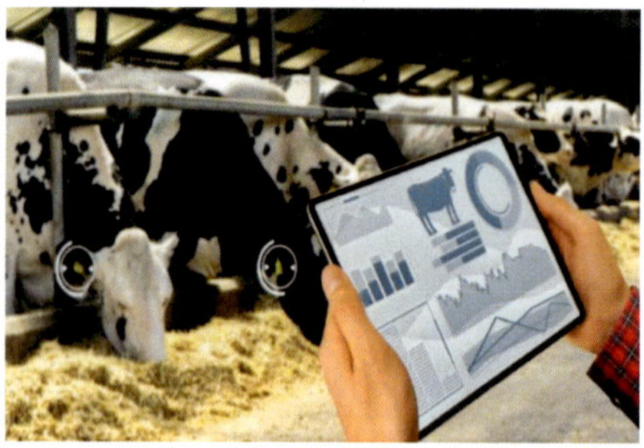

Ketosis and AI

Cow side tests for negative energy balance markers are available but are labor-intensive. Milk sample analysis using Fourier transform infrared spectroscopy (FTIR) allows for sampling numerous cows simultaneously. FTIR prediction models have moderate accuracy for hyperketonemia diagnosis (beta-hydroxybutyrate (BHB) $\geq$ 1.2 mmol/L).

Most research using FTIR has focused on homogenous datasets and conventional prediction models, including partial least squares, linear discriminant analysis, and ElasticNet.

Challenges and India Specific Constraints

When an animal visit a veterinarian, the doctors scribbles down the observations in to a case sheet or paper. And it is not always happening in every practice; many a times many constraints prevents such dedicated veterinary medical record maintenance. If its well-equipped clinic with dedicated manpower support, he/she type out notes in paragraph form in a computer or similar devices to document the visit; there's no systematic or widespread infrastructure in place for animal electronic health records. And while hand-captured notes work fine to document that one visit, in that one clinic, it limits how the data can be used and shared.

Where We Lack?

Unlike the human electronic health records, there aren't standardized ways to capture and map free text typed on a computer into codes that denote a specific type of disease and many experts find it as a major constraint in veterinary sector. All these factors leads to loss of millions of vet clinical records; these are essentially wasted as they're so cumbersome to work with due to non-coding. Clinics don't have the infrastructure to extract information from these veterinary medical records, while there's a lot of really interesting information in these medical records and once used properly and exploited their medical utility, they might even help advance not only animal health , but also human health.

Current Leads

A Stanford Medicine Team had devised a solution rooted in artificial intelligence, called DeepTag. DeepTag is an algorithm that essentially reads the typed-out notes from a vet and predicts specific diseases that are relevant for the animal. It boils the paragraph of medical notes into codes that represent certain ailments, symptoms or diseases.

In India, we need to develop such eVMR and Codification Tools and Practices to ensure early adoption to advanced technologies like AI and exploit them to improve our animal health and veterinary patient care.

Potentials for India

Veterinarians and researchers at the University of California, Davis had discovered a technique to predict leptospirosis in dogs through the use of artificial intelligence. They had developed one that outperformed traditional testing methods and provided accurate early detection of the disease. Traditional testing for Leptospira lacked sensitivity early in the disease process. Detection can take more than two weeks because of the need to demonstrate a rise in the level of antibodies in a blood sample. The AI model eliminated those two roadblocks to a swift and accurate diagnosis.

Their research involved historical data of patients at the UC Davis Veterinary Medical Teaching Hospital that had been tested for leptospirosis. Routinely collected blood work from 413 dogs was used to train an AI prediction model. Over the next year, the hospital treated an additional 53 dogs with suspected leptospirosis. The model correctly identified all nine dogs that were positive for leptospirosis (100% sensitivity). The model also correctly identified approximately 90% of the 44 dogs that were ultimately leptospirosis negative. The goal for the model is for it to become an online resource for veterinarians to enter patient data and receive a timely prediction. Such AI tools will help India.

Current Developments in India

The Indian Council for Agricultural Research under its National Agricultural Science Fund has supported an advanced research programme on developing Artificial Intelligence Tools for Applications in Veterinary Medicine at the Tamil Nadu Veterinary and Animal Sciences University (TANUVAS), Chennai.

This frontier research program is a multi-institutional project involving lead institutions like Indian Institute of Technology, BHU, Varanasi (Cooperating Centre CC-1), ICAR-Indian Veterinary Research Institute, Izatnagar (CC-2), Indian Institute of Information Technology, Design & Manufacturing, Chennai-600127 (CC-3) and Sri Sivasubramaniya Nadar (SSN) College of Engineering, Chennai – 603110 (CC-4) with TANUVAS, Chennai as the Lead Centre. The Project is titled as “Artificial Intelligence & IoT based Smart Vet Ecosystem for Animal Health, Patient Care & Precision Farming”, and is led by Dr.P.Selvaraj, a Senior Faculty in the field of Veterinary Medicine. Interested Veterinarians can contribute and collaborate in this programme.

It will develop a smart e VMR System applicable for India on its first phase and will work on developing AI Tools for health care and patient care applications on its next phase, besides developing IoT Tools and Smart Tools for Precision Livestock Farming and Health Care Applications. Ultimately there will be development of Veterinary Telemedicine Support Tools for real-time animal helath care support. It is envisioned that these smart tools will enable more than 70 plus veterinary colleges, 100s of research centers in veterinary and animal sciences and more than 35000 field institutions across India, may ultimately able to transform and improve the quality of veterinary medical care all over India.

TANUVAS Team is already working on AI-IoT Tools for applications in Vaccinations, Precision Farming & Health Care, AI driven for eVMR Development, AI in Disease Diagnosis, Monitoring and Surveillances, and Smart Medicine. Diseases like Mastitis, Metabolic diseases & Dairy Production Medicine, Common Infectious Diseases, Cardiology and Dermatology Issues are being under active research for AI tools development and applications.

2

Animal Oncology: A Road Map to Diagnosis and Management

P. Chaudhari*, C.N. Galdhar[1] and S.R. Upadhyay[2]

Professor and Head, Comparative Oncology Program & Translational Preclinical Imaging and Radiotherapy Facility, Animal Oncology Group Advanced Centre for Treatment, Research & Education in Cancer (ACTREC), Tata Memorial Centre Sector-22, Kharghar Navi Mumbai-410 210

[1]Professor Bombay Veterinary College, Maharashtra

[2]Professor, Veterinary Medicine, Sher-e-Kashmir University of Agricultural Sciences & Technology of Jammu, Jammu and Kashmir

Veterinary oncology is an upcoming field in recent years due to the integration of the importance of spontaneous canine cancers in understanding and developing novel strategies for human cancer management. We are stepping towards a very exciting era in veterinary oncology, where comparative oncology has played a significant role for many decades in understanding the molecular basis of cancer in companion animals. The comparative animal models have generated remarkable interest in both academia and industry. Studies have demonstrated the utility of comparative oncology in understanding drug resistance and tumor biology, contributing to the translational research[1]. This has yielded breakthrough discoveries, from advanced diagnostics to novel therapies, providing opportunities to improve the longevity and quality of life of the pets. These inputs have led to advancements such as the first conditionally approved chemotherapeutic agent for lymphoma, novel BRAF testing for canine urothelial carcinoma, tyrosine kinase inhibitors for mast cell tumors, updates in stereotactic/FLASH radiation, and novel immunotherapeutics. As the understanding of cancer biology has advanced, the field of veterinary oncology has grown significantly, paralleling developments in human oncology. Veterinary oncologists treat a variety of cancers in domestic animals, particularly dogs and cats, but also in exotic animals, horses, and even zoo animals. While the types of cancers in animals share similarities with human cancers, treatment strategies can differ significantly due to species-specific differences in anatomy, physiology, and response to therapies [2, 3].

Cancer in animals can occur in many forms, including lymphoma, mammary gland tumors, osteosarcoma, and various types of sarcomas. Common treatment modalities in animal oncology include surgery, chemotherapy, radiation therapy, immunotherapy, and palliative care. In many cases, a multidisciplinary approach is used, combining different therapies to improve quality of life and extend survival. Animal oncology is essential not only for improving the health and well-being of pets but provides insights into the understanding of cancer in humans. Studies have shown that canine osteosarcoma provides an effective model for understanding human bone cancer[1]. Similarly, canine lymphoma research has significantly contributed to advancements in immunotherapy[2]. Comparative oncology trials, which include naturally occurring cancers in animals, which has facilitated the development of targeted therapies and improved diagnostic techniques[3]. The study of cancer in pet animals has led to advances in human cancer management.

Cancer Types in Animals

Cancer is a leading cause of death in both dogs and cats, particularly in older animals. According to the Veterinary Cancer Society, cancer accounts for 47% of deaths in dogs, especially those over age ten, and 32% of deaths in cats[4].

Common cancers in pets include lymphoma, osteosarcoma, mammary gland tumors, and mast cell tumors. Each cancer type has its own set of diagnostic methods and treatment protocols[5].

Lymphoma: Lymphoma is one of the most common cancers in dogs, accounting for around 7-24% of all canine cancers. It originates in the lymphoid tissue, which is part of the immune system. Clinical signs include enlarged lymph nodes, weight loss, lethargy, and decreased appetite. Medical management is often effective, and many dogs respond well to treatment. The prognosis varies based on the stage at diagnosis and response to treatment. Certain breeds, such as Golden Retrievers, Boxers, and Basset Hounds, are more prone to developing lymphoma[6].

Osteosarcoma (Bone Cancer): Osteosarcoma is the most common primary bone tumor in dogs and often affects large and giant breeds like Rottweilers, Great Danes, and St. Bernards. It is an aggressive cancer that typically metastasizes to the lungs. Clinical signs include lameness, swelling, or a noticeable mass on the bone. Surgical limb amputation is the first line of treatment when the disease is localized. Multidrug chemotherapy is recommended in cases of metastatic disease. Radiation treatment may also be used for both curative and palliative purposes[7].

Mammary Tumor: Mammary tumors are the second most common neoplasia in dogs, particularly those that have not been spayed or have had multiple oestrus cycles. These tumors can be either benign or malignant. Clinical signs include small, non-painful lumps in the mammary glands, which may become hard, immobile, or ulcerated/large lumps. Surgical removal of the tumor is the treatment of choice. Chemotherapy or radiation may be considered for malignant cases. Breeds like Dachshunds, Cocker Spaniels, and Poodles are more commonly affected [8].

Hemangiosarcoma: Hemangiosarcoma is a malignant tumor of blood vessel cells. It often affects the spleen, liver, and heart. Clinical signs include lethargy, collapse, abdominal swelling (if the spleen is affected), and anemia. Surgical removal of the spleen or affected organ is common, followed by chemotherapy for extended survival. German Shepherds, Golden Retrievers, and Boxers are more commonly affected breeds [9].

Mast Cell Tumor: Mast cell tumors are one of the most common skin cancers in dogs. Clinical signs include lumps and bumps on the skin that may be raised, red, or ulcerated. Surgical removal is the primary treatment, with chemotherapy or radiation used for malignant cases. Boxers, Bulldogs, and Schnauzers are particularly affected [10].

Oral Melanoma

Melanoma is the most common oral malignancy in the dog. Oral and/or mucosal melanoma has been routinely considered an extremely malignant tumor with a high degree of local invasiveness and high metastatic propensity. Primary tumor size has been found to be extremely prognostic. Median survival times for dogs with oral melanoma treated with surgery are approximately 17 to 18, 5 to 6, and 3 months with stage I, II, and III disease, respectively. Standardized treatments such as surgery, fractionated radiation therapy, and chemotherapy have afforded minimal to modest stage-dependent clinical benefits and death is usually due to systemic metastasis. Numerous immunotherapeutic strategies have been employed to date with limited clinical efficacy; however, the use of xenogeneic DNA vaccines may represent a leap forward in clinical efficacy. Oral melanoma is a spontaneous syngeneic cancer occurring in outbred, immunocompetent dogs and appears to be a more clinically faithful therapeutic model for human melanoma [11, 12].

Diagnostic and Treatment Approaches

Accurate and timely diagnosis of cancer type, grade, and staging plays a pivotal role in selecting appropriate treatment modalities, including surgery, chemotherapy, radiotherapy, immunotherapy, or combinations of these to control the disease and determine prognosis [10, 13, 14,].

The diagnostic process typically involves:

- **Patient History and Physical Examination**: A detailed history and thorough physical examination form the basis for understanding tumor behaviour and disease staging [10, 13, 14].
- **Basic Diagnostics**: Hematological and biochemical profiling, along with radiographic examination, provide initial insights into tumor nature but are not sufficient for a definitive diagnosis [8, 10, 13].
- **Advanced Diagnostics:** Histopathology and Immunohistochemistry [8, 10, 13, 14, 15]

Tumor histology can predict both risk of local recurrence and distant metastasis, and this varies widely across different subtypes. Histopathological grading gives insights for prognostic assessment. Hematoxylin and eosin staining makes it possible to see the structures of cells and tissues and is the most basic test for confirming whether a disease is primary or metastatic. The immunohistochemistry is employed in the case of complex and subtyping of the tumor. The concept of surgical margins is getting awareness in veterinary practice, and it is becoming a routine part of cancer surgeries.

Confirmation requires:

- Cytology and histopathology:
- Biomarker detection
- Immunohistochemistry
- Molecular diagnostics, such as PCR for Antigen Receptor Rearrangements (PARR) for lymphoma diagnosis
- Flow cytometry for tumor classification

Imaging Techniques for Staging

Advanced imaging is critical for precise staging and metastasis evaluation:

- **Ultrasound (USG)**: Commonly used due to affordability, availability, and procedural simplicity [8, 10, 15].
- **Contrast-Enhanced CT (CECT)**: Provides detailed information about tumor shape, size, vascularity, and metastatic spread [10, 15].
- **Magnetic Resonance Imaging (MRI)**: Particularly indicated for neurological, spinal, and soft tissue malignancies [10, 15].
- **Positron Emission Tomography (PET) and Single Photon Emission Computed Tomography (SPECT)**: Useful for functional imaging and whole-body surveys, though regulatory requirements and limited availability restrict their use in veterinary practice [8, 15].

Treatment Approaches

Treatments are tailored to the animal's specific condition and cancer type:

- **Surgery**: Effective for localized tumors [8, 10, 13].
- **Chemotherapy**: Suitable for hematologic cancers or metastatic disease [10, 13,15].
- **Radiation Therapy**: Preferred for tumors that are surgically inaccessible [10, 13, 15].

- **Palliative Care**: For terminal cases, focusing on improving quality of life [8, 13, 15].
- **Emerging Therapies**: Innovations like immunotherapy and radioisotope therapy are gaining traction [8, 10, 13, 15].

Outcomes and Prognosis

The prognosis varies depending on the type of cancer, stage at diagnosis, and the animal's response to treatment. While some cancers can be treated successfully, others are more challenging and may require long-term management [16, 17].

Challenges in Animal Oncology

- **Limited Treatment Options:** Although treatment options are expanding, they remain more limited than in human oncology.
- **High Treatment Costs:** Cancer treatment for pets can be expensive, particularly chemotherapy or radiation therapy.
- **Ethical Considerations:** Deciding whether to pursue aggressive treatment or opt for euthanasia can be emotionally challenging for pet owners.

This overview covers some of the most common cancers in dogs and cats, including both the clinical presentation and treatment options. The prognosis varies widely depending on factors like cancer type, stage at diagnosis, and individual animal characteristics.

References

1. Dobson, J. M. "Significant advances in veterinary oncology–60 years on." Journal of Small Animal Practice 60.12 (2019): 711-722.
2. Bergman, Philip J. "Immunotherapy in veterinary oncology." Veterinary Clinics: Small Animal Practice 44.5 (2014): 925-939.
3. Argyle, David. "Veterinary and Comparative Oncology, A decade in cancer research." Veterinary & Comparative Oncology 10.1 (2012).
4. FETCH a Cure (https://fetchacure.org/resource-library/facts/)
5. Rafalko, Jill M., et al. "Age at cancer diagnosis by breed, weight, sex, and cancer type in a cohort of more than 3,000 dogs: Determining the optimal age to initiate cancer screening in canine patients." PLoS One 18.2 (2023): e0280795.
6. Bennett, Peter, Peter Williamson, and Rosanne Taylor. "Review of canine lymphoma treated with chemotherapy—Outcomes and prognostic factors." Veterinary Sciences 10.5 (2023): 342.
7. Simpson, Siobhan, et al. "Canine osteosarcoma in comparative oncology: Molecular mechanisms through to treatment discovery." Frontiers in veterinary science 9 (2022): 965391.
8. Withrow, S. J., Vail, D. M., & Page, R. L. (2013). Withrow and MacEwen's Small Animal Clinical Oncology (5th Edition). Elsevier.
9. Suzuki, Tamami, et al. "Current understanding of comparative pathology and prospective research approaches for canine hemangiosarcoma." Research in Veterinary Science 167 (2024): 105120.

10. De Nardi, Andrigo Barboza, et al. “Diagnosis, prognosis and treatment of canine cutaneous and subcutaneous mast cell tumors.” Cells 11.4 (2022): 618.
11. Pazzi, Paolo, Gerhard Steenkamp, and Anouska J. Rixon. “Treatment of canine oral melanomas: a critical review of the literature.” Veterinary Sciences 9.5 (2022): 196.
12. Dagli, Maria Lucia Zaidan, et al. “Identification of mutations in canine oral mucosal melanomas by exome sequencing and comparison with human melanomas.” Scientific Reports 14.1 (2024): 24174.
13. Dias, Joana NR, et al. “Immunotherapeutic strategies for canine lymphoma: Changing the odds against non-hodgkin lymphoma.” Frontiers in veterinary science 8 (2021): 621758.
14. Dobson, Jane M. “Breed-predispositions to cancer in pedigree dogs.” International Scholarly Research Notices 2013.1 (2013): 941275.
15. Ettinger, S. N., & Feldman, E. C. (2017). Textbook of Veterinary Internal Medicine (8th Edition). Elsevier.
16. Ito, Daisuke, Aric M. Frantz, and Jaime F. Modiano. “Canine lymphoma as a comparative model for human non-Hodgkin lymphoma: recent progress and applications.” Veterinary immunology and immunopathology 159.3-4 (2014): 192-201.
17. Dobson, Jane M. “Breed-predispositions to cancer in pedigree dogs.” International Scholarly Research Notices 2013.1 (2013): 941275.

3

Clinical Decision Support using Animal Data, Artificial Intelligence and Tele. Veterinary Services in Food Animal Practice

Abdul Samad

Former Dean and Director, Maharashtra Animal and Fishery Sciences University Nagpur, Maharashtra

Opportunities

India is home to largest milch animal population, totalling around 100 million cattle and buffalo (out of total population of 300 million) spread over 6.5 million census villages. India is the largest milk producer with CAGR of 4.5%, likely to go up to 5%, which is likely to create around 20 million jobs every year. The most significant factor is that dairy industry is likely to exceed IT industry in employment generation. In year 2018, India produced 146 million tonnes of milk contributing 26% of the agriculture GDP.

But the foundation of dairy industry is economically vulnerable as per animal productivity and fertility are very low leading to meagre profits and frequent demands to enhance procurement price. National schemes like Operation Flood, National Dairy Plan-I and National Dairy Plan II, largely focussed on milk collection, processing, distribution and organising farmers but the animal component has been neglected. Enhancing per animal productivity by empowering farmers to scientific management and breeding to achieve genetic improvement needs urgent attention. Although numerous technologies to improve health and genetics are available but the single most important gap is failure to deliver these to farmers. Unlike western world, India has not been able to develop modern veterinary service delivery models. In order to cater to breeding and health services of cattle and buffalo (300 million in numbers) and also pet animals in rural areas and small towns, huge manpower and infrastructure will be required.

Model Veterinary Services

It will be essential first to understand the gaps in the present veterinary services so that it's improvement using modern technologies could be understood. Lot has been written and published on veterinary service delivery models in the western countries, but in India this topic, although extremely critical, has not received due attention from the researchers and the policy makers. In this paper I will attempt to describe in brief a model which we have tested and found to be suitable to India's needs and then discuss the information technology tools required to implement this model. As a general rule a model veterinary service should fulfil following criteria:

Continuous and not ad hoc: the involvement of service provider should not be only to attend sickness or insemination

Predominantly Preventive: The service set up should be to keep animals healthy and productive. This is important in food animal practice, but equally necessary in pet animal practice.

Protocol based: The services should be scheduled and not based only on farmers' perception and observation.

Integrated with breeding In case of food animal practice, services should include consultancy on nutrition, management, genetic improvement

Business Consultancy: Veterinarians should act like business consultant to advise farmers to maximise profits

Challenges

As per an estimate there are Only around 60,000 registered veterinarians out of which only 40,000 are active but predominantly employed in government, municipal corporations, pharma, university, feed industries and R & D laboratories. A chunk of veterinarians opts for poultry industry. Hence the most sufferer industry is dairy which is not able to retain veterinary graduates. Government continues to be major employer with attractive salaries, perks and working conditions which can't be matched by livestock industry. Large animal practice is physically demanding hence not favoured by female veterinarians. Since dairy animal health services this is a rural practice, qualified graduates prefer pet practice in urban areas. There is dismal ratio of availability of vets to number of large animals in the country. Whereas, the National Agricultural Commission has recommended the ratio to be one veterinarian for 5000 large animals, for 300 million bovine population alone 60,000 practicing vets would be required. Compare this with USA, as per American Veterinary Medical Association Report there are 1,20,652 veterinarians for dairy animal population of around 12% of Indian livestock population.

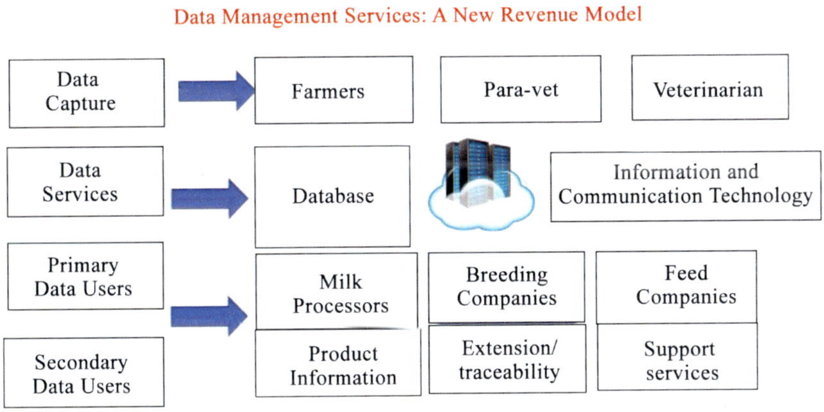

Team Approach

It is a fact that due to economic considerations the dairy animal to veterinarian ratio until next decade will not exceed 30,000:1. In order to fill the gap a large number of para-vets, village health workers and AI Technicians are working in rural areas. They are in fact the first farmer contacts in villages. These are not well-trained persons and as per legal provision, varying in different states, can provide minor veterinary services under the supervision of registered veterinarian. On an average, considering the cattle population density and intra-village distances a para-vet at the most can cater to AI and minor services to 1000 cattle units. This means that a team of 30 para-vet and one graduate vet will be able to cater to cluster of villages. The challenge is how to achieve functional supervision so that farmers get quality services at their doorstep when they need. This is where the information technology, big data analysis and penetration of services using televeterinary modules will play major role.

Reorient Services to Preventive

Currently most of the veterinarians are catering to clinical services as per the mandate given by the governments or the dairy companies. The dairy cooperatives continue to follow the 'Route System' of clinical services wherein on scheduled day the veterinarians visit villages in a route and treat sick animals. Drawback of this system is that there is no continuity in service and administration of drug or antibiotic is the only option open to the veterinarians. Animals falling sick and treatment is against the interest of the farmer (loss of production and cost of treatment), milk companies (compromised quality and quantity) and consumers (drug residues). In most of the western countries the veterinary services to the farmers are predominantly preventive. Such an approach requires strategic planning, such as, udder and uterine health programs, customised breeding to evolve better next generation heifers, optimized feeding to control cost of production and level of production and fertility. Hence the role of veterinarian in dairy practice is largely that of 'business consultant' which due to current orientation is largely clinical. In order to cater to large number of animals, the graduate veterinarians would need field workers who will work in tandem with him, both on the planned herd preventive program as well as administration of drugs and primary treatment as per the pre-decided protocols, communicated by the veterinarians.

ICT Enabled Breeding and Veterinary Services

Information and communication technology can play an important role in improving services to farmers as well as linking para-vets and vets for better monitoring and improvising quality of services. The author of this paper has been active in developing ICT tools to achieve the objective of modernizing veterinary services. The enterprise software Herdman developed by him is in use since last several decades. Currently, 17 lakhs cows and buffaloes are registered on the platform. On daily basis, >10,000 AI, 3000-3500 pregnancy checks, 1000 new registrations, 2000-2500 calvings and 5000-6000 treatments are recorded and updated. This huge data is analysed routinely and instantly to convey the problem areas to the concerned veterinarian and para-veterinarians. The treatment records consist of diagnosis, laboratory test data, drugs administered and cost of treatment. The system also records the mobility of the veterinarians, inventory of semen, liquid nitrogen, medicines, vaccine, all breeding events and animal movements (from owner to another owner). The animals that are dead or culled and sold are also updated and moved to archive file. This is probably the largest active data in the country. Analysis of data has provided experience to develop decision support model in terms of diagnosis and treatment help to be provided to the veterinarians and para-veterinarians. The farmers are closely involved as they are served with sms messages on performance of their animals.

Sustainable model

Since in India 90% farmers' dairy animal holding is 3-5, hence they are not able to invest in modern technologies and IoT. The challenge therefore is to develop ICT devices affordable and suitable to Indian farmers. In western countries the farmers are required to pay heavily for data management services, which is not possible in India. We have therefore developed a sustainable model of animal identification, traceability and performance recording that can be accessed by the vets, farmers, para-vets and industry stakeholders for providing various types of services to the farmers.

The system comprises of:

1. ***QR coded or FRFID ear tags:*** These are our patented technologies. The unique feature is that the data can be captured after scanning th e tag with a

dedicated App installed on cell phone. The scanning leads to opening of the animal's file for registration or new data (service) update. Data can be sent only after scan hence can't be fudged and tracked on the dashboard.

2. ***Mobivet***-App: The App is a scanner cum herd data management system. App is available for farmers, para-vets and vets. It is a complete management system and includes Daily Action List, Alarm lists of under-performing anima ls, breeding, milk and health entries, tele-veterinary and milk recording. Value-addition is that historic data is available to the service provider for taking informed decision on interventions.

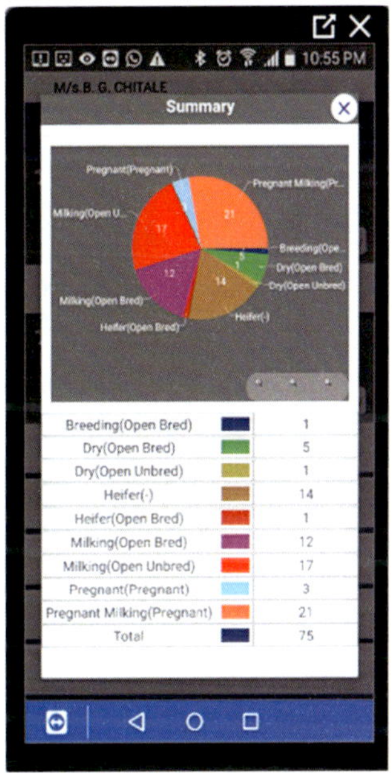

3. ***Herdman***-Server: This is server software for large data processing

4. ***Dashboard:*** the dashboard enables real time tracking of services by the para-vets and extension staff in field.

5. ***Tele*-veterinary service**: The concept here is that the para-vets or village animal health workers are used for capturing animal's physical examination data as video, images and sounds and the same then can be sent or streamed to the veterinarian for diagnosis and digital prescription.

6. ***Animal Health IoT:*** With strides in sensor technologies, we are focusing on collaboration to develop animal health IoTs suitable for small hold system. The data emanating from such devices can be linked to individual animal data file for correct diagnosis and advisory to the farmer, para-vet or vet.

Breeding Data Update and Decision Support

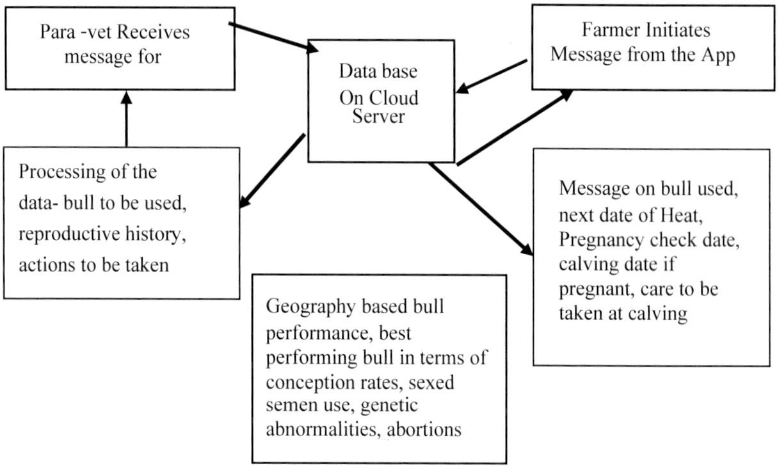

Decision Support in Clinical Management

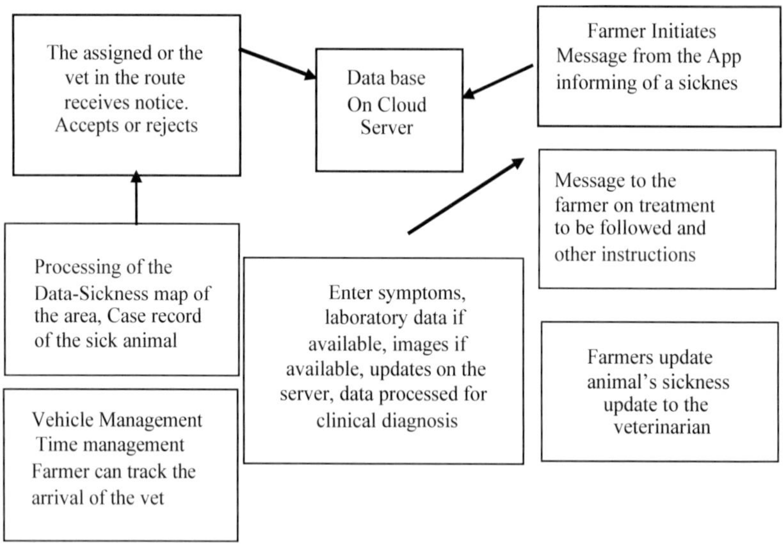

Generating Maps to Attend Disease Outbreaks

In areas where individual animal identification is still in infancy, premises can be registered with number of animals of each species with the farmers. We have developed a system for generating encrypted QR code for each premises tag which can be fixed to farmer premises. Each time a vaccinator or service provider visits the premises, he has to scan the premises code to generate list of species of animals and numbers owned by the farmer. The user then can update the vaccination record (with batch number for inventory management). Similar process is practiced in case a communicable or infectious disease is reported. This system enables generating premises maps for species, breeds, milking, breeding, vaccinated, unvaccinated animals. The system also enables generating maps of 'Hot' areas and premises list with contact details of adjoining high-risk areas.

Machine Interface

The system can be interfaced with data coming from various IoTs, such as, pedometer, milk parlour, tele-ECG, tele-stethoscope and tele-thermometer. These devices enable remote health monitoring, such as, rumination, time taken for feeding, number of active steps, behaviour changes, lying and resting time, etc. The diagnostic IoT-enables remote examination of animals.

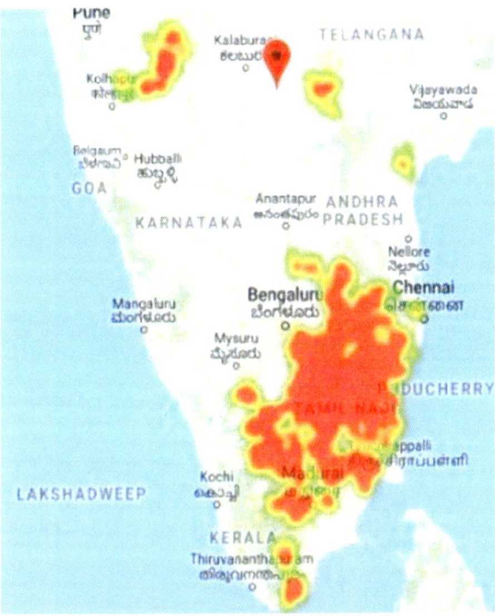

Artificial Intelligence -Driven Decision Support

AI-ML are now vital tools to analyse big data to generate trends and technical reports. Such reports are important from the point of view of macro-decisions, such as policy decisions. For example, if the system is linked to the milk collection centres, the system provides loyalty maps- that is farmers who are pouring regular milk, animals that are becoming high risk due to fertility and production issues, better performing animals, ranking of cows and bulls as per performance. An important insight Artificial intelligence gives is reports and maps on disease prevalence, disease frequencies, use of antibiotics and hormones, culling trends, reasons of culling and peak yield and their management in groups of animals. The Artificial intelligence also enables tracking movement of animals and infections.

Outbreak prediction and communication to the farmers.

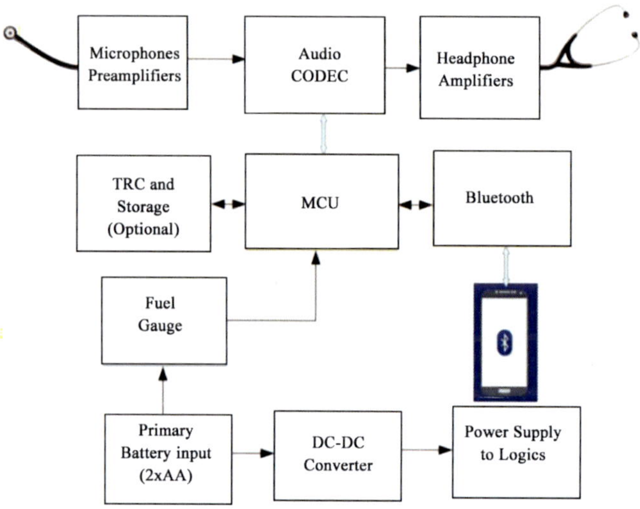

Tele.veterinary Services: We have recently launched tele.veterinary service for all species of animals. For dairy animals the software can be linked to Herdman / Mobivet software. Basic principle is that the veterinarian should be able to receive online the data of sick animal either from the owner or from the para-vet / vet in the field. For field vets and owners App is available, whereas for the consulting doctors, a dashboard is available. The doctor sitting from their home or district hospital can operate the system and provide services to any remote sick animals. There is facility of update of lab reports, images like x-ray MRI, sonography, ECG, heart, lung and rumen sounds (taken from stethoscope), images of the animals as well as videos. The Consultant also has facility of online video imaging of the animal. A digital prescription is shared with the para-vet or the owner who can take help of the local vet to administer.

4

Rabies in Livestock An Insight

Jyoti B Dutta

Professor & Head, Department of Veterinary Epidemiology & Preventive Medicine College of Veterinary Science, Assam Agricultural University, Khanapara Guwahati

Rabies is an ancient, dreadful disease known to mankind from the vedic ages. It is a zoonotic disease caused by Rabies virus, genus Lyssavirus family Rhabdoviridae, affecting all mammals including man. The WHO categorizes rabies as a neglected zoonotic disease that causes around 59,000 human deaths globally annually after onset of symptoms. It is a vaccine preventable disease reported from over 150 countries and territories barring the island nations like Australia, Brunei, Japan, Maldives, New Zealand, Papua New Guinea, Singapore, Timor Leste and the Pacific Island Countries. The Indian islands of Andaman Nicobar and Lakshadweep are rabies free so far.

On the other hand, Africa and Asia has the highest burden of human rabies including South-East Asia: Bangladesh, Bhutan, DPRK, India, Indonesia, Myanmar, Nepal, Sri Lanka, and Thailand. The Asia Pacific region having 60% of the world's population includes the world's most populous countries – India and China. Asia alone shares almost half of the global rabies deaths annually

Rabies in Asia is majorly transmitted by dog bites attributable to the higher density of dog population. Dogs are divided broadly to two categories: confined dogs i.e. owned dogs under leash, free-roaming dogs (FRDs) - may or may not be community owned and feral dogs - mostly abandoned and move without any restriction. The population of Free-roaming dogs (FRDs) is variable due to habitat, socio-cultural factors and human population density. The mean density of FRDs is 14 dogs/km^2 in Bangladesh, 42 in Bhutan, 468 in Philippines, 719 in rural Maharashtra in India. The status of zero human rabies in countries like Bhutan, Mongolia and Malaysia face a constant threat of rabies incursion from endemic countries through travel and trade activities with neighbouring endemic countries. On the same note, a few states in India like Goa and Sikkim are vulnerable for the high incidence of rabies in the neighbouring states. India has a large population of stray dogs, estimated at 62 million, and as per 2024 report, the pet dogs population stands at 36.85 million.

Rabies is sustained through two inter-related cycles: (i) urban; and (ii) sylvatic. In the former, domestic dog population harbours the rabies virus while in the latter, the wildlife such as jackal, fox, wolf, civet, mongoose and bats. India has reported rabies in species like foxes, bears, leopards, hyenas, civets including sambar deer due to spillover in the domestic-wild interface. Habitat loss, human encroachment into wildlife areas, tourism and changes in ecosystem dynamics are the major factors identified for such spillovers. The probability of rabies being found in a specific animal depends on regional control efforts and the prevalence of the virus in wildlife populations. Assam reported rabies in cattle, goat, pig, horses including dogs besides jackal and civet.

The disease causes an estimated 31,000 human deaths in Asia every year with an estimated expenditure of over 48,32,63,43,600.00 rupees for direct and indirect costs of post-exposure prophylaxis in human and dog rabies control efforts (Knobel *et al.* 2005). India on the other hand accounts for ~20,000 deaths annually, 40% of which are children aged 5-15 years with presumably a proportionate cost. Although no comprehensive surveillance data is available, the economic impact of rabies on livestock production is potentially high. A study in Assam estimated the economic impact of 40 dairy cows (average age 6 years) died of rabies to be Rs.36,96,000.00 (unpublished data). A number of published reports from India, Bangladesh, Nepal and Pakistan highlighted goats and dairy cattle amongst livestock to be the highest victim of dog bite cases.

The World Health Organization has set the goal of eliminating human rabies by 2030 (Zero by 2030). Having dog identified as the major animal reservoir of rabies to human and livestock, progress in preventing human rabies by culling of dogs was not acceptable to social, public, religious and animal welfare activists. Dog population management and mass dog vaccination alongside public awareness campaigns regarding post-exposure prophylaxis are the identified goals to inch towards elimination of dog-mediated human rabies from India.

Zero by 30 will be a herculean task for India with hardly four years to go. In this scenario, One Health approach with participation of stakeholders will be vital. Capacity building and laboratory infra-structure for brain sampling and early confirmed diagnosis, dog population management and vaccination coverage up to 70%, continuous sero-surveillance of vaccinated dogs are crucial. Both, human or animal rabies in a locality should be declared a notifiable disease after laboratory confirmation and mobilize the veterinary and human health departments to recruit adequate post-exposure prophylaxis, besides community awareness campaigns. Multi-sectoral convergence of human health, veterinary, forest and environment, municipal bodies and policy makers as well as media have immense role to play in combating a public health problem in a vast and diverse country like India. It will require a vision and full commitment from all the states of the country and the determination of the nation in getting freedom from dog–mediated rabies by controlling it at source - sustained mass dog vaccination campaign. The Government of India sponsored Action Plan for Rabies Elimination adopted at the national and state level (NAPRE and SAPRE) needs more steam to make the goal achievable within the set deadline.

The WOAH and WHO stipulate a step-wise approach for rabies elimination –

- Rabies is notifiable
- State of the art surveillance in operation
- 2 years of rabies cases (human and / or animal),
- Prevention of importation of rabies-infected animals, and
- An effective national rabies control strategy

Mexico has been successful in combating rabies, being an endemic country in 1991-95 controlled dog-mediated rabies during 1996-2001, achieved Zero human deaths during 2001-2007, elimination campaign – 2007-11 and maintained freedom 2011 onwards, through cross-sectoral collaboration by WHO and CDC with regional veterinary public health unit.

United against Rabies, the global partners – FAO, WOAH and WHO aim to end human and animal (livestock) death from dog-mediated rabies through a comprehensive One Health approach promoting mass dog vaccination, ensuring access to PEP, health worker training, improved surveillance, and bite prevention through community awareness. Combined with technical guidance from international organizations to strengthen the capacity for implementing rabies elimination programmes, sustained political will and community engagement are among the measures to reach the goal of 'Zero by 30' and, eventually freedom from dog-mediated rabies.

References

Balogh et al. 2023. One Health for Dog-mediated Rabies Elimination in Asia, *FAO, WOAH* and WHO *Working Together* in the *Asia Pacific* Region to Eliminate Dog-mediated Human Rabies by *2030*.

Knobel *et al*. 2005. Re-evaluating the burden of rabies in Africa and Asia. Bulletin of the World Health Organization 83(5), 360–368.

5

Veterinary Nuclear Medicine (VNM) & Targeted Drug Delivery System for Infectious Diseases: Can We Proceed with This in Veterinary Medicine?

Chandrakant N. Galdhar

Professor (CAS) and Radiological Safety Officer, Department of Veterinary Clinical Medicine, Mumbai Veterinary College (MAFSU), Parel- Mumbai, Maharashtra

Veterinary Nuclear Medicine (VNM)

Veterinary Nuclear Medicine (VNM) is a specialized field that uses radioisotopes to detect, diagnose, and treat diseases. Gamma scintigraphy involves injecting radioactive tracer pharmaceuticals into the animal's body and imaging them as they move through the body using a gamma radiation-sensitive camera. This technique provides a 2D or 3D image of the whole body or a specific organ, allowing for the estimation of the quantitative distribution within the region of interest (ROI). Advancements in gamma scintigraphy have allowed for the acquisition of information about both static and dynamic high-resolution images, such as heart wall motion, blood flow, and myocardial perfusion. Unlike other diagnostic modalities viz X-rays, ultrasonography, and CT; gamma scintigraphy offers functional information of specific organs. The most commonly used gamma radiation-emitting isotope is 99m-Technetium (^{99m}Tc), which emits a gamma energy of 98% 140-keV photon with only 10% internal conversion. Other radionuclides used in veterinary nuclear medicine facilities include iodine (^{123}I and ^{131}I), Gallium (^{67}Ga), and Thallium (^{201}Ti).

Targeted Drug Delivery System

Targeted drug delivery systems, based on nanoparticles, are novel methods that target specific organs or tissues to release therapeutic agents. These systems offer advantages such as good pharmacokinetics, precise infection targeting, reduced side effects, and reduced drug resistance in treatment.

Foot and Mouth Disease (FMD)

Foot and mouth disease (FMD) is a contagious disease affecting various species of cloven-hoofed animals, including cattle, buffaloes, pigs, sheep, goats, and many other species. The disease has seven serotypes, with O, A, C, Asia-1, SAT-1, SAT-2, and SAT-3 being prevalent in India. The global annual impact of FMD is estimated to be between US$ 6.5-21 billion in endemic countries, but India alone incurs Rs.20,000 Crores/annum. Vaccination is the most effective way to prevent FMD, but existing vaccines have limitations such as slow immune response development, short immunity duration, infected animals, and dependence on cold-chain immunization. In India, an oil adjuvant-based trivalent FMD vaccine is used in the ongoing FMD control program (FMDCP), which involves mass vaccination every six months to develop herd immunity and prevent the spread of the disease. However, logistical difficulties and inadequate manpower make it difficult for the program to be efficiently implemented. To address these issues and the short duration of immunity provided by inactivated FMD vaccines, a new generation of FMD vaccines should be produced safely and inexpensively. Nanocarriers have been considered a promising method for drug and vaccine delivery due to their structural stability, low cost, and tailorable properties. These nanoparticles can be processed potently by the immune system, prolonging the release of antigens, protecting it from degradation, and enhancing cell-mediated or humoral immunity. Department of Veterinary Nuclear Medicine, Mumbai Veterinary College has recently completed a research project on "Development and evaluation of a nanocarrier based novel foot-and-mouth disease virus vaccine for non-parenteral delivery" sponsored by the Department of Sciences and Technology, SERB Govt. of India. The project highlights the process of radiolabelling and examines the uptake of a conventional foot-and-mouth disease vaccine in the lymphoid organs of guinea pigs. This suggests the feasibility of radiolabelling various vaccine formulations, allowing for the exploration of antigen uptake. Such investigations provide valuable insights into the fate of the vaccine upon inoculation and its immunogenic potential.

Brucellosis

Brucellosis is a significant global issue affecting veterinary, public health, and economics, with over half a million cases reported annually. In India, 80% of people live in close contact with domestic livestock animals or wildlife, a risk factor for zoonotic disease transmission. The current national seroprevalence of brucellosis in cattle is around 13.5%, with test-and-slaughter being an effective strategy. However, socio-cultural constraints prevent cattle culling in India. Prevention of human brucellosis depends on managing existing brucella-infected animals and efficacious treatment. Despite extensive studies on disease in dairy cattle, data on the 'optimum antibiotic treatment' for brucellosis is either unavailable or disputed. Brucella's intracellular localization and adaptability to environmental conditions make treatment failure and relapse rates high. Department of Veterinary Nuclear Medicine, Mumbai Veterinary College has sanctioned a research project on "Macrophage Targeted Delivery System of Rifampicin for Effective Treatment of Brucellosis in Livestock" sponsored by Rajiv Gandhi Science and Technology Commission (RGSTC) Government of Maharashtra, Mumbai. Rifampicin, a broad-spectrum antibiotic, has been reported to be effective against Brucella species. In the present research project, our research group is developing a stable nano-drug delivery system of rifampicin with low macrophage cytotoxicity and high therapeutic efficacy.

Conclusions

Radiolabelling and nano-formulation have the potential for effective treatment in veterinary medicine. Therefore, the promotion of combining Veterinary Nuclear Medicine (VNM) and Targeted Drug Delivery Systems for the management of Infectious Diseases in the veterinary field is essential and needs to be encouraged.

Acknowledgments

The author expresses gratitude to the Science and Engineering Research Board (SERB) and Rajiv Gandhi Science and Technology Commission Government of Maharashtra (RGSTC) for funding their research project on FMD (grant no: CRG/2019/006547) and Brucellosis (Sanction Order/Project Proposal No. RGSTC/File-2024/DPP-327/CR-55/418; Dated: 29.11.2024) respectively. The author also thanks Maharashtra Animal and Fishery Sciences University- Nagpur and Mumbai Veterinary College for providing radiation facilities and the Board of Radiation and Isotope Technology and the Department of Atomic Energy for providing radioisotopes.

6

Piglets' Mortality and Remedies in Farm Conditions

Mondal, D. and Naskar, S.

Eastern Regional Station, Indian Veterinary Research Institute Kolkata, West Bengal

Being polytocous animal, sow give birth several (8-14) piglets in each farrowing, mother pig find several deficiencies and disorders during gestation, farrowing and postnatal conditions. Prior to birth intrauterine competition amongst the feotus piglets for nutrition and gas exchange is a big stress for abortion. Several infectious and non-infectious causes may hamper proper growth and pathological conditions resulting mortality (15-20%) in piglets than weaner and adults (Sarma, *et al*, 2012). Several risk factors are also responsible for piglet mortality.

Prenatal factors: Insults during pregnancy can impact a piglet's ability to survive after birth and regulate their body temperature. Some maternal aspects that affect survability and mortality amongst piglets are prolong farrowing duration more than 4 hours, number of parity of sow, usually first and second parity show high mortality than subsequent parities and also older sow lose more piglets.

Postnatal factors: Piglets after birth have to adjust to a new environment, that include outside temperature(thermal confort zone is 18-40C), humidity, nutritional status of vitamin and mineral level, suckling, and competing with littermates, litter size, mother health status. thermal stress, oxidative stress (oxidative stress is a condition that occurs when there is an imbalance of free radicals and antioxidants in the body). Oxidative stress can cause tissue damage and tissue malfunction reduces litter size and piglet survival.

Conditions that Limit Survibility of Piglets

Health status - where the production of milk is vital nutrient for piglets and any disease that cause agalactia or low milk production leads to piglet mortality. **Birth weight and body condition** indicate the survibility and susceptibility to diseases and protection from diseases. **Genetic make** - healthy piglets can be have from healthy parents and free from genetic illness. **Amount of colostrum** taken within hours after birth.**Season of farrowing** and envirnmental parameters- winter motality is more than summer and rainy season.**Fatty sow**

piglets may show high piglet mortality- there is chance of crushing, fatty sow gives more stillbirth and higher litter sizer. Thermoregulatory abilities of piglets- those piglets which can produce metabolic heat effectively is very important, piglets with low birth weight as heat loss per unit of body weight is inversely proportional to body size (Herpin et al 2002).Unlike other baby mammals, piglets don't have brown adipse tissue (BAT) that helps in convert energy from food, in piglets shivering thermogenesis from skeletal muscle has vital role, needs early skeletal muscle development. Male piglets are more vulnerable to mortality than females, although the body weight is higher in males with higher body mass index (weight/height, kg/m^2) than females, normal BMI in piglet 21.2kg,/m^2. Higher BMI indicates more fat. Ponderal index in male foetus is higher (PI) than females, PI method is used to diagnose impaired fetal development. It's an important indicator of fetal malnutrition and is easy to measure (weight in gram x100/length cm), PI noramally 2.5-3.

Non Infectious Causes of Piglet Mortality

Category of mortality are infectious origin and non infectious one. A wide range of both infectious and non infectious causes for piglet mortality. Non infectious causes of piglet mortality occurs within few weeks of birth is big hurdle for pig industry (Muns, *et al,* 2015)

Starvation: It is a condition when scanty amount of nutrients is available in the system to full fill the required energy. This may either unavailable of nutrients or cannot engulf right amount by the piglets coupled with othe factors like hypothermia, weak piglet tends to crushing, immature immune system (colostrum within 36 hrs feeding), littersize that competes for suckling competition and anaemic condition.

Physical injury: During piglet life, several physical injury can cause piglet mortality such as biting, fighting amongst litermates leads to infection and maggot formation,crushing by the over healthy sow and weak piglets when a sow rolls, sits to lie, or try to stands. Infantophagia is another rare condition, gilt can devour its piglets due to deficicy of phosphorus, Sodium and salt. And even within simple boredom in farm conditions.

Inherited and neonatal defect: Hernia(ubalical, inguina,scrotal), cryptorchidism, splay legs(genetic, floor,trauma,deficiency-Vit A and Manganese, intersexuality, hermaphrodism, epitheliogenesis imperfecta, and anal atresia are some of the most common genetic defects in piglets.

Porcine Stress Syndrome (PSS) - Porcine Stress Syndrome is a genetic defect with halothane gene (rynodine receptor 1 gene, RYR1 gene). It is an inherited, autosomal recessive disorder.This cause defective mechanism of Calcium and storing, release taking up in muscle fibre. This condition causes a progressive increase in body temperature, muscle rigidity, and metabolic acidosis, which can lead to sudden death. Several condition also aggravate the PSS with prolong farrowing process, cold exposure, neonatal diarrhoea,piglet anaemia etc.

Crushing- When mother sow like to rolls, sits to lie, or try to stands on of a sudden as a result some piglets particularly weak piglet get crushed. Factors that moderate crushing by the sow are habitual or behaviour of sow who did same earlier, piglets factor which are weak, anaemic and unadaptable piglets in farrowing pen.Harse wether that can irritate the sow, higher litter size, numbers of parity

Umbilical herniation: This occurs when the body wall adjacent to umbilicus and navel area doesn't fuse properly, causing intestinal parts protrution through the intrstinal wall to form 'ball like" structure outside.the frequency of this condition may be 0.5-1.2%. It is a familial matter and some report found due to specific genes (Du, *et al.*, 2009). Single nucleotide polymorphisms (SNPs) found strongly associated with these congenital defects.

Inanition or starvation (2.7%)- Insufficient amount of colostrum transfer to piglet in the early childhood may lead to inanition and infection as antibody transfer in piglets throgh blood is scarce.Other causes of inanition are sow may be suffering from agalactia or mastitis, premature piglets, peripartum asphyxia during birth, deformity of organs of piglets (atresia ani,cardiac abnormalities, teratogenic chemical and drugs etc)

Non viable piglets (NVP)- A non-viable piglet is a piglet that is born with such significant deficiencies that it has a low chance of survival, Low birth weight (less than 700gram),congenital defects,no suckling reflex, placental infarction, umbilical cord rupture, dystocia, vitamin B_2 deficiency, and poor sow nutrition. High numbers of piglet under this condition goes mortality 5-12% .

Perinatal Asphyxia- In-utero fetuses are evidently exposed to several factors that cause an interruption of the oxygen supply through the umbilicus to foetus causing asphyxia leading to hypoxia and metabolic acidosis. These conditions are important causes of intra-partum and neonatal mortality. Some studies have shown that at the time of birth piglets are quite immature compared with puppies, kittens and bunnies (Stanton and Carroll, 1974). Pigs are a polytocous species so piglets born at the end of the litter are likely to suffer asphyxiation to a greater extent.

Piglet anaemia: Piglet anaemia is a well established condition with deficiency of Iron in the blood and storage along with other ingredients needs for erythropoesis such as copper, cobalt, vitamin B_6, B_9 and B_{12}. Pig milk is poor source of Iron to produce required RBC formation more over the piglet growth rate is very high with 3:1 feed conversion ratio. Heritable trait of high prolificacy with higher litter size are vulnerable to anaemia, Intensive farming system feed contains less amount of Iron and related nutrients for erythropoeisis. Iron stored as ferritin in liver, kidney, spleen, muscle tissues, and large bone marrow like humerus, femur etc., piglets are borne with 40-60mg of iron including hemoglobin content.

Savaging (Cannibalism) by the sow: Sometimes a sow may be aggressively bites to her piglets lead to death due to fatal injury and haemorrahge. Breeds like white landrace, Ghoonru, Agonda goan show much infantophagia 1-3%. This may happen in gilts that first time farrowed i.e primiparous gilt. Several risk factors for piglets savaging include harse irritating environment, poor sympathy between the sow and the farm attendants, nutritional deficiency like Ca, P, vitamins, salt, fiber, water, first time confinded in defined area or farrowing pen. Breed of sow that have aggressive nature in congested population in herd.

Abdominal organ torsion or volvulus: In growing pigs it is prevalent 1-3%, clinical signs of swollen abdomen, anemia, painfull and bluish skin.Risk factors are rapid ingestion of large amount of feed/water, over crowded pens, feed ingradients are highly fermentable, stress hust before feeding. Divided feeding with small quantity, good quality feed/ straw,large quantity of fibre along with concentrate, use bran in feed few days before farrowing that reduce fermentation of take feed.

Gastric ulceration: Gastric ulcers, also known as gastroesophageal ulceration, are a serious health issue in pigs. The condition may occur when pars esophagia (non glandular part of esophagus into stomach) is destroyed leads to bleeding and ulceration.The condition may occur when dietary particle are fine, gastric fluidity is more, high dietary carbohydrates and more environmenta stress. Signs of ulceration are roughened, bile stained pars esophagia,fissures of pars esophagea, hyperkeratosis etc.

Cold exposure/chilling: Cold exposure due to season change, hail strome, sudden weather change, transport in cold environment and torrential train etc cause sudden drop of environmental temerature as a result young piglets are tend to get chilled, hypothermia, negative energy balance, crushing. Usually, after birth piglets hide under sow's udder to beat the cold exposure but sudden abrupt weather and ill piglets may be exposed to morality.

Transport stress: Transporting of animal for long journey in different adverse seasons affect pig healtht. Winter and hot weather transport, vehicular designs (loading system, floor type, level of congestion, avilability of drinking water, ventillation, vibration and jerking during transport, interval of every 60 minutes of journey for long trips, journey injury and porcine stress syndrome can affect the piglet mortality.Transport sickness cause 0.5-2% mortality (Voslarova, *et al*.,2017)

Toxins related mortality: Pigweed plant poisoning (nitrate, oxalate), Argot alkaloid exposure, Ochratoxin, Fumonsin, *E.coli* siga toxin and Clostridial toxin(botulinum)

Infectious Causes of Piglet Mortality

Several infectious agents are responsible for disease production particularly in piglets prior to weaning. Viral, bacterial, fungal, parasitic both coccidia and helminths also cause disease that may lead to some mortality

Viral Infection

Porcine circovirus- Piglets **are** affected with this four serotypes of virus (PCV1-4). It shows mortality, poor growth, progressing to the level of severe thinning 5 to 14 weeks of age. Pigs can develop enlarged lymph nodes, skin rashes, difficulty breathing, pneumonia jaundice, fever, stomach ulcers, diarrhea, or sudden. Both direct and indirect transmission in India along with other countries with incubation period of 2-4 weeks.

Corona virus (RNA): Like human (SARS, MERS, Covid-19), animals Corona viruses are prevalent in swine population. Four genera of corona virues are alfa, beta, gamma, and delta varaeities. (i) Transmissible gastroenteritis (TGE) virus in all age group (ii) porcine respiratory coronavirus (PRCV) in piglets (4-10wk). TGE charetized by diarrhoea with fowl smell, vomiting in high healthy piglets, anus wet and paste with foamy yellow feces and cud like,dehydration, shunken eye, rough coat, thirsty and weakness. Incubation perid 16 to 30 hours and virus transmission through milk, feces and inhalation.morbidity and mortality 50-60% and 10-20% respectively. (iii) Porcine epidemic diarrhoea virus : Cosely related to TGE in nursing piglets.Also a corona virus undergenus Alphacoronavirus. transmission through direct and indicrect contact,faeco-oral,cont*act,fomites,feed ,aerosol etc. IP-1-4days, clinical signs of* diarrhoea,vomiting dehydration and metabolic acidosis.Small intestine thining,undigested milk in stomach and water intestinal content. Morbidity upto 100& and mortality 10-100%.

Porcine Reproductive and respiratory Syndrome virus(Corona): Clinical signs of PRRS are wasting, coughing and pneumonia, and reproductive losses pale skin, inappetance, mild coughing, sneezing and pneumonia withincreased respiratory rates. Chrnoic cases with arthritis. Reproductive signs are fever, weak piglets, late term abortion with mammfied foetus, ear discolouration, prolong return to estrous, agalactia,infertility, mastitis, early farrowing, Transmission through secretion,urine, feces, air borne, vectored by flies, birds, animals. Morbidity 50-100 & and mortality 20-80%

Classical swine fever CSF (12wk): Highly contagious virus with Pestivirus (Flaviviridae, RNA).Transmission through ouronasal routes and semen. Incubation period 3-8 days. Clinical signs high fever, huddling, weakness, drowsiness, anorexia,conjunctivitis, crusty eyelids, constipation with pelated feces followed by watery diarrhea and yellow vomition, incoordination, unsteady, staggeringt, sometimes progressive posterior paresis. Skin hyepemic, abdominal haemorrhage, in theigh, ears, snout, and blotching of ear. The disease course 1-3 weeks, chronic cases characterized by anorexia, depression, elevated temperature, leukopenia, and periods of constipation and/or diarrhea. Poor reproductive performance with stillborn, mummified, malformed, weak or dead piglets. In boar with fever, anemia, prolonged clotting times,, diarrhea and conjunctivitis (Brown and Bevin, 2018). Morbidity in CSF is 80-100 while mortality not less than 20 but may reaches to 100%.

African swine fever (ASF): It is a ASFV is a double-stranded DNA virus of Asfarviridae family. The virus first identified in the 1920s in Kenya and now it is available world wide, in India in 2020 outbreaks occurred in Assam and runachal pradesh leads to death of thousands pigs.Transmission through infectious animals,fomites, food, ingestion of contaminated pig products and tick bites etc. Incubation period 5-20 days with clinical stages of peracute (virulent strains, high fever (42C), anorexia, lethargy and sudden death without much signs, mortality 100. Acute case with fever 40-42C, lethargy, anorexia, animals show centripetal cyanotic lesions at ears, snout, limbs, abdomen, tail and perianal area, epistaxis, nasal discharges,vomiting, diarrhoea, haemorrhagic splenomegaly and lymphadenitis, morality 80-100%. Subacute cases with multifocal necrosis in the skin and arthritis, panting, emaciation, abortion and chronic stages with mortality 30 to 70%.

Difference between CSF and ASF

Cause of CSF is Flaviviridae, RNA, IP-3-7days, transmission through garbage, direct, indirect contact to infected pigs, feed etc. Clinical forms are percaute, acute, subacute and chronic. Clinicopathological signs are more similar and differentiate can be done laboratory diagnosis

ASF, Asfarviridae, DNA, IP-5-21days, transmission throgh animals, fomites, food, ingestion of contaminated pig products and tick bite.Three clinical form percaute, acute and subacute and chronic. Clinicopathological signs are more similar and differentiate can be done laboratory diagnosis

Other viral diseases Pseudorabies in young mostly characterized by tremor, paddling, anorexia, couhing, dyspnoea, weight loss, fever 41-42C, mortality1-2%, lesions mostly respiratory involvement. FMD (8wk), Nipah virus (pig is amplified host, respiratory and Neurological, fever), Japanese encephalitis (still birth, weak piglet, neurological signs, piglet edema, reduced brain tissue and wasting piglet

Bacterial Diseases

Streptococcus suis: A common cause septicaemia and localization of bacteria in piglets, with mortality rates of up to 21.2%. Piglet show lateral recumbency and paddling with CNS disturbance. Older pigs also show include ataxia, opisthotonus, incoordination, tremors, convulsions , blindness and deafness. Pigs with polyarthritis have swollen joints and are lame.Pneumonic and fibrinopurulent meningitis..

Neonatal septicaemia: A disease that can cause high mortality in piglets. This could be due to both *Klebsiella pneumonae* and enterotoxigenic *Escherichia coli,* extraintestinal pathogenic *E. coli,(UTI,* biofilm bacteria localized bacteria),, beta-haemolytic streptococci. Piglets of 15-25 days with good body condtion auffer from this disease.The pigglets of a litter mostly suffer with clinical signs of recumbency,cyanosed and mouth breathing during summer months. They may also cause septicemia, meningitis, arthritis, and endocarditis. Mortality due to it 1-4%

Umbilical infections: It can lead to umbilical hernias, omphalitis (umbilicus, an enlarged umbilicus, and pain) and other systemic conditions which can cause mild to moderate mortality. Also can cause baterenia, septic arthriris, uveitis and peritonitis

Abortion and Still Birth (lungs not opened)

Abortion is *the termination of a pregnancy by removal or expulsion of an embryo or fetus from the uterus before full gestation period. Still birth is after 28 week to terminal of pregnancy may be due to O2 deprivation,large litter size, stress and nutrition, infection, poisoning of CO, asphyxia during birth, intrauterine competitionamongst foetus. Bacterial causes Brucellosis, Leptospirosis Monocytogenes, Leisteriosis, Staphylococcus aureas, Pasturella multocida,* Erysipelothrix rhusiopathiae, Protozoa- like Toxoplasma, Neosporiosis, trypanosoma, Trichomonus, babesia but rare in pigs (Edward and Baxter, 2014), ***viral*** *(CSF, ASF, Japanese B Encephalitis, porcine circovirus, PRRS, Pseudorabies etc), non infectious causes (heat stress, heavy metal, pesticides).*

Other causes of death in piglets include: bacterial polyserositis, chronic atrophic enteritis, salmonellosis, pneumonia, chronic atropic enteritisand colibacillosis, Porcine epidemic diarrhoea, Transmissible gastroenteritis, Actinobacillosis, Erysipelosis.

How to reduce piglet mortalities: Adapt effective management practice that reduce mortality due to stillbirth, dystocia, abortion, hypothermia, starvation, disease, crushing, and savaging etc. Keep good farrowing pen hygiene, warm microenvironment for newborn piglets, careful rearing of supernumerary piglets, colostrum feeding, and care for crushing and savaging. Assist nest building with material.Most of the piglet death occurs within few days of birth (Kirkden, et al., 2013). Keep healthy during pregnancy, teat sucking training,Restrict oxytocin uese,

Some Ways to Reduce Piglet Mortality Include

- Keep the sow good health during gestation period and parturition
- Optimizing farrowing housing to improve maternal behavior, avoid heat stress

- Breeding strategies towards smaller litters 6-8
- Teat training to ensure piglets ingest colostrum
- Reduce oxytocin use – induced farrowing-rupture umbalic cord, dystocia, more muconium causes O2 deprivation,
- Equalizing litters within 48 hours after farrowing to keep away post parturient agalacia
- Restraining the sow in a crate- to avoid crushing and savaging
- Creating a safe area for the sow-for minimum disturbance to piglet and sow
- Vaccination, health care and hygienic condition in farm

References

Brown, V.R.,, Bevins, S.N., (2018) A Review of Classical Swine Fever Virus and Routes of Introduction into the United States and the Potential for Virus Establishment. Front Vet Sci. Mar 5;5:31.

Du, Z.Q, Zhao, X, Vukasinovic, N, Rodriguez, F, Clutter, A.C., Rothschild, M.F. (2009). Association and haplotype analyses of positional candidate genes in five genomic regions linked to scrotal hernia in commercial pig lines. doi: 10.1371/journal.pone.0004837.

Edward and Baxter (2014) The gestating and lactating sow.Chantal and Farmer eISBN: 978-90-8686-803-2https://doi.org/10.3920/978-90-8686-803-2

Kirkden, R.D., Broom,D.M and I L Andersen, I.L (2012) Invited review: piglet mortality: management solutions, J Anim Sci 2013 Jul;91(7):3361-89. doi: 10.2527/jas.2012-5637.

Menegatt, J.C.O, Perosa, F.F, Gris, A.H, Piva, M.M., Serena, G.C., Bordignon, D.L, Reck, C, Menin, Á., Watanabe, T.T.N, Driemeier, D. Main, (2023) Causes of Death in Piglets from Different Brazilian Nursery Farms Based on Clinical, Microbiological, and Pathological Aspects. Animals. 13(24):3819. https://doi.org/10.3390/ani13243819

Nielsen NC, Bille N, Larsen JL, Svendsen J. Preweaning mortality in pigs. 7. Polyarthritis. Nord Vet Med. 1975 Nov;27(11):529-43. PMID: 1105403.

Sarma, N.K. Saharia, J and. Roychoudhury, R (2012) pre-weaning mortality of piglet in organized farm. Indian J. Anim. Prod. Mgmt. Vol. 28 (3-4) 245–250 (2012)

Muns, R., Nuntapaitoon,M. and Tummaruk, P.(2016) Non-infectious causes of pre-weaning mortality in piglets. Livestock Science,184(2):46-57

Voslarova, E., Vecerek, V., Passantino, A., Chloupek, P., Bedanova, I.(2017) Transport losses in finisher pigs: impact of transport distance and season of the year. Asian-Australas J Anim Sci. Jan;30(1):119-124. doi: 10.5713/ajas.16.0265.

7

Climate Change Impact on Animal Health and Diseases

S.K. Sharma[1] and Monika Joshi[2]

[1]Professor and Dean, College of Veterinary & Animal Science, Jodhpur- 342037
[2]Incharge, Department of Animal Nutrition, College of Veterinary & Animal Science, Navania, Rajasthan University of Veterinary & Animal Sciences, Bikaner

Introduction

Climate change, a global phenomenon of present time, has emerged as the greatest challenge of the world in the twenty-first century. Rising earth's surface temperature is one of the most threatening factors coming into view. The substantial changes in the earth's climate have an impact on ecosystems, economics and societies in a variety of ways (Sharma *et al.*, 2024). It is one of the important environmental, agricultural, human and animal health issue. Climate change is an association of multidimensional effects involving physical characteristics, causes and consequences (Visschers, 2018). The climate change has resulted in to increasing global average temperature of air and ocean, melting of snow, rising of ocean level, change in the rainfall pattern and extreme whether events such as drought, flood, heat waves, storms etc.

Increased pressure on the earth in the form of industrialization, modernization of agriculture and increased populations of livestock and human is responsible for climate change. Human activities are contributing to climate change by generation of greenhouse gases such as carbon dioxide, methane, nitrous oxide and fluorinated gases. The carbon dioxide is generated through uses of huge amount of fossil fuels as coal and oils. Methane and nitrous oxide are produced by city landfills, rice fields, use of nitrogen fertilizers in agriculture and livestock farming. Methane and nitrous oxide have shorter half-life in atmosphere therefore instead of powerful greenhouse gas effect carbon dioxide has major role for climate change (Sharma *et al.*, 2024).

Climate Change Scenario at Global and National Level

Human activities, principally through emissions of greenhouse gases, have unequivocally caused global warming, with global surface temperature increasing 1.1°C in 2011-2020. Rise in temperature is more over land (1.59°C) than over the ocean (0.88°C). Global greenhouse gas emissions have continued to increase. There is largest share in gross GHG emissions occurring in CO2 from fossil fuels combustion and industrial processes followed by methane, whereas the highest relative growth occurred in fluorinated gases (F-gases), starting from low levels in 1990. Average annual GHG emissions during 2010–2019 were higher than in any previous decade on record (IPCC, 2023).

In developing nations, like India, there is rapid population expansion, economic reform, rapid urbanization, industrial infrastructure development and environmental degradation; global warming and climate change is more challenging to manage. The Indian Meteorological Department recorded temperature increase over the Indian region is almost similar to the global average in its "Statement on Climate of India during 2018" report. India's average temperature increased by roughly 0.7°C between 1901 and 2018 and it is anticipated to increase by approximately 4.4°C by the year 2100.

Indian-Gangetic plains and the Western Ghats, monsoon rainfall decreased by around 6% between 1951 and 2015. In contrast, in central India, the intensity of heavy rainfall rose by over 75% over the same period. From 1951 to 2016, droughts' frequency and geographic area greatly increased particularly regions across central India, the southwest coast, the southern peninsula and northeastern India. The east coast of India had more frequent and intense, very severe cyclonic storms than the west coast during 2000-2018 (Krishnan *et al.*, 2020). These changes have far-reaching consequences, not only for human societies but also for the vast array of animal species inhabiting diverse ecosystems across the planet (Sharma *et al.*, 2024).

Climate Change and Animal Resources

There is a complex and multi-directional inter-relationship of climate change and animals. Emissions of methane into the atmosphere by the livestock is responsible for the climate change. On the other hand, climate change impacts the animal health and diseases. Animal health is adversely affected by changing climate particularly extreme climatic conditions such as heat waves, drought, flood etc. and emergence and reemergence of infectious diseases mostly vector borne diseases (VBD). Vectors and parasites are highly dependent on climatic conditions. The disease complexes under changing climate scenario comprises insects, vectors, parasites, micro-organisms and arthropod borne diseases. Climate change is believed to play a role in redistribution of hosts, vectors and pathogens worldwide. The host- pathogen-environment interplay is significantly affected by climate change (Lubroth, 2015). Temperature plays a central role by affecting health, production, and reproductive performance of animals. Forage production is also influenced by temperature and rainfall variation (Sawalhah *et al.*, 2019).

India's livestock sector is largest in the world. India's animal resources are considered an important part of food security for the nation, and with one of the world's largest growing economies, the impacts of climate change are exacerbated.

Climate Change and Animal Health and Diseases

A changing climate can have devastating impacts on the animal health. It can also affect disease patterns and making outbreaks harder to control. The climate change led to major biological changes. In the healthy and disease process, there is a constant fluctuation, where change from one to the other is determined by change in the balance between three components i.e. host, agent (pathogen and vector) and environment (Oyhantcabal *et al.*, 2010). The change in the environment / climate will undoubtedly affect the host as well as agent. Climate change affects incidence, spread and predictability of animal diseases.

Diseases occurrence is mainly affected by an increase in temperature and variation in rain fall pattern. The effects of climate change on animal health may be considered into two categories direct and indirect (Sharma *et al.*, 2024). The direct health impacts include temperature-related illness, changes in metabolic functions and morbidity due to extreme weather events (Nardone *et al.*, 2010). Indirect impacts are associated with pathogens, their transmission patterns, effect on intermediate hosts and vectors.

Direct Effects

The direct effect of climate change on animal health has been described as a reduced competence of the host to mount a response to infection (Bett *et al.*, 2017). Climate change in the form of changes in the quantity and distribution pattern of rainfall, increase in the average atmospheric temperatures, heat waves, extreme weather conditions etc. affect the animal health. Heavy rains and drought lead to failure of fodder and grain production due to either water logging or water scarcity. Animal health is adversely affected due to nutrient shortage. Poor nutrition not only causes deficiency and metabolic diseases but decrease immunity in the body. Immuno-compromised animals are more susceptible to various infections. Depending on the degree, duration and severity of heat exposure, livestock health can be affected by causing heat stroke, metabolic disorders, oxidative stress, immune suppression, decreased reproductive performance and even death.

Heat Stress / Heat Stroke

The impact of ambient conditions on animals' health can be estimated by calculating temperature–humidity index (THI) by considering ambient air temperature and humidity. Exotic and cross-bred cows are less tolerant to heat stress than our indigenous cows. Exotic cattle such as Holstein–Friesian dairy cows are predominantly susceptible to heat stress (West, 2003). When the ambient temperature is over 25°C, high yielding dairy cows become heat stressed with primary signs as increased rectal temperature and respiration rates (Staples and Thatcher, 2011). Panting is commonly observed in heat stroke and sequel to FMD.

Production Diseases

Production disorders such as SARA, ketosis, milk fever, fat cow syndrome and various deficiency disorders may be outcome of changing climate and improper nutrition (Sharma *et al.*, 2024). The heat-stressed animal eats less frequently during hotter times of the day leading to reduced feed intake, followed by increased feed intake at below ambient temperature of the day, which is considered as a major cause of SARA by increased output of bicarbonate, resulting in lameness (Stone, 2004).

Ketosis is a production disease characterized by a relatively high concentration of ketone bodies such as acetone, β-hydroxybutyrate, and acetoacetate with a concurrent decrease of blood glucose levels (Dann *et al.*, 2005). It is mainly due to negative energy balance, forceful lipo-mobilization and accumulated ketone bodies (Lacetera, 2019). During heat stress, animals' reduced feed intake combined with increased energy requirement for fulfillment of body physiological demand may is responsible to cause negative energy balance that influences the mobilization of adipose tissue consequently, resulting in the development of ketosis (Abuajamieh, 2015). The climate change also affects livestock health by hampering endocrine status, liver function, glucose, protein and lipid metabolism (Bernabucci *et al.*, 2006) leading to production diseases.

Reproductive Disorders

Reproductive performance in animals is affected due to thermal stress mainly by changing blood flows and production of different hormones, with reductions of 20%–30% in conception rates and anoestrus in ruminants during summer seasons (Talukder *et al.*, 2018). The pig industry suffers considerably due to impaired reproductive disturbances during late summer and early autumn months. It is called seasonal infertility in pigs influenced by photoperiod and temperature (Auvigne *et al.*, 2010). Temperature also adversely impacts semen quality (Nichi *et al.*, 2006), oestrus cycle (Wolfenson *et al.*, 2000) and oocyst and embryo development (Stewart *et al.*, 2011).

Indirect Effects

Indirect effect of climate change on livestock health is associated with climate-driven ecosystem changes and physiological adaptations which could trigger pathogen virulence and vector–pathogen–host exposure (Bett *et al.*, 2017). The emergence and re-emergence of vector borne pathogens have globally provided evidence for the relationship between climate change and effects on the pathogen interface (Caminade *et al.*, 2019). In the disease process, three epidemiological factors such as the agent, host and environment are closely entangled and persist in ecosystems. The climate change could enhance pathogen replication and/or virulence which can negatively affect livestock health (Harvell *et al.*, 2002).

Changes in the climate provide favourable environment for vector reproduction as well as pathogenic micro-organisms. There are chances of emergence and re-emergence of new strains and serotypes and inter-species infection. Changes in climate can result in alteration of disease patterns and the emergence of new disease syndromes particularly those spread by vectors. Vector borne diseases are especially susceptible to changing environmental conditions due to the impact of temperature, humidity and the demographics of vectors. Climate can directly influence arthropod survival and spread and virus replication.

Climate change, through complex interactions with hosts, vectors and environment, has facilitated the spread of the bluetongue virus into Europe, Rift Valley fever in Africa, and highly virulent influenza viruses in Asia including India. The temperate regions may become more suitable for tropical vector-borne diseases such as Rift Valley fever, African horse sickness, West Nile virus and schistosomiasis. Continuing uncertainty about how climate changes will affect livestock disease, leads to greater difficulty in preparing for and reducing disease impact. The interplay with other global changes such as land use, globalization of trade and population movement add to unpredictability.

Vector-borne Pathogen

Climate change positively affect the reproduction and spread of vector-borne pests such as midges, flies, ticks and mosquitoes (Thornton *et al.*, 2009). This intern has the potential to increase the geographic spread of vector-borne diseases such as bluetongue, lumpy skin diseases (LSDs), anaplasmosis, babesiosis and theileriosis. Global climate change patterns could positively affect the spatial distribution of vectors such as mosquitoes and ticks (IPCC, 2007). Arthropod vectors are very fragile to fluctuations in temperature and humidity. A model simulated by Wittmann *et al.* (2001) demonstrated that an increase of 2°C of environmental temperature can extensively spread *Culicoides* spp, which is responsible for the transmission of bluetongue virus in ruminants including wild ruminants. Bluetongue virus is identified in the India (Rao *et al.*, 2016; De *et al.*, 2019).

Haemo-protozoan infection is an important health hazard of livestock in tropical countries that can be transmitted by ticks and flies. As a tropical country, the livestock of India suffers severely with haemo-protozoan and ricketsial infection such as *Babesia* spp., *Anaplasma* spp. and *Theileria* spp. Tick and fly reproduction has been demonstrated to increase as humidity increases to 85% (Caminade *et al.*, 2019). Recently India has seen the outbreaks of LSD in cattle and notified the OIE. Generally arthropod vectors are markedly increased in numbers during the hot, humid weather condition and animals are worst affected by them during these favrouable climatic conditions (Sridhar *et al.*, 2020).

Few Other Pathogens

Climate change play a substantial role on pathogens that maintain a part of their lifecycle outside of the final host such as black quarter, anthrax and dermatophiloses. Anthrax is a deadly zoonotic disease caused by *Bacillus anthracis* spores. Temperature and other climatic conditions such as humidity, rainfall, pH, water activity of soil and availability of nutrients all affect the germination of anthrax spores. Heavy rainfall, soil erosion and drought may stir up the dormant spores and increase the exposure of livestock (WHO, 2008). Global climate change affects the seasonal temperature variation of migratory birds traveling from the Arctic area to a tropical area. Evidence exists that during migration, they carry and disperse avian influenza virus during the winter season therefore the migratory birds are identified as the potential source of avian influenza virus spread.

Parasites

Climatic change directly affect prevalence, severity and geographical distribution of parasites mainly helminths. It has been observed that the development rates of free-living larval stage of the *Haemonchus contortus* become increased in the tropical regions with increased temperature (Fox *et al.*, 2015). Global climate change could influence the rapid development of parasites in their invertebrate intermediate hosts like snails. The lifecycle of lungworms is also reliant on weather conditions and increases incidence in the summer/autumn than the winter season. Fascioliasis, schistosomiasis and nematodiasis parasitic diseases that are mostly influenced by climatic changes (Fox *et al.*, 2012). Parasitic diseases like trematodiasis (fascioliasis and schistosomosis) became endemic in water logging area due to increased humidity. Incidence of parasitic diseases in India and abroad explore the relationship between the incidence and climate change.

Conclusion

Animal health and diseases should be considered as an integral part of climate change strategies globally. There is need to reduce impacts of climate change on animal health and diseases and work to mitigate effects and adaptations to climate changes. New livestock systems should be developed to cope with changing climate and reduce disease incidence. There is need to improve diagnostics for prevention, early detection and early response to livestock health and disease threats and emergencies that could be triggered by climate change. National capacities in livestock disease should be strengthened by surveillance, preparedness and control through supporting and delivering workforce development and training.

References

Abuajamieh, M.K.A. 2015. Effects of heat stress or ketosis on metabolism and inflammatory biomarkers in ruminants and monogastrics. Graduate Theses and Dissertations. Iowa State University, Ames, Iowa, p 14762. Available via https://lib.dr.iastate.edu/ cgi/ viewcontent.cgi?article=5769&context=etd (Accessed 23 September 2019)

Auvigne, V., Leneveu, P., Jehannin, C., Peltoniemi, O. and Sallé, E. 2010. Seasonal infertility in sows: a five year field study to analyze the relative roles of heat stress and photoperiod. Theriogenology 74, 60–66.

Bernabucci, U., Lacetera, N., Basiricò, L., Ronchi, B., Morera, P., Serene, E. and Nardone, A. 2006. Hot season and BCS affect leptin secretion of periparturient dairy cows. Dairy Sci. 89, 348–349.

Bett, B., Kiunga, P., Gachohi, J., Sindato, C., Mbotha, D., Robinson, T., Lindahl, J. and Grace, D. 2017. Effects of climate change on the occurrence and distribution of livestock diseases. Prev. Vet. Med. 137, 119–129.Forastiere, F. 2010. Climate change and health: a challenge for epidemiology and public health. Int. J. Public Health 55, 83–84.

Dann, H.M., Morin, D.E., Bollero, G.A., Murphy, M.R. and Drackley, J.K. 2005. Prepartum intake, postpartum induction of ketosis and periparturient disorders affect the metabolic status of dairy cows. J. Dairy Sci. 88, 3249–3264.

De, A., Das, T.K., Chand, K., Debnath, B.C., Dey, S., Hemadri, D., Barman, N.N., Chaudhary, J.K., Muthuchelvan, D., Saxena, A. and Tewari, N. 2019. Seroprevalence of bluetongue and presence of viral antigen and type-specific neutralizing antibodies in goats in Tripura, a state at Indo-Bangladesh border of northeastern India. Trop. Anim. Health Prod. 51, 261–265.

Fox, N.J., Marion, G., Davidson, R.S., White, P.C. and Hutchings, M.R. 2012. Livestock helminths in a changing climate: approaches and restrictions to meaningful predictions. Animals 2, 93–107. Fox, N.J., Marion, G., Davidson, R.S., White, P.C. and Hutchings, M.R. 2015.Climate-driven tippingpoints could lead to sudden, high-intensity parasite outbreaks. Royal. Soc. Open Sci. 2, 140296.

Harvell, C.D., Mitchell, C.E., Ward, J.R., Altizer, S., Dobson, A.P., Ostfeld, R.S. and Samuel, M.D. 2002. Climate warming and disease risks for terrestrial and marine biota. Science 296, 2158–2162.

IPCC (Intergovernmental Panel on Climate Change) (2007): Climate Change 2007: Synthesis report. Contribution of Working Groups I, II and III to the Fourth Assessment Report of the Intergovernmental Panel on Climate Change [Core writing team: Pachauri, R.K. and Reisinger, A. (Eds.)]. IPCC, Geneva, Switzerland.

IPCC (Intergovermental Panel on Climate Change), (2023). Climate Change 2023, Synthesis Report, Summary for Policymakers, IPCC, Geneva, Switzerland.

Krishnan, R., Gnanaseelan, C., Sanjay, J., Swapna, P., Dhara, C., Sabin, T.P., Jadhav, J., Sandeep, N., Choudhury, A.D., Singh, M. and Mujumdar, M. 2020. Introduction to climate change over the Indian region. Assessment of climate change over the indian region: A report of the ministry of earth sciences (MoES), Government of India. 1-20.

Lacetera, N. 2019. Impact of climate change on animal health and welfare. Anim Front. 9, 26–31

Lubroth, J. (2015). Climate change and animal health. Building Resilience for adaptation to climate change in the agriculture sector. Animal health services, FAO, Rome. pp 63-70.

Nichi, M., Bols, P.E.J., Züge, R.M., Barnabe, V.H., Goovaerts, I.G.F., Barnabe, R.C. and Cortada, C.N.M. 2006. Seasonal variation in semen quality in Bos indicus and Bos taurus bulls raised under tropical conditions. Theriogenology 66, 822–828.

Oyhantcabal, W., Vitale, E. and Lagarmilla, P. (2010). Climate change and links to animal diseases and production. Conf. OIE, pp 179-186.

Rao, P.P., Hegde, N.R., Reddy, Y.N., Krishnajyothi, Y., Reddy, Y.V., Susmitha, B., Gollapalli, S.R., Putty, K. and Reddy, G.H. 2016. Epidemiology of bluetongue in India. Transbound. Emerg. Dis. 63, e151–e164.

Sawalhah, M.N., Holechek, J.L., Cibils, A.F., Geli, H.M. and Zaied, A. 2019. Rangeland livestock production in relation to climate and vegetation trends in New Mexico. Angeland Ecol. Manag. 72, 832–845.

S.K. Sharma, Garima Rathore and Monika Joshi. 2024. Impact of Climate Change on Animal Health and Mitigation Strategies: A Review. *Indian Journal of Animal Research*, DOI. 10.18805/IJAR.B-5303.

Sridhar, J., Kumar, K.K., Murali-Baskaran, R.K., Senthil-Nathan, S., Sharma, S., Nagesh, M., Kaushal, P. and Kumar, J. (2020). Impact of climate change on communities, response and migration of insects, nematodes, vectors and natural enemies in diverse ecosystems. Global Climate Change: Resilient and Smart Agriculture. pp. 69-93.

Staples, C.R. and Thatcher, W.W. 2011. Heat stress: effects on milk production and composition. In: Encyclopedia of dairy sciences, 4 vols, 2nd edn. Oxford, UK, Academic Press, pp: 561–566.

Stewart, B.M., Block, J., Morelli, P., Navarette, A.E., Amstalden, M., Bonilla, L., Hansen, P.J. and Bilby, T.R. 2011. Efficacy of embryo transfer in lactating dairy cows during summer using fresh or vitrified embryos produced in vitro with sex-sorted semen. J. Dairy Sci. 94, 3437–3445.

Stone, W.C. 2004. Nutritional approaches to minimize subacute ruminal acidosis and laminitis in dairy cattle. J. Dairy Sci. 87, E13–E26.

Talukder, M.A., Rahman, S.M., Miah, M.A., Shahjahan, M., Ali, M.Y., Alam, M.A., Kabir, M.H., Munira, S., Billah, M.M. and Habib, M.R. 2018. Prevalence of different dairy cattle diseases in selected dairy areas and farms of Bangladesh. Asian-Australas J. Biosci. Biotechnol. 3, 331–336.

Visschers, V.H. 2018. Public perception of uncertainties within climate change science. Risk Anal. 38, 43– 55.

West, J.W. 2003. Effects of heat-stress on production in dairy cattle. J. Dairy Sci. 86, 2131–2144.

WHO. 2008. Anthrax in humans and animals. Geneva, Switzerland: World Health Organization. Available via https://www.who.int/csr/resources/publications/ AnthraxGuidelines2008/en/ (Accessed 23 September 2019).

Wittmann, E.J., Mellor, P.S. and Baylis, M. 2001. Using climate data to map the potential distribution of *Culicoides imicola* (Diptera: Ceratopogonidae) in Europe. Rev. Sci. Tech. OIE 20, 731–740.

Wolfenson, D., Roth, Z. and Meidan R. 2000. Impaired reproduction in heat-stressed cattle: basic and applied aspects. Anim. Reprod. Sci. 60, 535–547.

8

A Closer Look at Livestock Health Cattle and Buffalo Disease Diagnosis in Punjab

Ashwani Kumar Sharma

Department of Veterinary Medicine, Guru Angad Dev Veterinary and Animal Sciences University, Ludhiana

Punjab, known as the "breadbasket of India," relies heavily on livestock, particularly cattle and buffalo, for its agricultural prosperity. These animals play a crucial role in the region's dairy industry, contributing significantly to milk production and rural livelihoods. However, like all livestock, cattle and buffalo in Punjab are susceptible to a range of diseases that can impact their health, productivity, and overall well-being. Timely and accurate diagnosis is essential for effective treatment and prevention. This article explores some of the most common diseases affecting cattle and buffalo in Punjab, along with the diagnostic procedures used to detect and manage these health issues, ensuring the sustainability and growth of the dairy sector.

Hydatidosis

Hydatidosis is a zoonotic disease caused by metacestode stages of parasite *Echinococcus granulosus* and is recognized as a major public health problem worldwide. This tapeworm is found in small intestine of the canid (definitive host) where it produce proglottids containing eggs. Upon shedding through faeces the later are ingested by the cattle, buffaloes and other intermediate hosts including man. These hatch in their intestine and the oncosphere invade circulatory system and lodge in various organs (liver, lung, brain etc.) where they develop into large thick walled unilocular cavity called hydatid cyst, which expands and can reach very large size and buds hundreds and thousands of protoscoleces endogenously. In a survey on hydatid cysts, a prevalence rate of around 5% has been recorded in more than 4000 meat samples of different animals in Punjab. Presence of large population of stray dogs in India is associated with high incidence of hydatidosis. Until now, tapeworms and its intermediate stages were not considered to cause primary disease in ruminants and presence of one or two hydatid cysts in viscera on post-mortem or radiography was usually taken as an incidental finding. As surgical removal is difficult a chemotherapeutic agents including praziquantel @ 5 mg/kg body wt. help in clinical recovery of affected animals.

Reticulo-ruminal and Abdominal Disorders

Chronic Reticuloperitonitis or reticulo-ruminal impaction in Cattle and Buffaloes are major referral cases at University Large Animal Veterinary Hospital in Punjab. These cases pose an intense diagnostic challenge in comparison to diseases of small and large intestine. However, from diagnostic point of view forestomach diseases can be categorized into primary indigestion due to fermentative disorders and reticulo-ruminal wall diseases. Most common clinical presentations of reticulo-ruminal diseases and their management are described below.

Traumatic Reticulo-peritonitis

Traumatic reticulo- peritonitis (TRP) is a long recognized syndrome and one of the major maladies responsible for reticulorumen dysfunction in cattle and buffaloes. It is caused by ingestion and entrapping of sharp penetrating foreign bodies in the reticular mucosa which may penetrate its wall leading to different manifestations of the disease. The disease occurs mainly in stall fed animals. The clinical symptoms of these cases need to be interpreted in term of stage of disease when the animal is presented. In per acute cases there is acute tympany, followed sometimes by rise in temperature which fall subsequently depending upon severity of damage. In chronic TRP cases, pain is manifested commonly in different forms. There is arched back condition and anxious expression, or/and frequently more abduction of fore limbs than in normal posture. Disinclination to sit or standing tendency with stiffness or guarded gate on exercise are usually evident.

Ruminal stasis leading to impaction has been observed as being a feature of chronic traumatic reticulitis. Absence of motility in 50 per cent and reduced motility in other 50 % of cases was recorded. Tympany is variably seen in these cases. Decreased or a sudden fall in milk production is an important sign in lactating animals. Mild to moderate depression in general behavior and attitude of affected cows is observed. Radiograph of carnioventral abdomen of bovines is an essential tool for diagnosis of these cases. Now a days two methods are in vogue for treatment of this malady. One is conservative treatment by immobilization of animal along with elevation of forequarter and other laparorumenotomy. Best option is to treat animal conservatively for three days and if no recovery is imminent then go for laparorumenotomy. Conservative treatment is effective and frequently results in recovery. It also help to differentiate TRP with primary indigestion. Now administration of magnet followed by broad spectrum antibiotics and immobilization are recent important part of conservative treatment. Magnet attach to free ferric foreign bodies. If foreign bodies had mild penetration and major part is in the reticulum, chances are that further penetration ceases after administration of magnet. Choice of antibiotic is important. Long acting penicillin and its derivatives twice daily for seven days are good choice for initial treatment of TRP cases.

Abomaso-duodenal Ulcerations

Abomasal ulcer or erosion is a break in the continuity of gastric mucosa that may vary in depth from the surface to a limit of the muscularis mucosa. In cattle abomasal ulcers are located mainly in the pyloric region. Abomasal ulceration in dairy cattle may occur at any age and may result into abomasal haemorrhage, melena, indigestion and even abomasal perforations leading to localized or generalized peritonitis and death. Abomasal ulcers and peritonitis resulting due to their perforation may account for 15% of natural deaths in cattle and buffaloes. Irrespective of the etiology, gastric ulcers seems to be sequel of the gastric erosions that fails to heal for a long time. Gastric erosions and ulcers develop naturally in man and animals and different theories have been proposed for defining their etiology in cattle. The involvement of abrasive agents, such as, roughages, geo sediments, and trichobezoars appears to be the most plausible theory especially in calves. Other incidental affections causing stress like penetrating foreign bodies, other periparturient diseases and different bacteria are some of the factors incriminated for abomasal ulceration. Different abrasive agents like, feedstuff and trichobezoars, abrade abomasal mucosa and cause erosions. Hyperacidity and decreased gastric mucus production that may be primary in chronic stress conditions or secondary due to excessive administration of corticosteroids may also result into development of gastric erosions and later on ulcers. This may be the possible reason behind high prevalence of abomasal ulcers in adult animals within 6 weeks of parturition or during peak milk production period.

The clinical signs of abomasal ulcers are variable and depend upon the severity and complications of the diseases. Abdominal pain, melena, intermittent diarrhea, pale mucus membranes, atony of the rumen, anorexia and fall in milk yield are common clinical signs associated with abomasal ulcers. However, in cases where ulcers are perforating and associated with localized or diffuse peritonitis, more advanced clinical signs, including complete anorexia, fever, increased heart and respiration rate, stasis of gastrointestinal tract and signs of severe abdominal pain may be apparent. At the terminal stages of the disease clinical sings may resemble septic shock. Occult faecal blood test has been found of good diagnostic significance. Other haematological and clinical signs can supplement it. There is anaemia and sometimes the affected cows die peracutely by exsanguinations into the abomasal lumen. Anaemia is manifested by pale mucous membrane, tachycardia, muscle weakness and the fall of PCV to less than 15 per cent. Treatment choices depend upon stage and severity of the diseases. If there is severe haemorrhagic ulceration and PCV is below 12 per cent, blood transfusion is required to save the animal. Administration of antibiotics and antacids are also required alongwith dietary changes. Locally acting antacids, like magnesium oxide (500-800 g/ 450 kg body weight once daily for 2 to 4 days) appears to be more useful and practically applicable for adult cattle. Use of antibiotics, effective against *Clostridium* spp., *Streptococcus* spp., *Bacillus* spp. and *Pseudomonas* spp. seems to be rational keeping in view the reports of their possible involvement in abomasal ulcers in cattle and buffaloes.

Peritonitis

Apart from causes mentioned above the etiology of inflammation of peritoneum is so diverse that at times it become difficult to identify the cause. Common causes include perforation of other abdominal viscera like uterus while doing AI or spontaneous idiopathic rupture of gravid uterus before or at time of delivery, penetrating abdominal injuries, chemical irritants like bile, urine etc. and other disease processes that allow trans mural migration of bacteria (neoplasia, visceral ischemia, prolonged gut stasis). Animal exhibit generalized pain, stiffness of gait and guards its abdomen. There is abdominal distension either due to accumulation of peritoneal exudates or paralytic ileus and is accompanied by septicemia, toxemia, paralytic ileus, shock and adhesions. There is sequestration of electrolytes and protein in abdominal cavity and atonic gut and therefore development of shock. Abdominal paracentensis post xiphoid and parallel to milk vein in abdominal region should be used in large animals to obtain fluid for examination.

Apart from these various diseases like right displacement of abomasum, left displacement of abomasum, intestinal obstruction, congestive heart failure, diaphragmatic hernia, caecal dilatation and torsion, diseases of liver (liver abscess) and pancreas etc. also possess similar signs and are considered while diagnosing cases of GIT stasis in ruminants.

Transtracheal wash (TTW) and Bronchoalveolar Lavage (BAL) for Diagnosis of Respiratory Affections in animals

Respiratory diseases have been causing losses to dairy cattle industries for many years, in terms of mortality, the cost of metaphylactic and therapeutic uses of antibiotics, and reduced growth performance of affected cattle.

Bovines are more susceptible to respiratory diseases because of anatomical and physiological features specific for this species; the absence of inter-alveolar and inter-bronchiolar collateral ventilation, the high ventilation rate and strong resistance to airflow within the respiratory conducts.

In Veterinary Practice, identification of specific pathogen causing lower respiratory tract infections continued to be a problem due to inadequate diagnostics. Most respiratory diseases are treated with empiric therapy; antimicrobials are used irrespective of its sensitivity to infections leading to its side effects and resistance. Many of these cases are treated on the basis of clinical signs, blood pathology, radiographs etc. Many a time final diagnosis is difficult and hence these cases require a lot of time to recover.

Under the present clinical setup, diagnosis of respiratory diseases is based on detailed and targeted history and thorough physical examination and clinical examination, hematology and radiography. With these modalities, the etiological diagnosis sometimes remains difficult and thus leads to treatment failures. Etiological diagnosis can be better achieved if lower respiratory samples are available for laboratory examination. In recent past, novel techniques *viz.* tracheal wash and bronchoalveolar lavage have been introduced for collection and examination of respiratory secretions in various species.

Transtracheal wash is a reliable technique for diagnosis of lower respiratory tract affections in animals. It gives a complete picture of pathological features of lower respiratory tract. The technique is most sensitive for detection of diseases of the tracheobronchial tree and is least sensitive for detection of interstitial lung disease. It is a commonly employed procedure for culture of pathogens of lower respiratory tract. Bacteriological evaluation of a transtracheal aspirate may provide useful information on antimicrobial sensitivity & aid in the selection of appropriate drugs. In animals with pneumonia, the nasal flora may not reflect that in the lung and cultures are best taken as transtracheal aspirates of the lower respiratory system. The cytological analysis of transtracheal wash is also useful for diagnosis and differentiation of lower respiratory diseases of inflammatory and non inflammatory origin. Cytology can be a useful diagnostic tool. Inflammation, neoplasia and specific pathogens can be differentiated with cytologic procedures. Transtracheal wash cytology provides a relatively simple technique for obtaining information regarding disease processes occurring in the trachea and bronchial tree.

Transtracheal Wash

Transtracheal wash is a simple diagnostic technique to collect tracheo-bronchial secretions for cytological and microbiological examination. Tracheo-bronchial secretions are collected percutaneously in a standing conscious animal. At ventral midline of neck, trachea is grasped, steel canula (10 G) is inserted through a small incision into the tracheal lumen between two tracheal rings. Infant feeding tube (7 Fr) is threaded through the steel canula towards the lungs so as to reach the thoracic inlet. Normal saline (50 ml) is infused and aspirated back immediately while withdrawing the catheter. If first attempt is unsuccessful, procedure can be repeated to a maximum of four times.

Nutritional Hemoglobinuria in Cattle and Buffaloes

Adult cattle and buffaloes are susceptible to the non-infectious hemolytic condition known as nutritional hemoglobinuria, which affects numerous animals each year during pregnancy and the first few months of lactation. Severe anaemia, hemoglobinuria, intravascular hemolysis, and mortality from anoxia and anaemia are its hallmark symptoms. In the native parlance, nutritional hemoglobinuria is known as "Post Parturient Hemoglobinuria" "Lahu mutna" or "Rakth mutna."

Despite the fact that the aetiology of nutritional hemoglobinuria is unknown, several risk factors have been connected to it, including the consumption of cruciferous plants, berseem saponin, dietary phosphorus insufficiency, decreased serum copper and selenium, and excessive molybdenum. The low phosphorus content of berseem, lucerne, sugar cane tops, sugar beets, kale, mustard as well as the presence of inhibitory factors like metallic ions interfere with dietary phosphorus absorption and assimilation, all contribute to a precipitous phosphorus deficiency. As a result of hypophosphatemia, red blood cell glycolysis and ATP generation is reduced causing an increase in fragility and hemolysis, all of which can lead to hemoglobinuria and hemoglobinemia. Within 20±10 days before or after parturition, infected buffaloes generally show the first noticeable evidence of passing red to coffee-coloured urine. Faeces might be solid, dry, and bile-coloured.

The diagnosis of nutritional hemoglobinuria is made using the clinical history, along with clinical signs like pale mucous membrane, tenesmus, and coffee to red brown urine. Keeping in view the economic losses due to high mortality, marked decrease in milk yield and long convalescent period in few survivors due to poor response to treatment, makes this an important disease.

As berseem is main fodder available in Punjab during the winter months so most of the cases are associated with berseem feeding. PPH is strongly associated with berseem feeding in the winter season. By virtue of its hemolytic saponin contents, the berseem feeding is thought to predispose the animals to nutritional hemoglobinuria however no saponin has been reported till date causing PPH in animals. Berseem is a rich source of calcium, with wide Ca ; P ratio that results in imbalance and deficiency of phosphorus. The recent parturition predisposes the animals to phosphorus deficiency.

9

Antimicrobial Resistance in Livestock Sector: An Update

Samiran Bandyopadhyay[1], Indranil Samanta[2]

[1]*ICAR-Indian Veterinary Research Institute, Eastern Regional Station Kolkata, West Bengal*

[2]*Department of Veterinary Microbiology, West Bengal University of Animal and Fishery Sciences, 37, K.B. Sarani, Kolkata, West Bengal, India*

AMR is undoubtedly the most serious challenge ever faced by the world health community because of its multifaceted complex nature and its overwhelming impact over the human and veterinary communities. Livestock sector is no exception to have the serious and devastating impact from the emergence and spread of AMR. Because of a steady shift towards intensive farming and increased stocking density there has been increase occurrence of infectious diseases. Growing world population, rapid urbanization, and deforestation, shrinkage of grazing land all aided to this process. This leads to increased usage of antimicrobials in food animals – cause of concern for the scientific community as AMU is known the single most important driver of AMR.

Antimicrobial Usage in Livestock

Antibiotics are used for three main purposes in food animals

1. Therapeutic purpose for treatment of sick/diseased animals.
2. Control treatment or metaphylaxis when exposed but apparently healthy animals are treated during any outbreak to reduce the spread of infection and sometimes to reduce morbidity in animals already incubating the disease.
3. Prophylactic treatment.

Nevertheless, apart from that antibiotics are often used as growth promoter in medicated feed and this has always been a controversial issue held responsible for emergence and spread of AMR in livestock sector.

Antibiotics at low or sub-therapeutic dosage are believed to improve feed conversion ratio by modifying the gut flora [8,9]. It is also propounded that antimicrobials protect intestinal epithelial lining, suppress the infections and toxins produced by the opportunistic pathogens and enhance the growth of healthy flora. However, recent studies showed that the growth promotion is only apparent when animals are kept in absence of proper biosecurity measures, which rise critical doubts about non-therapeutic use of AM (Prior, 1999).

While antimicrobials are necessary for treating sick animals, non-therpeutic usage remained a controversial issue for its purported role in the emergence of AMR. In food animals, it was estimated that about 131,109 tons of antimicrobials were used in 2013 and by 2030 this figure will reach to 200,235 tons (Van Boeckel *et al.*, 2017). A large proportion of it will be due to the non-therapeutic purposes as revealed from several reports (US Food and Drug Administration, 2016; European Medicines Agency, 2017). It is noteworthy that data of such kind is very limited when it comes to the developing parts of the globe; however, anecdotal reports suggested that non-therapeutic usage is no less in LMICs. About 3838 tons of antimicrobials were used in Vietnam, as emerged from a recent reports and more than 70% of it was used in animal sector. Nevertheless, when the calculation corresponds to biomass, the figure remained parallel referring to 261.7 mg and 247.3 mg per kg of human and animal biomass, respectively (Carrique-Mas *et al.*, 2020)we estimated AMU in Vietnam (human population 93.4 M in 2015. Actually, the LMICs are expected to face more challenges due to rapid urbanization, increase population, deforestation, and change in the ecosystem and increase in the demand of animal protein. It has been estimated that AMU in food animals is going to increase by 99% only among the BRICs. We have scarcity of data on AMU in animals in India. However, a study in dairy sector conducted by ICAR and ILRI in few selected areas revealed that over-the-counter access of antibiotics without prescription, and direct marketing of drugs to the dairy farmers are common and dairy farmers often take advice from untrained “animal health workers” and para-veterinarians for treatment. Mastitis is the most common condition where antimicrobials are frequently used (Mutua *et al.*, 2020; Sharma *et al.*, 2020)particularly the dairy sector, is important for food and nutritional wellbeing of communities in India, it supports livelihoods of many farmers, and contributes to the economy of the country. India is a high consumer of antibiotics and antimicrobial resistant (AMR. Nonetheless, on farm antibiotic use is low [10%] and only a small proportion of the milk samples (8%) contained antibiotic residue (Kumar *et al.*, 2021).

Other Factors Causing AMR

There are other factors which are known to promote AMR. This fact can be substantiated by the recent observations on resistance of the animal pathogens to certain groups of drugs which are not used in animals like carbapenem and glycopeptide. As resistance genes are often carried in the form of gene cassettes in plasmid or transposons, AMs in at sub-therapeutic concentrations of any antibacterial agent may give rise to multiple groups of antimicrobials. Several antiseptics like sodium hypochlorite, benzalkonium chloride, quaternary ammonium compounds, which are used for various household purposes may also give rise to AMR (Kampf, 2018)antibiotic resistance, horizontal gene transfer, and efflux pump. In cells adapted to benzalkonium chloride a new resistance was most frequently found to ampicillin (eight species. Heavy metals like, mercury (Hg), cadmium (Cd), copper (Cu), and zinc (Zn) in environment and exposure of the animals to such compounds through animal feed and water may trigger the animal pathogens to acquire AMR genes (Seiler & Berendonk, 2012)

AMR in Livestock Sector

Livestock Associated MRSA

Livestock associated MRSA has been known to emerge in animal/livestock sector and genotypically differs from HA-MRSA or CA-MRSA and these strains belong to clonal complex CC398. However, about 10% of the CA-MRSA infections were attributed to LA-MRSA. Although LA-MRSA infections are asymptomatic in animals they can cause severe infections in human like animal handlers, veterinarians and farmers (Cuny, Wieler & Witte, 2015)MRSA infections may occur outside and independent of hospitals, caused by community associated MRSA (CA-MRSA. Several reports suggested that animals are not permanently but transiently colonized by LA-MRSA and infection to human often depends on frequency and duration of animal contact (Anjum *et al.*, 2019)recent reports suggest a possible increasing trend in the zoonotic transmission of LA-MRSA in Europe. Since its emergence in the early 2000's, several investigations have indicated that persons in prolonged, repeated contact with affected livestock are at a higher risk of becoming colonized with LA-MRSA. LA-MRSA monitoring in livestock is voluntary under current EU legislation, and not all member states, including the UK, participate. UK LA-MRSA isolates have been detected through scanning surveillance, where samples are submitted from clinically diseased livestock for diagnostic investigation, and research studies. Surveys conducted on retail beef, pig and poultry meat on sale in the UK have also detected LA-MRSA. Taken together these results suggest that LA-MRSA is present in the UK, possibly at low prevalence level, as suggested by available evidence. In this review, we examine the data available from UK livestock and animal products, and make recommendations for future. We also review the findings from whole genome sequencing (WGS. LA-MRSA were reported in pigs (24–86%), cattle (31-37%) and farmers (9-37%) and veterinarians having contact with pigs (44-45%) in the European countries (Goerge *et al.*, 2017)cattle or poultry is very frequent. In Europe, LA-MRSA mostly belong to the clonal lineage CC398. Since colonized persons have an increased risk of developing MRSA infections, defining the burden of work-related infection caused by LA-MRSA CC398 is of interest to exposed personnel, insurance companies and infection control staff. This review summarizes data on the types of occupation-related infections caused by LA-MRSA CC398, the incidence of such infections as well as potential preventive strategies. We identified twelve case reports on infections among livestock-exposed persons. Overall, there is a lack of data describing the incidence of occupation-related infections due to MRSA CC398. Currently, no specific guidance towards the prevention of LA-MRSA CC398 colonization of persons with routine exposure exists. In vitro, MRSA CC398 strains are susceptible (>95%. Usually LA-MRSA are considered to be resistant to a number of antibiotics like β-lactams, macrolides, lincosamides, streptogramines, tetracyclines, fluoroquinolones and cotrimoxazole. Although glycopeptide is often selected for treating LA-MRSA infections, our study revealed the presence of vancomycin-resistant LA-MRSA from bovine and caprine milk (Bhattacharyya *et al.*, 2016). Further, two of these strains have the genotype (MRSA-SCC*mec*-V-spa*t267*) previously reported to cause human and animal infections.

Carbapenem Resistance

Carbapenems are considered last resort therapy for treating the infections caused by critical pathogens like ESBL producing *Enterobacteriaceae.* Carbapenem resistance has been reported among various health care associated infections world-wide including India, especially in the ICU or CCU wards. Nonetheless, such pathogens have been sporadically reported in animals. This is not surprising as carbapenems are rarely or not used in animals. But their usage is quite frequent in human to treat increasing burden of infections caused by ESBL producers. Of various carbapenem resistance determinants, KPC, OXA-48 and NDM have been more frequently detected among the *enterobacteriaceae*. The carbapenem resistance determinants along with other resistant gene(s) are often carried on plasmid, integrons or other mobile genetic elements with insertion sequences. Such genetic architecture make the pathogen a true superbug because of their non-susceptibility to all the common antibiotics . While NDM and OXA-48 were more commonly detected in *E. coli* and *K. pneumoniae* both in hospital and community acquired infections, KPC producing *K. pneumoniae* was frequent cause of nosocomial infections in USA, Israel, Greece and other countries. Because of high morbidity and mortality associated with CRE infections, CRE are also known as 'killer bacteria" or nightmare bacteria". CRE (*Escherichia* and *Klebsiella*) with several carbapenemase like VIM, KPC, NDM, OXA, and IMP were reported from diverse animal species (pigs, poultry, cattle, seafood, dogs, cats, horses, pet birds, swallows, wild boars, wild stork, gulls, and black kites) in Africa, America, Asia, Australia, and Europe (Köck *et al.*, 2018). In India, carbapenem resistance has been reported from pigs (Pruthvishree *et al.*, 2017; Tamta *et al.*, 2020)fecal sample (n = 673, diarrhoeic cattle (Bandyopadhyay *et al.*, 2021b)72 MDR isolates, including 35 E. coli (DC: 27; HC 8 and companion animals (Bandyopadhyay *et al.*, 2021a)no systemic study has been carried out on CRE in companion animals in Indian subcontinent. In total, 237 canine specimens collected from five veterinary polyclinics in and around Kolkata were analyzed for isolation, antimicrobial resistance profiling and molecular characterization of carbapenem-resistant (CR. In recent past, Tewari *et al.*, 2019AmpC lactamase- and/or metallo-β-lactamase (MBL reported MBL (IMP, SIM) resistance determinants among 6% of the *E. coli* isolates from bovine and poultry in North-eastern regions.

Cephalosporin Resistance

A spectrum of β-lactam deactivating enzymes - β-lactamses are often employed by bacteria for developing resistance to cephalosporins and cephalosporinase or AmpC type β-lactamse (ACBL) and extended spectrum β-lactamse (ESBL) are possibly the most common variants. While narrow spectrum β-lactamse producers exhibit resistance towards first and second generation cephalosporins, ACBL and ESBL can exhibit resistance to newer generation or higher generation cephalosporins as well. Whereas ESBLs can be inhibited by β-lactamse-inhibitor like clavulinic acid or sulbactum, ACBL can remain active even in the presence of β-lactamse inhibitors. A study carried out in three states of India –Jharkhand, West Bengal and Mizoram, revealed that more than 50% of the *Klebsiella* isolated from bovine milk have reduced susceptibility to at least one cephalosporin and occurrence of ESBL was higher among the cows with clinical (13.4%) and subclinical mastitis (7.5%) than the healthy one (1.5%) and about 30% of the isolates were AmpC β-lactamse producers (Koovapra *et al.*, 2016)isolated from milk samples (n=340. Further, nearly 6% of the poultry and 3% of the bovine milk were found to harbor ESBL producing *E. coli* as revealed in a separate study conducted in Odisha (Kar *et al.*, 2015)India. Of 316 E. coli isolated from 305 samples (170 fecal samples from poultry and 135 milk samples from cattle. About 3.2% of the buffalo milk samples were found to carry ESBL (Bandyopadhyay *et al.*, 2018). Likewise, a recent study conducted in healthy and diarrhoeic cattle from different agro-climatic zones of West Bengal found that about 70% of the multi-drug resistant *E coli* and *Klebsiella pneumoniae* harboured *bla*CTX-M-15 ESBL gene (Bandyopadhyay *et al.*, 2021b)72 MDR isolates, including 35 E. coli (DC: 27; HC 8.

Colistin-resistance

Polymixin or colistin, which had been previously disserted because of toxicity and advent of relatively safe drugs like aminoglycosides, has now gained attention because of their effectiveness against various multi-resistant super bugs like carbapenem-resistant pathogens and now is considered in preserved drug category. It is effective against a range of pathogens like including *Escherichia coli*, *Enterobacter* spp., *Klebsiella* spp., *Citrobacter* spp., *Salmonella* spp., and *Shigella* spp including the nonfermentative Gram-negative bacteria, such as *Acinetobacter baumannii*, *Pseudomonas aeruginosa*, and *Stenotrophomonas maltophilia* (Aghapour et al., 2019). However, uninterrupted use of colistin as monotherapy in CRE infections and use of colistin in animals led to emergence of colistin resistance (Li *et al.*, 2020). In general, colistin-resistance is imparted by modification of outer membrane lipopolysaccharide leading to change of surface charges (Bandyopadhyay, 2020)an age old drug which lost attention following introduction of more effective and less toxic drugs, has again been favoured by the clinicians for its supremacy over the modern drugs for treating infections caused by refractory pathogens like carbapenem-resistant Enterobacteriaceae. However, emergence of plasmid-mediated colistin resistance came as a major setback. Animal sector, which had long history of colistin use as growth promoter, particularly in countries like China and Vietnam, has been blamed for emergence and spread of colistin-resistance across the globe. This paper describes various aspects of colistin resistance and its spread across the animal sector.","container-title":"Indian Journal of Animal Health","DOI":"10.36062/ijah.59.1.2020.29-32", "ISSN": "0019-5057", "issue": "1","journalAbbreviation": "Indian Journal of Animal Health", "language": "en", "page": "29","source": DOI.org (Crossref. Furthermore, plasmid mediated colistin resistance (*mcr*) which was first detected in China possibily due to its exuderant usage in pig and poultry farming (Liu *et al.*, 2016)polymyxin resistance has involved chromosomal mutations but has never been reported via horizontal gene transfer. During a routine surveillance project on antimicrobial resistance in commensal Escherichia coli from food animals in China, a major increase of colistin resistance was observed. When an E coli strain, SHP45, possessing colistin resistance that could be transferred to another strain, was isolated from a pig, we conducted further analysis of possible plasmid-mediated polymyxin resistance. Herein, we report the emergence of the first plasmid-mediated polymyxin resistance mechanism, MCR-1, in Enterobacteriaceae.\nMETHODS: The mcr^{1} gene in *E coli* strain SHP45 was identified by whole plasmid sequencing and subcloning. MCR-1 mechanistic studies were done with sequence comparisons, homology modelling, and electrospray ionisation mass spectrometry. The prevalence of mcr-1 was investigated in E coli and Klebsiella pneumoniae strains collected from five provinces between April, 2011, and November, 2014. The ability of MCR-1 to confer polymyxin resistance in vivo was examined in a murine thigh model.\nFINDINGS: Polymyxin resistance was shown to be singularly due to the plasmid-mediated mcr-1 gene. The plasmid carrying mcr-1 was mobilised to an E coli recipient at a frequency of 10(-1 became a cause of concern world-wide because of their rapid spread across the food animals ad human being. Recent past, it was also recorsed from India (Ghafur *et al.*, 2019)including poultry meat, mutton meat, fish, fruit and vegetables, collected from food outlets in Chennai, India, were processed to identify Col-R bacteria using eosin methylene blue agar supplemented with colistin. Colistin minimum inhibitory concentrations (MICs. Apart from pigs and poultry, colistin resistance was reported in cows (Hernández *et al.*, 2017)although colistin resistance was non-mobilisable. The isolate was producing extended-spectrum beta-lactamases and belonged to serotype O9:H10 and sequence type ST533. Here we report an mcr-3 gene detected in Europe following earlier reports from Asia and the United States.”,”container-title”:”Euro Surveillance: Bulletin Europeen Sur Les Maladies Transmissibles = European Communicable Disease Bulletin”,”DOI”:”10.2807/1560-7917.ES.2017.22.31.30586”,”ISSN”: ”1560-7917”,”issue”:”31”,”journalAbbreviation”: ”Euro Surveill”, ”language”: ”eng”, ”note”: ”PMID: 28797328\nPMCID: PMC5553059”,”page”:”30586” ,”source”:”PubMed”,”title”:”Co-occurrence of colistin-resistance genes mcr-1 and mcr-3 among multidrug-resistant Escherichia coli isolated from cattle, Spain, Septemberndez”, ”given”: ”Marta”}, {“family”: ”Iglesias”, ”given”: ”M. Rocío”}, {“family”:”Rodríguez-Lázaro”, ”given”: ”David”}, {“family”: ”Gallardo”, ”given”: ”Alejandro”}, {“family”:”Quijada”, ”given”: ”Narciso”}, {“family”: ”Miguela-Villoldo”, ”given”: ”Pedro”}, {“family”:”Campos”, ”given”: ”Maria Jorge”}, {“family”: ”Píriz”,”given”:”Segundo”},{“family”: ”López-Orozco”,”given”:”Gema”}, {“family”: ”Frutos”, ”given”: ”Cristina”, ”non-dropping-particle”: ”de”}, {“family”: ”Sáez”, ”given”: ”José Luis”}, {“family”: ”Ugarte-Ruiz”, ”given”: ”María”},{“family”: ”Domínguez”, ”given”:”Lucas”}, {“family”: ”Quesada”,”given”: ”Alberto”}], ”issued”:{“date-parts”: [[“2017”,8,3]]}}}], ”schema”:”https://github.com/citation-style-language/schema/raw/master/csl-citation.json”} and pet animals (Rumi *et al.*, 2019) plasmid-mediated AmpC (pAmpC. Of late, Government of India banned use of colistin in animals as growth promoter.

Quinolone Resistance

In human quinolones are often prescribed for treating urinary and respiratory tract infections, while in animals quinolones indicated for soft tissue and urinary tract infections in pet animals, colibacillosis in poultry and bovine respiratory disease. As quinolones are semisynthetic molecules, it was assumed that quinolone resistance will not emerge easily. However, the picture is quite opposite as resistance to quinolones has been quite frequently reported in this part of the globe. Screening about 862 clinical *E coli* isolates collected from chickens, ducks, pigs, and cows from Jiangsu, China revealed that resistance to ciprofloxacin and enrofloxacin may range from 13.1% and 16.4% in cows to as high as 95.4% and 100% in ducks (Yassin et al., 2017). In contrast, Kaspersen *et al.*, 2018 recorded that only 1.6% of the animal *E. coli* isolates were quinolone-resistant. In addition, several studies conducted through out the globe indicated increasing detection of quinolone resistance among poultry (de Jong, Stephan & Silley, 2012)there are a number of veterinary monitoring programmes that collect bacteria in food-producing animals at slaughter and determine their susceptibility against antibiotics relevant for human medicine. The data generated are part of the risk analysis for potential food-borne transmission of resistance. There has been much debate about the use of fluoroquinolones in veterinary medicine, and so, this review will consider the fluoroquinolone data from two surveys and compare them to national surveillance programmes. At the outset, it must be pointed out that there is, however, a lack of agreement between several programmes on what is meant by the term ‘fluoroquinolone resistance’ through use of different definitions of resistance and different resistance breakpoints. An additional aim of this paper is to clarify some of those definitions. Despite the debate about the contribution of antibiotic use in veterinary medicine to the overall resistance development in human pathogens, the data suggest that clinical resistance to fluoroquinolones in Escherichia coli and nontyphoidal Salmonella is generally uncommon, except for a few countries. Ongoing surveillance will continue to monitor the situation and identify whether this situation changes within the respective animal populations. For the benefit of both the epidemiologist and the clinician, it would be strongly advantageous that national monitoring surveys report both percentages of clinical resistance and decreased susceptibility.”,”container-title”:”Journal of Applied Microbiology”,”DOI”:”10.1111/j.1365-2672.2011.05193.x”,”ISSN”:”1365-2672”,”issue”:”2”,”language”:”en”,”note”:”_eprint: https://onlinelibrary.wiley.com/doi/pdf/10.1111/j.1365-2672.2011.05193.x”,”page”:”239-245”,”source”:”Wiley Online Library”,”title”:”Fluoroquinolone resistance of Escherichia coli and Salmonella from healthy livestock and poultry in the EU ”,”volume”:”112”,”author”:[{“family”:”Jong”,”given”:”A.”,”non-dropping-particle”:”de”},{“family”:”Stephan”,”given”:”B.”},{“family”:”Silley”,”given”:”P.”}],”issued”:{“date-parts”:[[“2012”]]}}}],”schema”:”https://github.com/citation-style-language/schema/raw/master/csl-citation.json”}

Future Course of Action

India’s national action plan on AMR came into force in 2017 and it aims at substantial reduction in the burden of AMR pathogens prevalent in human and animal sector and it calls for a holistic and over-arching approach for its effective implementation. At the same time NAP on AMR also included several meticulous plans to optimize AMU in these sectors in order to counter the burgeoning problem of AMR. However, effective implementation of NAP on AMR is yet to achieve due to lack of adequate resources. The recent pandemic curtailed fund and fund allocation is still not sufficient, at least in animal sector for timely and successful implementation of NAP. Although ICAR has started a surveillance programme in network Region wise estimation of AMU in food animals may add information upon the specific role of AMU in animals on spread of AMR. It is well understood that poor and marginal farmers who keep livestock in backyard farming system rarely use antibiotics. However, this may not be the scenario in organized or intensive rearing system. ICAR-INFAAR, A PAN-India network started by ICAR to understand the status of AMR in food animals may adopt an AMU estimation protocol in near future to have country wise data on AMU in livestock sector in India. Although the therapeutic use of antibiotics is necessary, the nutritional or prophylactic usage of antimicrobials needs to be regulated. Government of India banned the use of colistin in food animals for growth promotion. Systemic phasing out of the non-therapeutic use of antibiotics and ban of medically important antibiotics may diminish AMU in animals. Stringent abidance of antibiotic residue limit in raw or processed food of animal origin should be another criteria to reduce the unnecessary usage of antibiotics. Infection prevention control with adequate biosecurity measures, promotion of alternatives to antimicrobials, financial incentives and awareness on AMR and AMU among various stakeholders can reduce the unscrupulous usage of antimicrobials in animal farming and thereby the problem of AMR.

References

Aghapour, Z., Gholizadeh, P., Ganbarov, K., Bialvaei, A.Z., Mahmood, S.S., Tanomand, A., Yousefi, M., Asgharzadeh, M., Yousefi, B. and Kafil, H.S. (2019) Molecular mechanisms related to colistin resistance in Enterobacteriaceae. Infect Drug Resist. 12, 965–975.

Anjum, M.F., Marco-Jimenez, F., Duncan, D., Marín, C., Smith, R.P. and Evans, S.J. (2019) Livestock-Associated Methicillin-Resistant Staphylococcus aureus From Animals and Animal Products in the UK. Front Microbiol. 10, 2136.

Bandyopadhyay, S. (2020) Emergence of colistin-resistance- An update. Indian Journal of Animal Health. 59, 29.

Bandyopadhyay, S., Banerjee, J., Bhattacharyya, D., Samanta, I., Mahanti, A., Dutta, T.K., Ghosh, S., Nanda, P.K., Dandapat, P. and Bandyopadhyay, S. (2018) Genomic Identity of Fluoroquinolone-Resistant blaCTX-M-15-Type ESBL and pMAmpC β-Lactamase Producing Klebsiella pneumoniae from Buffalo Milk, India. Microb Drug Resist. 24, 1345–1353.

Bandyopadhyay, S., Banerjee, J., Bhattacharyya, D., Tudu, R., Samanta, I., Dandapat, P., Nanda, P.K., Das, A.K., Mondal, B., Batabyal, S. and Dutta, T.K. (2021a) Companion Animals Emerged as an Important Reservoir of Carbapenem-Resistant Enterobacteriaceae: A Report from India. Curr Microbiol. 78, 1006–1016.

Bandyopadhyay, S., Bhattacharyya, D., Samanta, I., Banerjee, J., Habib, M., Dutta, T.K. and Dutt, T. (2021b) Characterization of Multidrug-Resistant Biofilm-Producing Escherichia coli and Klebsiella pneumoniae in Healthy Cattle and Cattle with Diarrhea. Microb Drug Resist.

Bandyopadhyay, S. and Samanta, I. (2020) Antimicrobial Resistance in Agri-Food Chain and Companion Animals as a Re-emerging Menace in Post-COVID Epoch: Low-and Middle-Income Countries Perspective and Mitigation Strategies. Frontiers in Veterinary Science. 7, 620.

Bhattacharyya, D., Banerjee, J., Bandyopadhyay, S., Mondal, B., Nanda, P.K., Samanta, I., Mahanti, A., Das, A.K., Das, G., Dandapat, P. and Bandyopadhyay, S. (2016) First Report on Vancomycin-Resistant Staphylococcus aureus in Bovine and Caprine Milk. Microb Drug Resist. 22, 675–681.

Carrique-Mas, J.J., Choisy, M., Van Cuong, N., Thwaites, G. and Baker, S. (2020) An estimation of total antimicrobial usage in humans and animals in Vietnam. Antimicrobial Resistance & Infection Control. 9, 16.

Cuny, C., Wieler, L.H. and Witte, W. (2015) Livestock-Associated MRSA: The Impact on Humans. Antibiotics (Basel). 4, 521–543.

de Jong, A., Stephan, B. and Silley, P. (2012) Fluoroquinolone resistance of Escherichia coli and Salmonella from healthy livestock and poultry in the EU. Journal of Applied Microbiology. 112, 239–245.

European Medicines Agency (2017) Sales of Veterinary Antimicrobial Agents in 30 European Countries in 2015.

Ghafur, A., Shankar, C., GnanaSoundari, P., Venkatesan, M., Mani, D., Thirunarayanan, M.A. and Veeraraghavan, B. (2019) Detection of chromosomal and plasmid-mediated mechanisms of colistin resistance in Escherichia coli and Klebsiella pneumoniae from Indian food samples. J Glob Antimicrob Resist. 16, 48–52.

Goerge, T., Lorenz, M.B., van Alen, S., Hübner, N.-O., Becker, K. and Köck, R. (2017) MRSA colonization and infection among persons with occupational livestock exposure in Europe: Prevalence, preventive options and evidence. Vet Microbiol. 200, 6–12.

Hernández, M., Iglesias, M.R., Rodríguez-Lázaro, D., Gallardo, A., Quijada, N., Miguela-Villoldo, P., Campos, M.J., Píriz, S., López-Orozco, G., de Frutos, C., Sáez, J.L., Ugarte-Ruiz, M., Domínguez, L. and Quesada, A. (2017) Co-occurrence of colistin-resistance genes mcr-1 and mcr-3 among multidrug-resistant Escherichia coli isolated from cattle, Spain, September 2015. Euro Surveill. 22, 30586.

Kampf, G. (2018) Biocidal Agents Used for Disinfection Can Enhance Antibiotic Resistance in Gram-Negative Species. Antibiotics (Basel). 7, 110.

Kar, D., Bandyopadhyay, S., Bhattacharyya, D., Samanta, I., Mahanti, A., Nanda, P.K., Mondal, B., Dandapat, P., Das, A.K., Dutta, T.K., Bandyopadhyay, S. and Singh, R.K. (2015) Molecular and phylogenetic characterization of multidrug resistant extended spectrum beta-lactamase producing Escherichia coli isolated from poultry and cattle in Odisha, India. Infect Genet Evol. 29, 82–90.

Kaspersen, H., Urdahl, A.M., Simm, R., Slettemeås, J.S., Lagesen, K. and Norström, M. (2018) Occurrence of quinolone resistant E. coli originating from different animal species in Norway. Veterinary Microbiology. 217, 25–31.

Koovapra, S., Bandyopadhyay, S., Das, G., Bhattacharyya, D., Banerjee, J., Mahanti, A., Samanta, I., Nanda, P.K., Kumar, A., Mukherjee, R., Dimri, U. and Singh, R.K. (2016) Molecular signature of extended spectrum β-lactamase producing Klebsiella pneumoniae isolated from bovine milk in eastern and north-eastern India. Infect Genet Evol. 44, 395–402.

Kumar, N., Sharma, G., Leahy, E., Shome, B.R., Bandyopadhyay, S., Deka, R.P., Shome, R., Dey, T.K. and Lindahl, J.F. (2021) Understanding Antibiotic Usage on Small-Scale Dairy Farms in the Indian States of Assam and Haryana Using a Mixed-Methods Approach-Outcomes and Challenges. Antibiotics (Basel). 10, 1124.

Köck, R., Daniels-Haardt, I., Becker, K., Mellmann, A., Friedrich, A.W., Mevius, D., Schwarz, S. and Jurke, A. (2018) Carbapenem-resistant Enterobacteriaceae in wildlife, food-producing, and companion animals: a systematic review. Clin Microbiol Infect. 24, 1241–1250.

Li, B., Yin, F., Zhao, X., Guo, Y., Wang, W., Wang, P., Zhu, H., Yin, Y. and Wang, X. (2020) Colistin Resistance Gene mcr-1 Mediates Cell Permeability and Resistance to Hydrophobic Antibiotics. Frontiers in Microbiology. 10, 3015.

Liu, Y.-Y., Wang, Y., Walsh, T.R., Yi, L.-X., Zhang, R., Spencer, J., Doi, Y., Tian, G., Dong, B., Huang, X., Yu, L.-F., Gu, D., Ren, H., Chen, X., Lv, L., He, D., Zhou, H., Liang, Z., Liu, J.-H. and Shen, J. (2016) Emergence of plasmid-mediated colistin resistance mechanism MCR-1 in animals and human beings in China: a microbiological and molecular biological study. Lancet Infect Dis. 16, 161–168.

Mutua, F., Sharma, G., Grace, D., Bandyopadhyay, S., Shome, B. and Lindahl, J. (2020) A review of animal health and drug use practices in India, and their possible link to antimicrobial resistance. Antimicrob Resist Infect Control. 9, 103.

Pokharel, S., Shrestha, P. and Adhikari, B. (2020) Antimicrobial use in food animals and human health: time to implement 'One Health' approach. Antimicrobial Resistance & Infection Control. 9, 181.

Prior, S. (1999) Use of antibiotics in livestock production and antimicrobial resistance. Royal Society of Medicine, London, UK

Pruthvishree, B.S., Vinodh Kumar, O.R., Sinha, D.K., Malik, Y.P.S., Dubal, Z.B., Desingu, P.A., Shivakumar, M., Krishnaswamy, N. and Singh, B.R. (2017) Spatial molecular epidemiology of carbapenem-resistant and New Delhi metallo beta-lactamase (blaNDM)-producing Escherichia coli in the piglets of organized farms in India. J Appl Microbiol. 122, 1537–1546.

Roth, N., Käsbohrer, A., Mayrhofer, S., Zitz, U., Hofacre, C. and Domig, K.J. (2019) The application of antibiotics in broiler production and the resulting antibiotic resistance in Escherichia coli: A global overview. Poultry Science. 98, 1791–1804.

Rumi, M.V., Mas, J., Elena, A., Cerdeira, L., Muñoz, M.E., Lincopan, N., Gentilini, É.R., Di Conza, J. and Gutkind, G. (2019) Co-occurrence of clinically relevant β-lactamases and MCR-1 encoding genes in Escherichia coli from companion animals in Argentina. Vet Microbiol. 230, 228–234.

Schar, D., Sommanustweechai, A., Laxminarayan, R. and Tangcharoensathien, V. (2018) Surveillance of antimicrobial consumption in animal production sectors of low- and middle-income countries: Optimizing use and addressing antimicrobial resistance. PLoS Med. 15, e1002521.

Seiler, C. and Berendonk, T. (2012) Heavy metal driven co-selection of antibiotic resistance in soil and water bodies impacted by agriculture and aquaculture. Frontiers in Microbiology. 3, 399.

Sharma, G., Mutua, F., Deka, R.P., Shome, R., Bandyopadhyay, S., Shome, B., Goyal Kumar, N., Grace, D., Dey, T.K., Venugopal, N., Sahay, S. and Lindahl, J. (2020) A qualitative study on antibiotic use and animal health management in smallholder dairy farms of four regions of India. Infect Ecol Epidemiol. 10, 1792033.

Tamta, S., O R, V.K., B S, P., R, K., Rupner, R.N., G E, C., Dubal, Z.B., Sinha, D.K. and Singh, B.R. (2020) Faecal carriage of extended spectrum beta-lactamase (ESBL) and New Delhi metallo beta-lactamase(NDM) producing Escherichia coli between piglets and pig farmworkers. Comp Immunol Microbiol Infect Dis. 73, 101564.

Tewari, R., Mitra, S., Ganaie, F., Das, S., Chakraborty, A., Venugopal, N., Shome, R., Rahman, H. and Shome, B.R. (2019) Dissemination and characterisation of Escherichia coli producing extended-spectrum β-lactamases, AmpC β-lactamases and metallo-β-lactamases from livestock and poultry in Northeast India: A molecular surveillance approach. J Glob Antimicrob Resist. 17, 209–215.

US Food and Drug Administration (2016) 2016 Summary Report on Antimicrobials Sold or Distributed for Use in Food-Producing Animals.

Van Boeckel, T.P., Glennon, E.E., Chen, D., Gilbert, M., Robinson, T.P., Grenfell, B.T., Levin, S.A., Bonhoeffer, S. and Laxminarayan, R. (2017) Reducing antimicrobial use in food animals. Science. 357, 1350–1352.

Yassin, A.K., Gong, J., Kelly, P., Lu, G., Guardabassi, L., Wei, L., Han, X., Qiu, H., Price, S., Cheng, D. and Wang, C. (2017) Antimicrobial resistance in clinical Escherichia coli isolates from poultry and livestock, China. PLoS One. 12, e0185326.

10

Diagnosis and Management of Inflammatory Spinal Diseases in Dogs

Prathmesh Deshmukh

BVSc & AH, CVA., Acumed Veterinary Specialty, Mumbai, Referral Veterinary Neurology Clinic, Swapnapurti CHS, Thakur Village, Kandivali East ,Mumbai, Maharashtra, India

The Central Nervous System not only consists of the Brain but also involves the Spinal cord.

The spinal cord is responsible for conveying information from the Brain to the rest of the body via the peripheral nervous system. The spinal cord can be divided into 4 functional segments.

1. C1-C5 (Upper Cervical Segments)
2. C6-T2 (Brachial Plexus)
3. T3-L3 (Thoraco - Lumbar)
4. L4-S3 (Lumbo-Sacral Plexus)

It is important to note that the motor and sensory function of the pelvic limbs are not only controlled by the Lumbo-Sacral plexus but also involve the Thoraco-Lumbar segments (T3-L3) of the spinal cord. It is important to understand not only the neuroanatomy, but also the functional anatomy before approaching a neurological patient.

The field of neurology has been evolving over the past few decades and with the lack of access to advanced diagnostics such as Magnetic Resonance Imaging (MRI) scans, it has been noted that clinicians over the years often developed what is commonly called a "Confirmation Bias".

A few decades ago, in India, the only available diagnostic for neurological patients was Myelography and it was the most widely used diagnostic for neurological patients. Myelography involved injecting a small amount of a radio-opaque contrast material into the subarachnoid space of the spinal cord which was followed up by a radiograph. The flow of contrast material stopped at a particular region which was considered as the area of the spinal cord affected by a compressive lesion

(Intervertebral Disc Disease) or a Spinal cord neoplasm (tumors). The ones who did not show any abnormalities in the spinal cord were presumed to be from a vascular event such as an Aortic Thromboembolism. The differential diagnosis thus got restricted to one or more than one of these etiologies i.e. Intervertebral Disc Disease (IVDD), Spinal cord Neoplasm or Aortic Thromboembolism.

Over the period, owing to the limitations and the risks associated with myelography, it was phased out and was replaced by advanced imaging such as Magnetic Resonance Imaging (MRI) and Computed Axial Tomography (CAT) scans (Barone, Ziemer et al. 2002).

We now know better that there exist several differential diagnoses outside our previous three common suspects, which fall in the VITAMIN-D system. The VITAMIN-D system is a very important tool in every clinician's pocket. It helps prevent Confirmation Bias and improves patient care.

V - Vascular

I - Infectious / Inflammatory.

T- Trauma.

A - Anomalous.

M - Metabolic.

I - Idiopathic / Idiosyncratic.

N - Neoplastic / Nutritional.

D - Degenerative.

Vascular: The common vascular spinal cord diseases in dogs involve Fibrocartilaginous Embolism(FCE) / Ischemic Myelopathy which occurs due to a small fragment of the disc material entering the blood vessels supplying the spinal cord. After extensive research we have now established that FCE does not need surgical intervention, nor does it benefit from Thrombotics such as Heparin, Streptokinase or Warfarin. The recommendations for patients suffering from FCE are Physical therapy and rehabilitation. Aortic Thrombo-Embolism although more common in Feline patients, based on a multicentric international study which involved studying dogs from 1997 to 2014 we know now that Aortic Thromboembolism is uncommon in Dogs (Ruehl, Lynch et al. 2020). With the easy access to Ultrasound machines it is recommended that the patients who suffer from a suspicious Aortic Thrombo-Embolism undergo a thorough abdominal ultrasound, complete cardiac examination including an Echocardiography and a full medical workup before an appropriate treatment option is chosen (Lake-Bakaar, Johnson and Griffiths 2012).

MRI scans can also be used to diagnose thromboembolism. If the clinicians suspect this, they should ensure to include a wider field of view (FOV) during the imaging of the Lumbar spinal cord so that the abdominal aorta is covered.

Infectious / Inflammatory

Living in a tropical country in India, we do have a fair share of infectious and inflammatory diseases present. Several tick-borne diseases are known to trigger inflammation in the nervous system. Other infectious diseases such as Toxoplasma, Neospora have been diagnosed and reported in the Cerebrospinal fluid. A common infectious disease in Cats known as Feline Infectious Peritonitis (FIP) has been commonly known to cause neurological disease.

The inflammation which is triggered off in the Central Nervous System is called Meningoencephalitis which is noted in the Brain and Myelitis in the Spinal cord.

Trauma

Traumatic spinal cord diseases involve vertebral fractures and subluxation secondary to Accidents, automobile trauma. Certain small breed predispositions to Atlanto-Axial subluxation / luxation can lead to spinal cord trauma.

Anomalous

Certain anomalous conditions such as Syringomyelia are common in breeds such as King Charles Cavalier Spaniels. French Bulldogs, Pugs are predisposed to hemivertebrae and Subarachnoid Diverticulum (SAD).

Metabolic - Hypoglycemia can trigger seizures in some pets.

Idiopathic

Idiopathic Epilepsies are more common in dogs as compared to cats. They do not have a known etiology.

Neoplasms

Primary spinal cord tumors include Spinal meningiomas, Peripheral Nerve sheath tumors. Can often be diagnosed on a Contrast MRI.

Degenerative

The most common degenerative disease in clinical practice is Intervertebral Disc Disease commonly referred to IVDD. German Shepherds suffer from Degenerative Myelopathy which has an onset of progressive paraparesis in middle to senior age groups.

Inflammatory Spinal Cord Diseases in Dogs

Infection or Inflammation in the spinal cord is often referred to as Myelitis.

The inflammation can either be localized /focal or widespread/multifocal (Gonçalves, De Decker et al. 2022).

Inflammation in the spinal cord can lead to either weakness in one or more than one limbs commonly referred to as paresis or loss of function paralysis.

The affection of Cervical spinal cord C1-C5 and C6-T2 will cause paresis/ paralysis in all four limbs, it is important to remember that you have to first rule out the Brain involvement before calling it a tetraparesis/ tetraplegia originating from the Cervical spinal cord. The affection of the Thoraco-Lumbar T3-L3 and Lumbo-Sacral L4-S3 can cause affection of only the pelvic limbs.

The next challenge a clinician has to face is to differentiate between the Paraplegia originating from the Thoraco-Lumbar Segment (T3-L3) and Lumbo-Sacral Segment (L4-S3). Since both the segments will cause paresis/paralysis of the pelvic limbs and similarly tetraparesis/tetraplegia originating either from Upper Cervical (C1-C5) or Brachial Plexus (C6-T2).

The C1-C5 and T3-L3 segment affection will involve normal to exaggerated spinal reflexes, normal muscle tone and are associated with lesser degree of muscle atrophy, whereas the C6-T2 and the L4-S3 segment affection are associated with reduced to absent spinal reflexes, weaker muscle tone and muscle atrophy is often noted.

After the neuro-localization the next step involves the differential diagnosis using VITAMIN-D. The basic work up for such patients should involve complete blood test Hematology, Biochemistry including Electrolytes. Survey Spinal Radiographs. The next step would involve a MRI scan of the Spine with Contrast.

It is important to note that a Gadolinium contrast study should be involved in patients suspected to have an Inflammatory/ Infectious disease process or a Neoplasm. The neurolocalization is very important before taking the patients in for an MRI scan as some inflammatory spinal cord diseases may be completely normal or have very subtle signs which can be only visualized in thin sections of the MRI, For example a 5 year male Beagle with Cervical Hyperaesthesia, Tetraparesis and Pain may have a normal looking cervical spine MRI but upon screening of his lumbar spine one may fine a mild disc bulge or a desiccated disc and the clinician may be tempted to perform a dedicated study of the lumbar spinal cord. Neurolocalization is thus extremely important. If the patient is exhibiting Tetraparesis, Cervical pain the clinician should be well aware of the fact that a lumbar disc bulge is unlikely to do so and then perform a dedicated study of the Cervical spine preferably with Contrast if no signs of disc compression are noted.

It is very important to keep in mind that the MRI should be used to confirm your suspicion and not something to put the patient under hoping to get a diagnosis. The MRI scan may not always give us a complete diagnosis , it can only help us diagnose certain diseases or rule out certain pathologies (Lamb, Croson et al. 2005).

A CerebroSpinal Fluid (CSF) Tap is very useful in diagnosing or ruling out Inflammatory spinal diseases in dogs. As opposed to the human counterparts, a CSF collection in veterinary science always requires the patient to be completely anaesthetised. The CSF tap can be performed at two locations - The Cisterna Magna which is space located between the occipital protuberance and the Atlas bone or the Lumbar puncture which is located between L5-L6 for dogs and L6-L7 for cats (Fentem, Nagendran et al. 2023).

The CSF collection site needs to be aseptically prepared, and the fluid is collected while the patient is being monitored under general anaesthesia. The CSF primary analysis needs to be performed soon since the CSF being low in proteins, the cellular count can get affected with passing time. The normal WBC count in the Cisterna magna CSF should be less than 5 cells whereas in the lumbar tap can be upto 11 cells.

The Cisterna Magna CSF should normally have protein count less than 25mg/dl and the lumbar spinal CSF may have normal protein count upto 35mg/dl (Mariani, Nye et al. 2019).

Any aberrations from these values may indicate inflammation in the CSF. It is always recommended that the CSF tap be performed before corticosteroid administration. The corticosteroid administration will reduce the cellular counts in the CSF and affect the interpretation of results.

The CSF should also be tested for infectious diseases. The most commonly occurring ones being Canine Distemper, Neospora, Toxoplasma, Cryptococcus, Trypanosoma , Ehrlichia canis (Lukács, Peters et al. 2020), (Bach, Cray et al. 2023). These can be diagnosed on the basis of CSF PCR tests.

Once the infections are ruled out, we have to consider the inflammation to be of Unknown Origin (Auto-immune) origin. The treatment for the infectious spinal disease would involve treating the underlying infectious disease along with an anti-inflammatory dose of prednisolone. The treatment for the auto-immune spine diseases may involve a higher dose of prednisolone (1-2mg/kg q12), but long-term monotherapy with corticosteroids may cause severe systemic adverse effects, hence an immunosuppressant drug can be introduced alongside to help minimize the dose and the adverse effects of the corticosteroids. The commonly used drugs in management of inflammatory spinal diseases are Cytarabine Arabinoside, Leflunomide, Cyclosporine. It is always recommended to test for the infectious diseases first and rule them out before using immunosuppressant drugs. Using an immunosuppressive dose of prednisolone or another drug with a pre-existing infection may sometimes be counterproductive to treating the patient (Jeffery and Granger 2023).

The prognosis for inflammatory spine diseases will depend firstly on the grade of the inflammation which can be found based on the WBC counts and the protein contents in the CSF and also the response to treatment (Elbert, Yau and Rissi 2022).

This disease can be very aggressive and has a high mortality if untreated, about 1/3rd of the pets will continue to get worse despite receiving the recommended treatments. A follow up MRI scan 3-4 months later is usually advised for patients with inflammatory neurological diseases (Cornelis, Van Ham et al. 2019).

References

Bach, F. S., et al. (2023). "A comparison between neurological clinical signs, cerebrospinal fluid analysis, cross-sectional CNS imaging, and infectious disease testing in 168 dogs with infectious or immune-mediated meningoencephalomyelitis from Brazil." Frontiers in Veterinary Science 10: 1239106.

Barone, G., et al. (2002). "Risk factors associated with development of seizures after use of iohexol for myelography in dogs: 182 cases (1998)." Journal of the American Veterinary Medical Association 220(10): 1499-1502.

Cornelis, I., et al. (2019). "Clinical presentation, diagnostic findings, prognostic factors, treatment and outcome in dogs with meningoencephalomyelitis of nknown origin: a review." The Veterinary Journal 244: 37-44.

Elbert, J. A., et al. (2022). "Neuroinflammatory diseases of the central nervous system of dogs: a retrospective study of 207 cases (2008–2019)." The Canadian Veterinary Journal 63(2): 178.

Fentem, R., et al. (2023). "Complications associated with cerebrospinal fluid collection in dogs." Veterinary Record 193(6).

Gonçalves, R., et al. (2022). "Inflammatory disease affecting the central nervous system in dogs: a retrospective study in England (2010–2019)." Frontiers in Veterinary Science 8: 819945.

Jeffery, N. and N. Granger (2023). "New insights into the treatment of meningoencephalomyelitis of unknown origin since 2009: a review of 671 cases." Frontiers in Veterinary Science 10: 1114798.

Lake-Bakaar, G. A., et al. (2012). "Aortic thrombosis in dogs: 31 cases (2000–2010)." Journal of the American Veterinary Medical Association 241(7): 910-915.

Lamb, C. R., et al. (2005). "Magnetic resonance imaging findings in 25 dogs with inflammatory cerebrospinal fluid." Veterinary Radiology & Ultrasound 46(1): 17-22.

Lukács, R. M., et al. (2020). "Ehrlichia canis infection in the cerebrospinal fluid of a dog characterized by morulae within monocytes and neutrophils." Veterinary Clinical Pathology 49(3): 470-475.

Mariani, C. L., et al. (2019). "Cerebrospinal fluid lactate in dogs with inflammatory central nervous system disorders." Journal of Veterinary Internal Medicine 33(6): 2701-2708.

Ruehl, M., et al. (2020). "Outcome and treatments of dogs with aortic thrombosis: 100 cases (1997-2014)." Journal of Veterinary Internal Medicine 34(5): 1759-1767.

11

Cytauxzoonosis in Domestic and Wild Cats: An Emerging Concern

Pallav Shekhar, Namrata, Vivek Kumar Singh and Mritunjay Kumar

Department of Veterinary Medicine and Veterinary Clinical Complex, Bihar Veterinary College, Bihar Animal Sciences University, Patna, Bihar

Cytauxzoonosis is an emerging tick-borne disease of domestic cats and wild felids caused by the protozoa of the genus Cytauxzoon. The common clinical findings in affected cats are similar to other hemoparasitic infections namely anorexia, depression, anemia, vomiting, icterus, and high fever. The first reporting of feline cytauxzoonosis with four fatal cases was done by Wagner in Missouri, USA in the year 1976.

Bobcats (*Lynx rufus*) are recognized as the natural wild reservoir of *Cytauxzoon felis* with prevalence reaching up to 100% in some enzootic areas (Zieman et al., 2017). This infection is highly fatal in domestic cats with 97% mortality without treatment (Meinkoth and Kocan, 2005). However, subclinical infection in some cats has also been evidenced i.e., they were infected with *C. felis* but did not display the acute clinical signs of the disease before diagnosis (Brown et al., 2010 and Rizzi et al., 2015).

Several other wild felids apart from bobcats and domestic cats have been found to be affected by fatal or nonfatal *Cytauxzoon* sp. infection. These include lions, jaguar, cougars, pumas, ocelots, Iberian lynx, meerkats, European wild cats and Asiatic wild cat, panthers, and tigers (Jakob and Wesemeier, 1996; Rotstein et al., 1999; Yabsley et al., 2006; Andre et al., 2009; Filoni et al., 2012 and Furtado et al., 2017).

Tick bite is the primary mode of transmission of this disease. Tick is an important ectoparasite of domestic animals, placed second after mosquitoes in terms of vector capability (Ghosh and Nagar, 2014). Two ixodid tick species have been involved in the transmission of *C. felis,* namely *Dermacentor variabilis* (the American dog tick) and *Amblyomma americanum* (the lone star tick) (Blouin et al., 1987 and Reichard et al., 2010). These ticks transmit the infective sporozoites during the blood meal either from bobcats or chronically infected domestic cats to naive cats (Allen et al., 2019). The larval, nymph, and adult forms of competent ticks are capable of taking *Cytauxzoon* spp. infection from the infected host during a blood meal. And after molting into the nymph or adult forms, these ticks transmit the organism to the next felid host.

Etiology

Cytauxzoonosis is caused by the protozoa belonging to the phylum Apicomplexa, class Sporozoasida, order Piroplasmorida, family Theileriidae and genus Cytauxzoon (Sherrill and Cohn, 2015). There are three genera; viz. Cytauxzoon, Babesia, and Theileria in the order piroplasmida having intraerythrocytic stage called piroplasm common in their lifecycles (Votypka et al., 2017). The diameter of the intraerythrocytic piroplasms is 1-2 μm and they may take several forms i.e., round "signet ring" form, bipolar oval "safety pin" form, round anaplasmoid or tetrads (Greene et al. 2006).

The three genera, Cytauxzoon, Babesia, and Theileria are classified based on morphological and parasite life cycle characteristics, such as host preference and the type of cell infected. Babesia sp. sporozoites directly enter the host erythrocytes and develop into merozoites after a suitable tick bite (Schnittger et al., 2012 and Sivakumar et al., 2014). Contrastingly, Cytauxzoon and Theileria protozoa first infect macrophages and/or lymphocytes, where they undergo schizogony, which results in the rupture of the infected host cells releasing numerous merozoites. Also, Babesia can be transmitted both transstadially and transovarially by the ticks but Cytauxzoon and Theileria are limited to transstadial transmission (Tarigo et al., 2013).

A total of five *Cytauxzoon* spp. have been recognized worldwide to date (Panait et al., 2021). These are *Cytauxzoon felis* from America, *Cytauxzoon europaeus*, *Cytauxzoon otrantorum*, and *Cytauxzoon banethi* from Europe, and *Cytauxzoon manul* from Asia. The taxonomic classification using the 18S rRNA genes has proven that all five species are related with < 2% identity variance between them (Wikander and Reif, 2023). *Cytauxzoon felis* infection for decades has been viewed as uniformly fatal in domestic cats, but recently increasing cases of survival have been documented (Brown et al., 2008; Haber et al., 2007; Rizzi et al., 2015).

Transmission

Tick bite is the primary mode of transmission of Cytauxzoon organism. Experimentally it was found that *Dermacentor variabilis* is capable of transmitting the protozoan *Cytauxzoon felis* from bobcats to domestic cats, between bobcats, and between domestic cats (Blouin et al., 1984, 1987). However, the study by Riechard et al. (2010) confirmed that primary vector of *C. felis* is *Amblyomma americanum*, although it does not rule out *D. variabilis* as a vector. These two ixodid ticks have been confirmed to be involved in transmission in USA, but no such identification could be made from other geographical regions. The sporadic occurrence, short disease process and high fatality rate of cytauxzoonosis in domestic cats make them to serve as incidental dead-end hosts (Greene et al., 2006). There is no transmission of *Cytauxzoon* sp. through physical contact between infected cats (Wagner et al., 1980). Inoculation of naive cats only with schizonts results in cytauxzoonosis and death and not with the RBCs containing piroplasms (Kier et al., 1987: Wagner et al., 1980). Blood transfusion can induce cytauxzoonosis only when schizonts are transmitted which is extremely unlikely because only sick cats harbor schizont stage and so would not be used as a donor. Transfusion from recovered cats could transmit piroplasms resulting in parasitemia of erythrocytes and not in cytauxzoonosis (Kier et al., 1987; Motzel and Wagner, 1990; Wagner et al., 1980). It is confirmed that all felidae family members are susceptible to infection but no infection in any non-felid animal has been reported (Shock et al., 2011). Vertical transmission of Cytauxzoon organism from mother to offspring is not possible (Lewis et al., 2012a). Transmission of the organism from chronically infected domestic cats to naive cats through tick bites has been observed thus proving that cats are competent reservoirs for *Cytauxzoon* sp. (Reichard et al., 2010). Further, it was found that for transmission of *C. felis* by an *A. americanum* tick a minimum of 36 hrs of attachment is required. Ingesting the infected ticks is not likely to transmit the infection to naive cats (Thomas et al., 2017).

Risk Factors

Cats of any sex and age may be infected, however, young adults are mostly infected. There is a significant association of infection to outdoor access and feral cats in tick-prevalent areas. The cats residing in thinly populated residential areas, urban edge habitats, and in close proximity to natural or unruly areas (i.e., areas with greater prevalence of ticks and reservoir hosts) were at greater risk of *C. felis* infection (Reichard et al., 2008). There is no association of disease with gender, breed, and age and no relation was found with FIV and/or FeLV status (Carli et al. 2012).

Chronology of Worldwide Reporting

Wagner (1976) for the first time reported feline cytauxzoonosis with four fatal cases in domestic cats in Missouri, USA. Earlier *C. felis* was assumed to be found only in North America, but this infection has also been detected in felines in South America, Europe and Asia. Garner et al. (1996), first time confirmed fatal cytauxzoonosis in a captive-reared white tiger in USA. Jakob and Wesemeier (1996) announced the microscopic identification of *C. felis* piroplasms in a captive Bengal tiger from Germany. Ketz-Riley et al. (2003) first time reported a case of *Cytauxzoon manul* in Pallas's cats (*Otocolobus manul*) from Mongolia. Criado-Fornelio et al. (2004) are credited for the first detection of *Cytauxzoon* sp. from a domestic cat in Madrid, Spain. Luaces et al. (2005) claimed to find the first report of intraerythrocytic piroplasm in Iberian lynx which was most likely the first report of a wild felid piroplasm infection from Europe. Millan et al. (2007) determined prevalence of *Cytauxzoon* spp. infection using 18S rRNA PCR to be 15% (3 of 20) in Iberian lynx (*Lynx pardinus*) of Spain. Mendes-de-Almeida et al. (2007) microscopically detected first Cytauxzoon infection in domestic cats in Brazil. Peixoto et al. (2007) reported a lethal case of cytauxzoonosis in a lioness (*Panthera leo*) reared in a zoo in the state of Rio de Janeiro, Brazil. Karaca et al. (2007) underwent a prevalence study, in Turkey, in which 7.5% of Van Cats had *C. felis* infection. Criado-Fornelio et al. (2009) detected *Cytauxzoon* sp. infection in France in one out of 116 tested domestic cats. Andre et al. (2009) detected the parasite in asymptomatic wild felids in captivity in zoos from Brasilia and cities located in the state of São Paulo using molecular techniques. Varshney et al. (2009) reported the first fatal case of feline cytauxzoonosis in India. The case was diagnosed solely based on clinical signs and microscopic demonstration of intra-erythrocytic piroplasms. Carli et al. (2012) were the first to describe *Cytauxzoon* sp. infection in cats in Italy. The infection was confirmed by both blood smear examination and molecular analysis. Kelly et al. (2014) claimed to report the first cytauxzoon organism in African wild felids, though cytauxzoonosis like disease in domestic cat had already been reported from Zimbabwe by Foggin, (1982). Rassouli et al. (2015) confirmed *C. felis* in a stray cat by blood smear and Zaeemi et al. (2015) found the infection in a wild cat (*Felis silvestris*) using molecular analysis, from Iran. Leclaire et al. (2015) conducted first molecular characterisation of *Cytauxzoon* sp. in South African meerkats. Sujay et al. (2016) reported seventy percent (14/20) of lion population housed in a rescue center of Bannerghatta Biological Park, India to be positive for *C. felis* using PCR. Alho et al. (2016) reported the first *Cytauxzoon* sp. infection in a domestic cat from Portugal. Veronesi et al. (2016) were the first to diagnose *Cytauxzoon* sp. infection in wildcats (*Felis silvestris silvestris*) of Italy. Legroux et al. (2017) were the first to document clinical case report of *Cytauxzoon* sp. infection in a domestic cat in France. Nentwig et al. (2018) gave the first case report of cytauxzoonosis in domestic cat in Switzerland. Zou et al. (2019) from Yunnan Province of China, found 21.5% of domestic cats harbored *C. felis*. Panait et al. (2020) microscopically and molecularly identified first Cytauxzoon sp. in a domestic cat in Germany. Panait et al. (2021) recognized three new species of Cytauxzoon in wild felids in Europe, viz. *C. europaeus*, *C. otrantorum*, and *C. banethi.* Guizelini et al. (2021) found to have fatal infection with *C. felis* in a captive-reared jaguar (*Panthera onca*) from Brazil. Malangmei et al. (2021) from India made prevalence study for hemoparasitic infection in apparently healthy cats in which infection with *Cytauxzoon* spp. accounted for 2.70%. Naidenko et al. (2022) found a captive serval (*Leptailurus serval*) to be infected with *Cytauxzoon* sp. and this was the first detection of the pathogen from Russia. Baitha et al. (2023) reported *Cytauxzoon* spp. in a 16 years old male tiger at Rajgir Zoo Safari, Bihar, India.

Clinical Findings

There is short duration of illness, lasting between 2 and 12 days in both natural and experimental infections (Birkenheuer et al., 2006; Cohn et al., 2011). Clinical signs usually appear at approximately 5-14 days after infection. These signs include inappetence, depression, lethargy, fever, dyspnea, vomiting, icterus, generalized pain, vocalization and tachycardia. Occasional occurrence of seizures also occured in some cases (Lloret et al. 2015). Disseminated Intravascular Coagulation was evidenced on studying hemostatic status of Cytauxzoon felis infected cats (Conner et al. 2015). The most common presenting ailments are anorexia, lethargy, fever and icterus (Cohn et al., 2012). The other common signs are tachycardia, ticks on body, vocalization, discomfort on abdominal palpation, splenomegaly, hepatomegaly and lymphadenomegaly. Ataxia, cardiac murmur, seizures, panuveitis and hypothermia are the less likely ones (Pacholec and Cohn 2020). Development of hypothermia and shock-like state is found to appear just prior to the death (Greene et al., 2006; Lloret et al., 2015; Miller and Davis, 2013; Sherrill and Cohn, 2015). A few instances of abortion in cytauxzoonosis positive cats has been reported (Weisman et al. 2007; Cohn et al. 2011). But there were no piroplasms or schizont-laden macrophages in the placenta, fetal muscle, or bone marrow though all the tissues couldn't be examined. Abortion associated with cytauxzoonosis has not been established in cats as with other hemoparasites in different species, including cattle, sheep, horses, primates, and mice (Correa et al., 1978; Espenoza et al., 2005; Nagore et al., 2004 and Potgieter et al., 1992).

Diagnosis

Microscopic Examination

Microscopic detection of intraerythrocytic piroplasms is widely used for the diagnosis of cytauxzoonosis (Birkenheuer et al., 2006b; Weisman et al., 2007). The piroplasms are round to oval structures, 1–2 μm in diameter, having a dark purple eccentric nucleus and a pale blue cytoplasm i.e., signet ring appearance. But in some cases they may be more elongated with a bipolar nucleus i.e., safety pin-like (Greene et al. 2006 and Holman and Snowden 2009). In endemic areas, the acute phase of the disease in domestic cats is diagnosed based on a combination of clinical signs and the intraerythrocytic piroplasms in a blood smear or the schizont-laden macrophages in fine-needle tissue aspirates (Holman and Snowden, 2009; Lloret et al., 2015; Sherrill and Cohn, 2015). The identification of piroplasms is not pathognomic for cytauxzoonosis as the cats that recuperate from the disease or develop subclinical infection frequently maintain low numbers of piroplasms for months, years or for life (Brown et al., 2010). Also, intraerythrocytic piroplasms may take few days to appear after the onset of clinical signs. Thus, the blood smear examination is less sensitive than that of tissue aspirates.

On the day of presentation sensitivity of erythrocytic piroplasms identification can be as low as 50%. This is because acute cytauxzoonosis is the result of schizogenous stage of the parasite (in mononuclear cells) and therefore illness can occur before piroplasms are identifiable within the RBCs (Reichard et al. 2009 and Reichard et al. 2010). The stain precipitant, Howell-Jolly bodies or artifacts can be mistaken for piroplasms and sometimes too low parasitaemia can be overlooked in micorscopic examination thus decreasing the sensitivity of this method of diagnosis.

Molecular Diagnosis

PCR assays are generally 1,000 times more sensitive than microscopic blood smear visualization and are especially relevant to confirm suspected cytauxzoonosis in the absence of microscopic piroplasms (Wang et al., 2017). Additionally, PCR assay can differentiate *Cytauxzoon* spp. from *Theileria* spp. and *Babesia* spp., as they are morphologically similar (Brown *et al.,* 2010; Schreeg *et al.,* 2016; Shock *et al.,* 2012). Molecular diagnosis of *Cytauxzoon* spp. using different targets in 18S rRNA (Diaz-Reganon et al., 2017, Grillini et al., 2023, Haber et al., 2007; Nentwig et al., 2018; Reichard et al., 2010), ribosomal internal transcribed spacer regions 1 and 2 (ITS1, ITS2) (Brown et al., 2008, 2009) and mitochondrial gene cox3, cytochrome b and cytochrome c oxidase subunit I genes (Panait et al., 2021; Schreeg et al., 2016) have been performed.

Serological Test

Commercial serological diagnostic kits are not available to detect cytauxzoonosis. It was found that though antibodies to *Cytauxzoon* spp. developed in experimentally infected domestic cats it was difficult to extract purified antigens (Shindel et al., 1978). And since antibodies take time to develop, antibody-based kits will not be much effective for diagnosis of this acute disease (Cowell et al., 1988). Meinkoth et al. (2000) have used fluorescent immunoassay to test three cats for serum antibodies to *C. felis*.

Summary and Conclusion

Cytauxzoonosis is an emerging and often fatal tick-borne disease affecting domestic and wild cats, caused by protozoa of the genus Cytauxzoon. First reported in Missouri, USA, in 1976, the disease has since been identified in various regions globally, including South America, Europe, and Asia. The primary vectors are the ticks Dermacentor variabilis and Amblyomma americanum, transmitting the infection primarily from bobcats, the natural reservoir, to domestic cats. The disease manifests with severe clinical signs such as anorexia, depression, anemia, and high fever, leading to high mortality in untreated cases. Although traditionally viewed as uniformly fatal, recent cases have shown some cats surviving the infection. Risk factors include outdoor exposure and proximity to tick-infested areas. Cytauxzoonosis poses a significant health threat to felids, highlighting the need for vigilant tick control and further research into effective treatments and prevention strategies.

References

Alho, A.M., Silva, J., Fonseca, M.J., Santos, F., Nunes, C., de Carvalho, L.M., Rodrigues, M. and Cardoso, L. 2016. First report of Cytauxzoon sp. infection in a domestic cat from Portugal. Parasit Vectors 9:220.

Allen, K.E., Thomas, J.E., Wohltjen, M.L. and Reichard, M.V. 2019. Transmission of Cytauxzoon felis to domestic cats by Amblyomma americanum nymphs. Parasit. Vectors. 12(28), 1–6.

Andre, M.R., Herrera, H.M., Fernandes, S.J., de Sousa, K.C., Gonçalves, L.R., Domingos, I.H., de Macedo, G.C. and Machado, R.Z. 2009. Tick-borne agents in domesticated and stray cats from the city of Campo Grande, state of Mato Grosso do Sul, midwestern Brazil. Ticks Tick Borne Dis 6:779 –786.

Antognoni, M.T., Rocconi, F., Ravagnan, S., Vascellari, M., Capelli, G., Miglio, A. and Tommaso, M.D. 2022. Cytauxzoon sp. infection and coinfections in three domestic cats in central Italy. Vet. Sci. 9, 50.

Aschenbroich, S.A., Rech, R.R., Sousa, R.S., Carmichael, K.P. and Sakamoto, K. 2012. Pathology in practice. Cytauxzoon felis infection. J. Am. Vet. Med. Assoc. 240:159 –161.

Baitha, D.K., Shekhar, P., Kumar, A., Kumar, B., Patil, M and Singh, V.K. 2023. Treatment and Care of an old tiger affected with seizures and Cytauxzoon sp. In Rajgir Zoo Safari, Nalanda. In 32nd National Congress of Veterinary Parasitology and National Symposium on Sustainable Control of Parasitic Diseases for Improved Productivity of Livestock in Current Scenario. pp. 65.

Birkenheuer, A.J., Le, J.A., Valenzisi, A.M., Tucker, M.D., Levy, M.G. and Breitschwerdt, E.B. 2006a. Cytauxzoon felis infection in cats in the mid-Atlantic states: 34 cases (1998 –2004). J Am Vet Med Assoc 228:568 –571.

Birkenheuer, A.J., Marr, H., Alleman, A.R., Levy, M.G., and Breitschwerdt, E.B. 2006b. Development and evaluation of a PCR assay for the detection of Cytauxzoon felis DNA in feline blood samples. Vet Parasitol 137: 144 –149.

Blouin, E.F., Kocan, A.A., Glenn, B.L., Kocan, K.M. and Hair, J.A. 1984. Transmission of Cytauxzoon felis from bobcats, Felis rufus (Schreber), to domestic cats by Dermacentor variabilis (Say). J Wildl Dis 20:241–242.

Blouin, E.F., Kocan, A.A., Kocan, K.M. and Hair, J.A. 1987. Evidence of a limited schizogonous cycle for Cytauxzoon felis in bobcats following exposure to infected ticks. J. Wildl. Dis. 23,499 –501.

Brown, H. M., Latimer, K. S., Erikson, L. E., Cashwell, M. E., Britt, J. O. and Peterson, D. S. 2008. Detection of persistent Cytauxzoon felis infection by polymerase chain reaction in three asymptomatic domestic cats. Journal of veterinary diagnostic investigation: official publication of the American Association of Veterinary Laboratory Diagnosticians, Inc. 20(4), 485–488.

Brown H.M., Lockhart J.M., Latimer K.S. and Peterson D.S. (2010). Identification and genetic characterization of Cytauxzoon felis in asymptomatic domestic cats and bobcats. Vet. Parasitol. 172:311–316.

Brown H.M., Modaresi S.M., J.L. C, Latimer K.S. and Peterson D.S. (2009). Genetic variability of archived Cytauxzoon felis histologic specimens from domestic cats in Georgia, 1995–2007. J. Vet. Diagn. Invest. 21:493–498.

Bruce, D. and Klink, V.M.D. 2003. Cytauxzoonosis: an emerging tick-borne disease of cats. Vet bulletin. Merial Limited, Duluth, pp 1–3

Carli E., Solano-Gallego L., De Arcangeli S., Ventura L., Ligorio E. and Furlanello, T. 2022. Clinicopathological findings and risk factors associated with Cytauxzoon spp. infection in cats: A case-control study (2008–2021). Front. Vet. Sci. 9,976173.

Carli E., Trotta M., Bianchi E., Furlanello T., Caldin M., Pietrobelli M. and Solano-Gallego, L. 2014. Cytauxzoon sp. infection in two free ranging young cats: clinicopathological findings, therapy and follow up. Türk Parazitol. Derg. 38(3), 185–189.

Carli, E., Trotta, M., Chinelli, R., Drigo, M., Sinigoi, L., Tosolini, P., Furlanello, T., Millotti, A., Caldin, M. and Solano-Gallego, L. 2012. Cytauxzoon sp. infection in the first endemic focus described in domestic cats in Europe. Vet. Parasitol. 183,343–352.

Clarke, L.L. and Rissi, D.R. 2015. Neuropathology of natural Cytauxzoon felis infection in domestic cats. Vet. Pathol. 52, 1167–1171.

Cohn, L.A., Birkenheuer, A.J., Brunker, J.D., Ratcliff, E.R. and Craig, A.W. 2011. Efficacy of atovaquone and azithromycin or imidocarb dipropionate in Cats with Acute Cytauxzoonosis. J. Vet. Intern. Med. 25, 55–60.

Cohn, L.A., Shaw, D., Shoemake, C. and Birkenheuer, A.J. 2020. Second illness due to subsequent Cytauxzoon felis infection in a domestic cat. JFMS Open Rep. 6:1-5.

Conner, B.J., Hanel, R.M., Brooks, M.B., Cohn, L.A. and Birkenheuer, A.J. 2015. Coagulation abnormalities in 5 cats with naturally occurring cytauxzoonosis. J Vet Emerg Crit Care (San Antonio) 25, 538 –545.

Cowell, R.L., Fox, J.C., Panciera, R.J. and Tyler, R.D. 1988. Detection of anticytauxzoon antibodies in cats infected with a Cytauxzoon organism from bobcats. Vet. Parasitol. 28, 43–52

Criado-Fornelio, A., Buling, A., Pingret, J.L., Etievant, M., Boucraut-Baralon, C., Alongi, A., Agnone, A. and Torina, A. 2009. Hemoprotozoa of domestic animals in France: prevalence and molecular characterization. Vet. Parasitol. 159 (1), 73–76

Criado-Fornelio, A., Gónzalez-del-Río, M.A., Buling-Sarana, A. and BarbaCarretero, J.C. 2004. The expanding universe of piroplasms. Vet. Parasitol. 119 (4), 337–345.

Diaz-Reganon D., Villaescusa A., Ayllon T., Rodríguez-Franco F., Baneth G., Calleja-Bueno, L., García-Sancho, M., Agulla, B. and Sainz, A. 2017. Molecular detection of Hepatozoon spp. and Cytauxzoon sp. in domestic and stray cats from Madrid, Spain. Parasites Vectors. 10,112.

Ferris, D.H. 1979. A progress report on the status of a new disease of American Cats: Cytauxzoonosis. Comp. Immunol. Microbiol. Infects. Dis. 1,269–276.

Filoni C., Catão-Dias J.L., Cattori V., Willi B., Meli M.L., et al. (2012). Surveillance using serological and molecular methods for the detection of infectious agents in captive Brazilian neotropic and exotic felids. J. Vet. Diagn. Invest. 24:166 –173.

Foggin, C.A.: A cytauxzoonosis-like disease in a cat in Zimbabwe. Zimbabwe Vet. J. 1982, 13, 28–30.

Franks, P.T., Harvey, J.W., Shields, R.P. and Lawman, M.J.P. 1988. Hematologic findings in experimental feline cytauxzoonosis. J. Am. Anim. Hosp. Assoc. 24, 395–401.

Frontera-Acevedo K. and Sakamoto K. 2015. Local pulmonary immune responses in domestic cats naturally infected with Cytauxzoon felis. Vet. Immunol. Immunopathol. 163, 1–7.

Frontera-Acevedo, K., Balsone, N.M., Dugan, M.A., Makemson, C.R., Sellers, L.B., Brown, H.M., Peterson, D.S., Creevy, K.E., Garner, B.C. and Sakamoto, K. 2013. Systemic immune responses in Cytauxzoon felis-infected domestic cats. Am. J. Vet. Res. 74,901–909.

Furtado M.M., Taniwaki S.A., Metzger B., Dos Santos Paduan K., O'Dwyer H.L., et al. (2017). Is the free-ranging jaguar (Panthera onca) a reservoir for Cytauxzoon felis in Brazil? Ticks and Tick Borne Dis. 8:470 – 476.

Garner M.M., Lung N.P., Citino S., Greiner E.C., Harvey J.W. and Homer, B.L. 1996. Fatal cytauxzoonosis in a captive-reared write tiger (Panthera tigris). Vet. Pathol. 33, 82–86.

Ghosh S. and Nagar G. (2014). The problem of ticks and tick-borne diseases in India with special emphasis on progress in tick control research: a review. J. Vector Borne Dis. 51: 259-270.

Greene, C.E., Latimer, K., Hopper, E., Shoeffler, G., Lower, K. and Cullens, F. 1999. Administration of diminazene aceturate or imidocarb dipropionate for treatment of cytauxzoonosis in cats. J. Am. Vet. Med. Assoc. 215, 497–500.

Greene, C.E., Meinkoth J. and Kocan, A.A. 2006. Cytauxzoonosis. In Infectious diseases of the dog and cat, Ed Greene CE, Saunders Elsevier, St. Louis, MO pp. 722–733.

Grillini, M., Beraldo, P., Frangipane di Regalbono, A., Dotto, G., Tessarin, C., Franzo, G., Marchiori, E., Modrý, D. and Simonato, G. 2023. Molecular survey of Cytauxzoon spp. and Hepatozoon spp. in felids using a novel real-time PCR approach. Front. Vet. Sci. 10, 1113681.

Haber, M.D., Tucker, M.D., Marr, H.S., Levy, J.K., Burgess, J., Lappin, M.R. and Birkenheuer, A.J. 2007. The detection of Cytauxzoon felis in apparently healthy free-roaming cats in the USA. Vet. Parasitol. 146,316– 320.

Holman, P.J. and Snowden, K.F. 2009. Canine hepatozoonosis and babesiosis, and feline cytauxzoonosis. Vet. Clin. North Am. Small Anim. Pract. 39, 1035–1053.

Jakob, W. and Wesemeier, H.H. (1996). A fatal infection in a Bengal tiger resembling cytauxzoonosis in domestic cats. J. Comp. Pathol. 114, 439 – 444.

Jalovecka, M., Hajdusek, O. and Sojka, D. 2018. The complexity of piroplasms life cycles. Front. Cell. Infect. Microbiol. 8, 248.

Karaca, M., Akkan, H.A., Tutuncu, M., Ozdal, N., Deger, S. and Agaoglu, Z.T. 2007 Cytauxzoonosis in Van Cats. YYU Vet. Fak. Derg. 18(1), 37–39.

Kastl B.C. and Springer N.L. 2023. Serum biochemical changes in cats with naturally acquired feline cytauxzoonosis. J. Am. Vet. Med. Assoc. 261(4):517-525.

Kelly, P., Marabini, L., Dutlow, K., Zhang, J., Loftis, A. and Wang, C. 2014. Molecular detection of tick-borne pathogens in captive wild felids, Zimbabwe. Parasit. Vectors 7:514.

Ketz-Riley, C.J., Reichard, M.V., Van den Bussche, R.A., Hoover, J.P., Meinkoth, J. and Kocan, A.A. 2003. An intraerythrocytic small piroplasm in wild-caught Pallas's cats (Otocolobus manul) from Mongolia. J. Wildl. Dis. 39 (2), 424–430.

Kier, A.B., Wagner, J.E. and Kinden, D.A. 1987. The pathology of experimental cytauxzoonosis. J. Comp. Pathol. 97,4

Kier, A.B., Wightman, S.R. and Wagner, J.E. 1982. Interspecies transmission of Cytauxzoon felis. Am. J. Vet. Res. 43, 102–105.

Leclaire, S., Menard, S. and Berry, A. 2015. Molecular characterization of Babesia and Cytauxzoon species in wild South African meerkats. Parasitol. 142, 543–548.

Legroux J. P., Halos L., René-Martellet M., Servonnet M., Pingret J.L., Bourdoiseau, G., Baneth, G. and Chabanne, L. 2017. First clinical case report of *Cytauxzoon* sp. infection in a domestic cat in France. BMC Vet. Res. 13, 81.

Levi M., Schultz M. and van der Poll T. 2010. Disseminated intravascular coagulation in infectious disease. Semin. Thromb. Hemost. 36(4), 367-77.

Lewis, K.M., Cohn, L.A. and Birkenheuer, A.J. 2012a. Lack of evidence for perinatal transmission of Cytauxzoon felis in domestic cats. Vet. Parasitol. 188, 172–174.

Lewis, K.M., Cohn, L.A., Marr, H.S. and Birkenheuer A.J. 2012b. Diminazene diaceturate for treatment of chronic Cytauxzoon felis parasitemia in naturally infected cats. J. Vet. Intern. Med. 26, 1490 –1493.

Lewis, K.M., Cohn, L.A., Marr, H.S. and Birkenheuer, A.J. 2014. Failure of efficacy and adverse events associated with dose-intense diminazene diaceturate treatment of chronic Cytauxzoon felis infection in five cats. J. Feline. Med. Surg. 16:157–163.

Lloret, A., Addie, D.D., Boucraut-Baralon, C., Egberink, H., Frymus, T., Gruffydd-Jones, T., Hartmann, K., Horzinek, M.C., Hosie, M.J., Lutz, H., Marsilio, F., Pennisi, M.G., Radford, A.D., Thiry, E., Truyen, U. and Möstl, K. 2015. Cytauxzoonosis in cats: ABCD guidelines on prevention and management. J. Feline Med. Surg. 17, 637– 641.

Luaces, I., Aguirre, E., García-Montijano, M., Velarde, J., Tesouro, M.A., Sánchez, C., Galka, M., Fernández, P. and Sainz, A. 2005. First report of an intraerythrocytic small piroplasm in wild Iberian lynx (Lynx pardinus). J. Wildl. Dis. 41 (4), 810–815.

Maia, L.M., Cerqueira Ade, M., de Barros Macieira, D., de Souza, A.M., Moreira, N.S., da Silva, A.V., Messick, J.B., Ferreira, R.F. and Almosny, N.R. 2013. Cytauxzoon felis and 'Candidatus Mycoplasma haemominutum' coinfection in a Brazilian domestic cat (Felis catus). Rev. Bras. Parasitol. Vet. 22 (2), 289–291.

Malangmei, L., Ajith, K.G., Nandini, A., Bora, C.A.F., Varghese, A., Amrutha B. M., Kurbet, P.S., Pradeep, R.K., Nimisha, M., Deepa, C.K., John, L. and Ravindran, R. 2021. Molecular characterization of hemoparasites and hemoplasmas infecting domestic cats of Southern India. Front. Vet. Sci. 7:597598.

Meier H.T. and Moore L.E. 2000. Feline cytauxzoonosis: a case report and literature review. J. Am. Anim. Hosp. Assoc. 36, 493– 496.

Meinkoth, J.H. and Kocan, A.A. 2005. Feline cytauxzoonosis. Vet. Clin. North Am. Small Anim. Pract. 35 (1), 89–101.

Meinkoth, J.H., Kocan, A.A., Whitworth, L., Murphy, G., Fox J.C. and Woods J.P. 2000. Cats surviving natural infection with Cytauxzoon felis: 18 cases (1997–1998). J. Vet. Intern. Med. 14: 521–5.

Mendes-de-Almeida, F., Labarthe, N., Guerrero, J., Faria, M.C., Branco, A.S., Pereira C.D., Barreira, J.D. and Pereira, M.J.S. 2007. Follow-up of the health conditions of an urban colony of free-roaming cats (Felis catus Linnaeus, 1758) in the city of Rio de Janeiro, Brazil. Vet. Parasitol. 147(1-2), 9-15.

Millan, J., Naranjo, V., Rodríguez, A., Pérez De La Lastra, J.M., Mangold, A.J., De La Fuente, J. 2007. Prevalence of infection and 18S rRNA gene sequences of Cytauxzoon species in Iberian lynx (Lynx pardinus) in Spain. Parasitol. 135:1–7

Miller, J. and Davis, C.D. 2013. Increasing frequency of feline cytauxzoonosis cases diagnosed in western Kentucky from 2001 to 2011. Vet. Parasitol. 198, 205–208.

Moghaddam, M.R., Zaeemi, M. and Razmi, G.R. 2020. Preliminary study of Cytauxzoon felis infection in outdoor cats in Mashhad, Iran. Parasitol. Res. 119, 4177–4183.

Motzel, S.L. and Wagner, J.E. 1990. Treatment of experimentally induced Cytauxzoonosis in Cats with Parvaquone and Buparvaquone. Vet. Parasitol. 35:131–138.

Naidenko S.V., Erofeeva M.N., Sorokin P.A., Gershov S.O., Yakovenko N.P., Botvinovskaya, A.S. and Alekseeva, G.S. 2022. The First Case of *Cytauxzoon* spp. In Russia: The Parasite Conquers Eurasia. Animals. 12:593.

Nentwig, A., Meli, M.L., Schrack, J., Reichler, I.M., Riond, B., Gloor, C., Howard, J., Hofmann-Lehmann, R. and Willi, B. 2018. First report of Cytauxzoon sp. infection in domestic cats in Switzerland: natural and transfusion-transmitted infections. Parasit. Vectors. 11(1), 292.

Panait L.C., Mihalca A.D., Modry D., Jurankova J., Ionica A.M., Deak, G., Gherman C.M., Heddergott M., Hodzic A., Veronesi. F., Reichard M., Zieman E.A., Nielsen C.K., Agustín Jimenez-Ruiz F. and Hrazdilovamn, K. (2021). Three new species of Cytauxzoon in European wild felids. Vet. Parasit. 290,109344.

Panait, L.C., Stock, G., Globokar, M., Balzer, J., Groth, B., Mihalca, A.D. and Pantchev, N. 2020. First report of Cytauxzoon sp. infection in Germany: organism description and molecular confirmation in a domestic cat. Parasitol. Res. 119, 3005–3011.

Peixoto, P.V., Soares, C.O., Scofield, A., Santiago, C.D., França, T.N. and Barros, S.S. 2007. Fatal cytauxzoonosis in captive-reared lions in Brazil. Vet. Parasitol. 145, 383–387.

Rassouli, M., Sabouri, S., Goudarzi, A. and Parsa, M. 2015. Cytauxzoon felis in a stray cat in Iran. Comp. Clin. Pathol. 24:75–77.

Reichard, M.V., Edwards A.C., Meinkoth, J.H., Snider T.A., Meinkoth, K.R., Heinz, R.E. and Little, S.E. 2010. Confirmation of Amblyomma americanum (Acari: Ixodidae) as a vector for Cytauxzoon felis (Piroplasmorida: Theileriidae) to domestic cats. J. Med. Entomol. 47, 890 – 896.

Reichard, M.V., Meinkoth, J.H., Edwards, A.C., Snider, T.A., Kocan, K.M., Blouin, E.F. and Little, S.E. 2009. Transmission of Cytauxzoon felis to a domestic cat by Amblyomma americanum. Vet Parasitol. 161,110 5.

Reichard, M.V., Rugg, J.J., Thomas, J.E., Allen, K.E., Barrett, A.W., Barrett, A.W., Murray, J.K., Herrina, B.H., Beam, R.A., King, V.L., and Vatta, A.F. 2019. Efficacy of a topical formulation of selamectin plus sarolaner against induced infestations of Amblyomma americanum on cats and prevention of Cytauxzoon felis transmission. Vet. Parasitol. 270 Suppl 1, S31-S37.

Reichard, M.V., Thomas, J.E., Arther, R.G., Hostetler, J.A., Raetzel, K.L., Meinkoth, J.H. and Little, S.E. 2013. Efficacy of an Imidacloprid 10%/Flumethrin 4.5% Collar (Seresto (R), Bayer) for Preventing the Transmission of Cytauxzoon felis to Domestic Cats by Amblyomma americanum. Parasitol. Res. 112, 11–20.

Rizzi, T.E., Reichard, M.V., Cohn, L.A., Birkenheuer, A.J., Taylor, J.D. and Meinkoth, J.H. 2015. Prevalence of Cytauxzoon felis infection in healthy cats from enzootic areas in Arkansas, Missouri, and Oklahoma. Parasit. Vectors 8(1):13

Rotstein D.S., Taylor S.K., Harvey J.W. and Bean J. (1999). Hematologic effects of cytauxzoonosis in Florida panthers and Texas cougars in Florida. J. Wildl. Dis. 35 (3): 613–617.

Schnittger L., Rodriguez A.E., Florin-Christensen M. and Morrison D.A. (2012). Babesia: a world emerging. Infect. Genet. Evol. 12:1788 –1809.

Schreeg, M.E., Marr, H.S., Tarigo, J.L., Sherrill M.K., Outi, H.K., Scholl, E.H., Bird, D.M., Vigil, A., Hung, C., Nakajima, R., Liang, L., Trieu, A., Doolan D.L., Thomas, M.E., Levy, M.G., Reichard, M.V., Felgner P.L., Cohn, L.A. and Birkenheuer, A.J. 2018. Identification of Cytauxzoon felis antigens via protein microarray and assessment of expression library immunization against cytauxzoonosis. Clin. Proteomics 15, 44.

Sherrill, M.K. and Cohn, L.A. 2015. Cytauxzoonosis: diagnosis and treatment of an emerging disease. J. Feline Med. Surg. 17,940–948.

Shindel, N., Dardiri, A.H. and Ferris, D.H. 1978. An indirect fluorescent antibody test for the detection of Cytauxzoon-like organisms in experimentally infected cats. Can. J. Comp. Med. 42,460 – 465.

Shock B.C., Birkenheuer A.J., Patton L.L., Olfenbuttel C., Beringer J., Grove, D.M., Peek, M., Butfiloski, J.W., Hughes, D.W., Lockhart, J.M., Cunningham, M.W., Brown, H.M., Peterson, D.S., Yabsley, M.J. 2012. Variation in the ITS-1 and ITS-2 rRNA genomic regions of *Cytauxzoon felis* from bobcats and pumas in the eastern United States and comparison with sequences from domestic cats. Vet. Parasitol. 190, 29 –35

Shock, B.C., Murphy, S.M., Patton, L.L., Beringer, J., Prange, S., Grove, D.M., Peek, M. and Butfiloski, J.W. 2011. Distribution and prevalence of Cytauxzoon felis in bobcats (Lynx rufus), the natural reservoir, and other wild felids in thirteen states. Vet Parasitol. 175, 325–330.

Sivakumar T., Hayashida K., Sugimoto C. and Yokoyama N. 2014. Evolution and genetic diversity of Theileria. Infect. Genet. Evol. 27:250 –263.

Snider, T.A., Confer, A.W. and Payton, M.E. 2010. Pulmonary histopathology of Cytauxzoon felis infections in the cat. Vet. Pathol. 47, 698 –702.

Sujay, C.S., Krishna, S., Gonathinayagam, S., Senthilkumar, S., Manjunatha, V and Thangaraj, M.J. 2016. Serological evidence of Cytauxzoon felis in captive lions of India. In Joint AAZV/EAZWV/IZW.

Tarigo, J.L., Scholl, E.H., Bird, D.M., Brown, C.C., Cohn, L.A., Dean, G.A., Levy, M.G., Doolan, D.L., Trieu, A., Nordone, S.K., Felgner, P.L., Vigil, A., Birkenheuer, A.J. 2013. A novel candidate vaccine for cytauxzoonosis inferred from comparative Apicomplexan genomics. PLoS One 8: e71233.

Thomas, J.E., Ohmes, C.M., Payton, M.E., Hostetler, J.A. and Reichard, M.V. 2017. Minimum transmission time of Cytauxzoon felis by Amblyomma americanum to domestic cats in relation to the duration of infestation, and investigation of ingestion of infected ticks as a potential route of transmission. J. Feline Med. Surg. 20, 67–72.

Varshney, J.P., Deshmukh, V.V. and Chaudhary, P.S. 2009. Fatal cytauxzoonosis in a kitten. Intas Polivet 10,392–393.

Veronesi, F., Ravagnan, S., Cerquetella, M., Carli, E., Olivieri, E., Santoroa, A., Pesaro, S., Berardi, S., Rossi, G., Ragni, B., Beraldo, P. and Capelli, G. (2016). First detection of Cytauxzoon spp. infection in European wildcats (Felis silvestris silvestris) of Italy. Ticks and Tick-Borne Diseases. 7(5), 853–858.

Votypka J., Modry D., Obornik M., Slapeta J., and Lukes J. (2017). "Apicomplexa," in Handbook of the Protists. Pp 1–58. Springer International Publishing AG.

Wagner, J.E. 1976. A fatal cytauxzoonosis-like disease in cats. J. Am. Vet. Med. Assoc. 168, 585–588.

Wagner, J.E., Ferris, D.H., Kier, A.B., Wightman, S.R.; Maring, E.; Morehouse, L.G. and Hansen, R.D. 1980. Experimentally induced cytauxzoonosis-like disease in domestic cats. Vet. Parasitol. 6, 305–311.

Walker, D.B. and Cowell, R.L. 1995. Survival of a domestic cat with naturally acquired cytauxzoonosis. J. Am. Vet. Med. Assoc. 206:1363–1365.

Wang J.L., Li T.T., Liu G.H., Zhu X.Q. and Yao C. 2017. Two tales of Cytauxzoon felis infections in domestic cats. Clin. Microbiol. Rev. 30:861–885.

Weisman, J.L., Woldemeskel, M., Smith, K.D., Merrill, A. and Miller, D. 2007. Blood smear from a pregnant cat that died shortly after partial abortion. Vet. Clin. Pathol. 36:209 –211.

Wikander Y.M. and Reif K.E. 2023. Cytauxzoon felis: An Overview. Pathogens. 12: 133.

Yabsley M. J., Murphy S. M. and Cunningham M.W. (2006). Molecular detection and characterization of Cytauxzoon felis and a Babesia species in cougars from Florida. J.Wildl. Dis. 42:366 –374.

Zaeemi, M., Razmi, G.R. and Khoshnegah J. 2015. The first detection of Cytauxzoon felis in a wild cat (Felis silvestris) in Iran. Comp. Clin. Pathol. 24: 181–184.

Zieman, E.A., Jimenez, F.A. and Nielsen, C.K. 2017. Concurrent examination of bobcats and ticks reveals high prevalence of Cytauxzoon felis in southern Illinois. J Parasitol. 103(4), 343-348.

Zou, F.C., Li, Z., Yang, J.F., Chang, J.Y., Liu, G.H., Lv, Y. and Zhu, X.Q. 2016. Cytauxzoon felis infection in domestic cats, Yunnan Province, China. Emerg. Infect. Dis. 25(2), 353–354.

12

Heart Failure Management in Cats

S. Prathaban

Department of Veterinary Clinical Medicine, Madras Veterinary College Chennai, Tamil Nadu

Cardiomyopathies in acts can be classified broadly as Hypertrophic cardiomyopathy and non-hypertrophic cardiomyopathies. Usually, no alarming clinical signs are detected during routine examination in the preclinical stage except cardiac murmurs in some cats with HCM. This is because, that the cats are sedentary and excellent in hiding the signs of illness from the pet parents. Hence the onset is often acute with the sudden appearance of the clinical signs linked to congestive heart failure like severe dyspnoea, cardiogenic shock, aortic thromboembolism, arrhythmias and even syncope and death

Cats with CHF will be presented with severe dyspnoea, due to fulminant pulmonary oedema and or pleural effusion. The pleural effusion associated with CHF is usually a modified transudate, some cases it may be chylous .In echocardiography ,the size of the left atrium should be determined .If the LA size is normal ,then the dyspnoea may not be of cardiac origin .The presence of B-lines in the lung area in association with LA enlargement confirms cardiogenic pulmonary oedema. Stress, anaesthesia, I/V fluids and steroids leads to decompensation and fulminant pulmonary oedema. Thoracocentesis is will be helpful if there is dyspnoea due to significant pleural effusion. At least 300ml of effusion can be usually removed. The dyspnoeic cat is very fragile and should be handled carefully. Butorphanol may be given for anxiolytic effect. Oxygen administration is beneficial. Furosemide when given intravenously has an initial venodilator effect and should be repeated as required monitoring the sleeping respiratory rate (SRR). Addition of nitro-glycerine (vasodilator) reduces preload, decreases left atrial pressure and help in reducing pulmonary oedema. If the clinical signs are suggestive of cardiogenic shock or myocardial failure, Pimobendan I/V or Dobutamine CRI should be considered.

Severe left sided congestive heart failure (stage C)	
Furosemide	• 1-2 mg/kg IV (or IM if IV access cannot be easily gained) • 2nddose after 30-60 minutes • Repeat (1 mg/kg IV) every 1-2 hours. Increase interval between doses once respiratory rate is <40-50 breaths/minute (e.g., to intervals of 4-6 hours)
Nitroglycerine–e.g., topical ointment (if available) or patches (e.g., 5 mg patch cut into quarters)	• Apply 0.25-0.5 cm ointment onto hairless, well perfused skin every 6 hours, for up to 3 days • ¼ patch applied to hairless skin once a day • Monitor blood pressure and discontinue if the patient becomes hypotensive
Butorphanol(anxiolytic effect)	• 0.2-0.3 mg/kg IM or IV
Mild or moderate heart failure; Chronic congestive heart failure (stage C)	
Furosemide	• Dose range: 1 mg/kg SID/BID up to 3 mg/kg TID PO; monitor sleeping or resting respiratory rate and renal biochemistry/electrolytes after dose adjustments • Aim to give minimum effective dose to control CHF (with owner monitoring SRR at home)
ACE (angiotensin converting enzyme) inhibitor 1. Benazepril 2. Enalapril 3. Ramipril 4. Imidapril	1. 0.25-0.5 mg/kg PO SID 2. 0.5 mg/kg PO SID 3. 0.125 mg/kg PO SID 4. 0.25 mg/kg PO SID
Telmisartan(angiotensin II receptor blocker)	• 1 mg/kg PO SID
Spironolactone(care with Maine Coon cats as risk of drug-induced facial dermatitis)	• 2 mg/kg PO SID
Pimobendan(care if suspected or known LVOTO)	• 0.1-0.25 mg/kg PO BID (e.g., 0.625 mg (½ tablet) or 1.25 mg (1 tablet) per cat PO BID
Refractory congestive heart failure (stage D)	
Torasemide	• 0.1-0.3 mg/kg PO SID/BID
Pimobendan(if not already used as above)	• 0.1-0.25 mg/kg PO BID. Consider TID administration
Hydrochlorothiazide(with amiloride in some preparations) (sequential nephron blockade)	• 1-2 mg/kg PO SI

Diuretics are essential in the management of CHF, with furosemide is the most commonly prescribed diuretic. During chronic therapy furosemide dose should be slowly down titrated, with home monitoring of sleeping respiratory rate(SRR).,to aim minimum effective daily dose which controls clinical signs. Serum electrolytes should be checked minimum one week after treatment

Reduced cardiac output will result in neuroendocrine activation, which results in progression of CHF. Initially reduced blood pressure results in sympathetic stimulation, with beta-receptor stimulus resulting in tachycardia, increased myocardial contraction and increased risk for arrhythmias. Alpha-receptor stimulation will result in vasoconstriction, increasing pre- and after-load. Renin release and activation of the renin-angiotensin-aldosterone system (RAAS) ultimately results in angiotensin II and aldosterone release. Both angiotensin II and aldosterone result in myocardial remodelling and fibrosis. Angiotensin II is a potent vasoconstrictor and triggers increased vasopressin and endothelin release. Aldosterone causes increased sodium and water retention and the CHF syndrome. There is evidence for RAAS activation in cats with HCM or after therapy with some drugs, including furosemide. Therefore, in cats with CHF requiring furosemide, it is logical to also start treatment to counteract the RAAS system, such as an angiotensin-converting enzyme (ACE) inhibitor (*e.g.*, benazepril) or an angiotensin II receptor (AT1) blocker (*e.g.*, telmisartan) and/or an aldosterone antagonist (spironolactone).

Telmisartan (AT1 blocker) was used earlier, and evidence in cats suggest a favourable effect on RAAS. The aldosterone antagonist spironolactone is a mild diuretic and its addition to cats receiving, furosemide and benazepril, reduced, morbidity and mortality.

Pimobendane is an inodilator drug, which improves pump function by calcium sensitization and phosphodiesterase III inhibition. It is also a balanced vasodilator, reducing afterload and preload, and improves myocardial function without increasing myocardial oxygen consumption. It is indicated in cardiomyopathies associated with impaired systolic function, especially dilated cardiomyopathy. Positive inotropes and arteriodilator drugs are theoretically contraindicated in HCM with left ventricular outflow tract obstruction (LVOTO), since the combination of increased contraction and arteriodilatation may increase the severity of LVOTO. However, a retrospective case-control study of cats treated with CHF associated with HCM including some with LVOTO showed an increased survival time in cats receiving pimobendan. LVOTO did not result in increased adverse events in another study; in contrast, a prospective study failed to show any survival benefit for cats with CHF receiving pimobendan.

Pimobendan may improve LA function, which may in turn reduce the risk for thromboembolic complications, and it has been reported to inhibit platelet aggregation, although this may only be at doses much higher than the clinical recommendation.

Diltiazem is licensed in some countries to treat feline HCM and has been advocated as a treatment to improve diastolic function, but interim analysis of one study showed no additional benefit of diltiazem compared with furosemide alone. Its major indication is an antiarrhythmic drug.

If a cat is receiving beta-blockers (*e.g.*, for previously diagnosed HCM with LVOTO), the dose should be carefully down-titrated or even stopped after a few weeks. This is because the intense neuroendocrine activation of CHF includes increased sympathetic drive to maintain cardiac output; beta-blockade may prevent some of this compensatory effort. However, the decision about discontinuing beta-blockers depends on each individual case (*e.g.*, if there is significant LVOTO).

Refractory CHF: Torsemide a much more potent ceiling loop diuretic can be used -Once a administration, with one I tenth dose furosemide is adequate. But renal function and electrolytes should be monitored, since the risk of causing acute kidney injury is high. Sequential nephron blockade with the addition of hydrochlorothiazide (often combined with amiloride) can be considered.

Cardiogenic shock (hypotension)	
Pimobendan (injectable or chewable tablets)	• 0.15 mg/kg IV • 0.625 mg (½ tablet) or 1.25 mg (1 tablet) per cat PO BID
Dobutamine	• 2-5 μg/kg/minute CRI
Tachyarrhythmias	
Atenolol (do not start if in uncontrolled CHF)	• 1 mg/kg PO SID/BID for ventricular or supraventricular arrhythmias
Diltiazem (modified release tablets)	• 1-3 mg/kg PO BID/TID for supraventricular arrhythmias
Sotalol	• 0.5-2 mg/kg PO BID for supraventricular or ventricular arrhythmias
Thromboembolism: treatment	
Methadone	• 0.1-0.3 mg/kg IV (q6-8 hours)
Clopidogrel	• 18.75 mg per cat PO SID • Initial loading dose for FATE: 37.5 mg or 75 mg PO
Low molecular weight heparin (dalteparin)	• Initial dose 200 U/kg, then 100 U/kg SC BID
Rivaroxaban	• 1.25-2.5 mg PO per cat SID/BID (pending data in affected cats)
Apixaban	• 0.2 mg/kg PO SID (pending data in affected cats)
Aspirin	• 18.75 mg per cat PO every 3 days (or twice a week) (anti-platelet dose)

Alteplase (tissue plasminogen activator, tPA)	• 1 mg/kg IV
Cyproheptadine	• 0.1-0.5 mg/kg PO BID/TID
Thromboembolism: prevention	
Clopidogrel	• 18.75 mg per cat PO SID
Aspirin	• 18.75 mg per cat PO every 3 days (or twice a week) (anti-platelet dose)

Cardiogenic shock is seen in end stage cardiomyopathies, precepted by the development of haemodynamically significant arrhythmias. There will be reduced cardiac output, and peripheral perfusion (prolonged CRT, cold extremities). Cardinal sign is systemic hypertension (systolic blood pressure < 100mmHg). Treatment is with pimobendan. Dobutamine CRI also used in emergency setting.

Cats with severe cardiomyopathies associated with LA dilatation and impaired LA function are at increased risk for formation of cardiac thrombi and subsequent systemic thromboembolism. This can be anywhere along the arterial tree, but typically distal aortic emboli result in severe pain, paralysis, loss of associated pulse (*e.g.*, femoral artery), pallor (*e.g.*, nail beds), and cold extremity of affected limbs. Muscles (*e.g.*, gastrocnemius) are often contracted and painful on palpation. Anticoagulant drugs listed in the table are used for the treatment and prevention.

Arrhythmias are common in feline myocardial disease and indicate worse prognosis. Increased wall stress results in ventricular arrhythmias. Atrio ventricular block reflect fibrosis. Atrial stretch may result in supraventricular premature complexes or atrial fibrillation. Tachy arrhythmias will compromise diastolic function

13

Advances in Practical Echocardiography in Small Animal Practice

K. Jeyaraja

Professor, Department of Veterinary Clinical medicine, Madras Veterinary College Chennai, Tami Nadu

Tissue Doppler Imaging

Doppler echocardiography relies on detection of the shift in frequency of ultrasound signals reflected from moving objects. With this principle, conventional Doppler techniques assess the velocity of blood flow by measuring high-frequency, low-amplitude signals from small, fast-moving blood cells. In TDI, the same Doppler principles are used to quantify the higher-amplitude, lower-velocity signals of myocardial tissue motion.

There are important limitations to TD interrogation. As with all Doppler techniques, TDI measures only the vector of motion that is parallel to the direction of the ultrasound beam. In addition, TDI measures absolute tissue velocity and is unable to discriminate passive motion (related to translation or tethering) from active motion (fiber shortening or lengthening). The emerging technology of Doppler strain imaging provides a means to differentiate true contractility from passive myocardial motion by looking at relative changes in tissue velocity.

TDI can be performed in pulsed-wave and color modes. Pulsed-wave TDI is used to measure peak myocardial velocities and is particularly well suited to the measurement of long-axis ventricular motion because the longitudinally oriented endocardial fibers are most parallel to the ultrasound beam in the apical views. Because the apex remains relatively stationary throughout the cardiac cycle, mitral annular motion is a good surrogate measure of overall longitudinal left ventricular (LV) contraction and relaxation.

To measure longitudinal myocardial velocities, the sample volume is placed in the ventricular myocardium immediately adjacent to the mitral annulus. The cardiac cycle is represented by 3 waveforms (Figure below) (1) Sa, systolic myocardial velocity above the baseline as the annulus descends toward the apex; (2) Ea, early diastolic myocardial relaxation velocity below the baseline as the annulus ascends away from the apex; and (3) Aa, myocardial velocity associated with atrial contraction. The lower-case "a" for annulus or "m" for myocardial (Ea or Em) and the superscripted prime symbol (E′) are used to differentiate tissue Doppler velocities from conventional mitral inflow. Pulsed-wave TDI has high temporal resolution but does not permit simultaneous analysis of multiple myocardial segments.

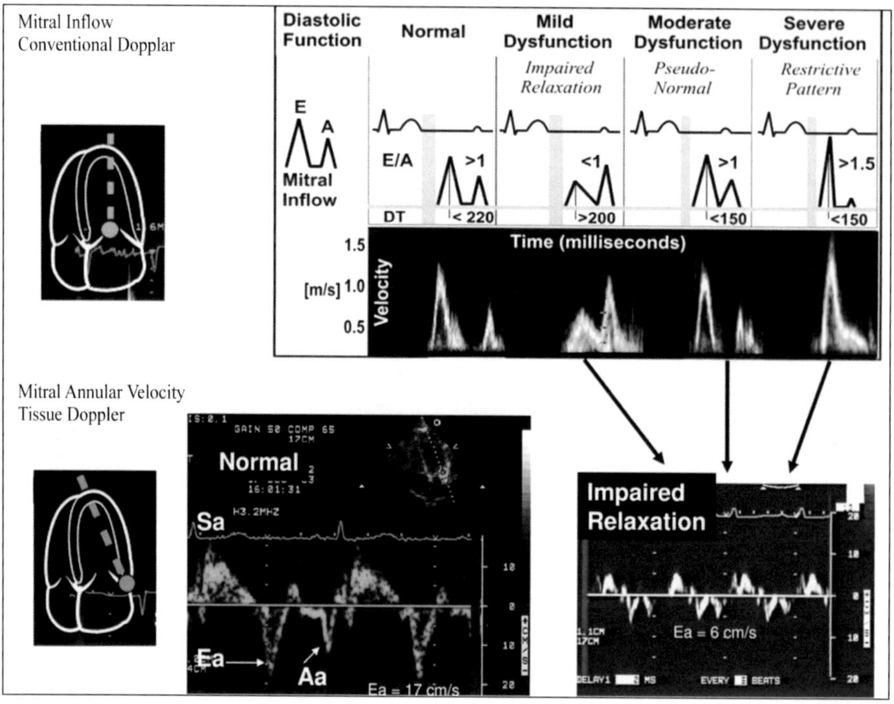

Tissue Doppler imaging is a relatively recently developed ultrasound technique which allows the quantification of both global and regional myocardial function from measurements of myocardial velocities in real time. Annular velocities can also be quantified using the TDI technique. The pulsed-wave TDI mode provides information on tissue movements from a single sample volume. The 2D color TDI mode is better than the pulsed-wave TDI mode for the evaluation of myocardial function because of its ability to simultaneously quantify velocities in several segments within a single myocardial wall or within different myocardial walls in order to calculate velocity gradients and to assess intra- or inter ventricular synchrony, respectively. The TDI technique has been shown to be more sensitive than conventional echocardiography in detecting systolic and diastolic myocardial alterations in humans as well as in experimental or spontaneous heart diseases in animals.

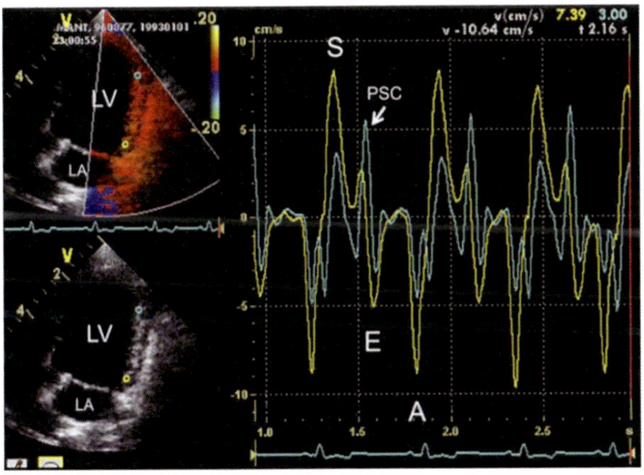

Longitudinal myocardial velocity profiles of the left ventricular free wall (LVFW) obtained from a dog with moderate mitral valve disease using two-dimensional color tissue Doppler imaging (left parasternal 4-chamber view). Simultaneous recordings of myocardial velocities are obtained in 2 segments of the LVFW (basal and apical segments, yellow and green curves respectively). A typical severe longitudinal dysfunction is observed, characterized in both segments by an inverted E/A ratio. A positive post-systolic contraction wave (PSC), confirmed by Strain Imaging (data not shown), occurring after aortic valve closure and greater than the S wave, is also present for the apical motion. The color display of velocity is superimposed on the two-dimensional view (left upper panel). S, E, and A are peak myocardial velocities during systole, early diastole, and late diastole, respectively. LA: left atrium.

Radial velocity profiles recorded within 2 segments of the left ventricular free wall using the twodimensional color tissue Doppler imaging (TDI) mode in 2 Cavalier King Charles Spaniels with severe mitral valve disease but "opposite" systolic myocardial performance (right parasternal transventricular short-axis views). These 2 simultaneous recordings of myocardial velocities in a sub-endocardial (yellow) and sub-epicardial (green) segment both indicate that the sub-endocardium is moving more rapidly than the sub-epicardium in systole and also in diastole,thus defining systolic and diastolic myocardial velocity gradients (white double arrows). However, for the dog the sub-endocardial and sub-epicardial velocity profiles are nearly superimposed in systole, thus indicating a very low systolic myocardial velocity gradient (0.9 cm/s versus 3.9 cm

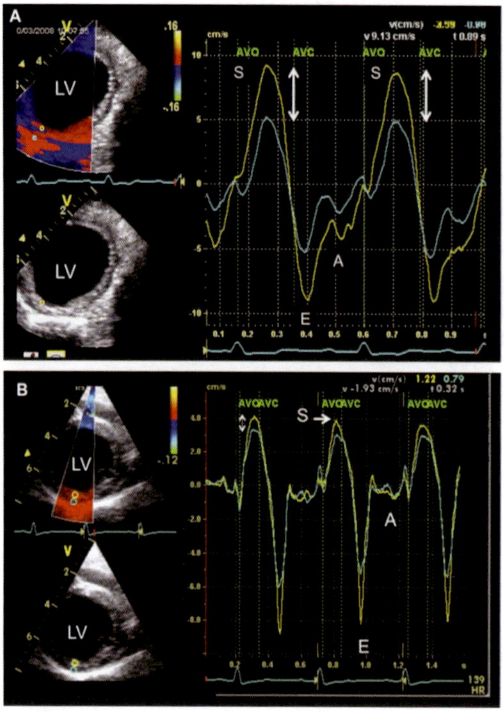

One important TDI application is the assessment of diastolic function, which may be impaired in aged dogs with MVD. Such diastolic alterations are usually more common and more pronounced for the longitudinal than for the radial motion. However, in one recent study, no decrease in radial or longitudinal early diastolic velocities or in TDI E/A ratio (suggesting an impaired diastolic function) was observed in dogs with MVD compared to healthy controls. Conversely several diastolic TDI variables (i.e., early TDI diastolic wave (E) and TDI E/A ratio in different segments) were significantly increased in dogs with congestive heart failure compared with those without any sign of decompensation and normal controls. However, the former had a significantly higher heart rate than the latter, which may have contributed to these diastolic findings to an unknown extent.

In addition, although TDI variables are less load dependent than conventional echocardiographic indices, a preload influence is highly likely, as a significant correlation has been found between the LA/Ao ratio and early diastolic velocities. Recent data from human studies have confirmed that both systolic and diastolic TDI velocities of the LV are preload-dependent. Alteration of myocardial synchrony may also be observed in dogs with MVD, using left parasternal long-axis views.

Tidholm et al. Demonstrated that the difference in longitudinal systolic velocity time-to-peak between the LV and the interventricular septum was significantly increased in dogs with MVD, with and without congestive heart failure, as compared to healthy control dogs, indicating intraventricular dyssynchrony. Whether such alteration is primarily related to MVD or represents an age-related finding remains however to be determined.

Lastly, the TDI technique may also be used to help identify systolic changes, revealing increased systolic velocities and gradients in the case of hyperkinesia and the opposite pattern in the case of hypokinesia. Systolic transmural gradients should be preferred because they are more reliable and sensitive indicators of regional LV dysfunction than isolated systolic velocity values. In the study by Tidholm et al. reported no decrease in systolic performance (but instead an increase in several systolic velocities) was evidenced in dogs with MVD using the TDI technique. Again a load effect and an influence of heart rate may partially explain these results.

Strain and Strain Rate Imaging

Strain and Strain Rate imaging are 2 quantitative TDI-derived imaging techniques, which can be used to measure myocardial segmental deformation (contraction or stretching) and rate of deformation, respectively. Myocardial strain represents the deformation of a myocardial segment over time, and is expressed as the % change from its original dimension. Myocardial strain rate is the temporal derivative of strain, and therefore describes the rate of myocardial deformation.

Unlike TDI, Strain and Strain Rate imaging provide true measures of local myocardial deformation, thereby separating active from passive myocardial motion and offering a more "representative" or direct evaluation of intrinsic myocardial function. Very few data are available regarding strain and strain rate alterations associated with canine MVD. Radial systolic LV strain was measured between the 2 papillary muscles by using the right parasternal ventricular short-axis view and longitudinal systolic LV strain was measured at the base using the left apical 4-chamber view. A significant decrease in the longitudinal absolute value of systolic strain was identified at the latest heart failure stage (ISACHC class 3) compared with healthy controls and dogs from other ISACHC classes.

Speckle Tracking Echocardiography

Two-dimensional STE is the most recently developed ultrasound technique and allows quantitative assessment of regional myocardial function. This non-Doppler technique is based on frame-by-frame tracking of the tiny echo-dense speckles observed within the myocardium on gray scale 2D echocardiographic images and subsequent measurement of myocardial motion. By analyzing speckle motion, STE offers the opportunity to assess myocardial tissue velocity, strain and strain rate, as well as the LV rotation independently of cardiac translation and beam angle, unlike the Doppler based techniques (TDI or TDI-derived techniques). The

STE technique may be used to assess systolic strain and regional synchrony in canine MVD. Longitudinal systolic strain may also be assessed by STE for the whole LV in 18 different segments using 3 different standard apical planes. The obtained bull's-eye representation of segmental systolic strain has been found to be closely correlated with coronary anatomy in humans.

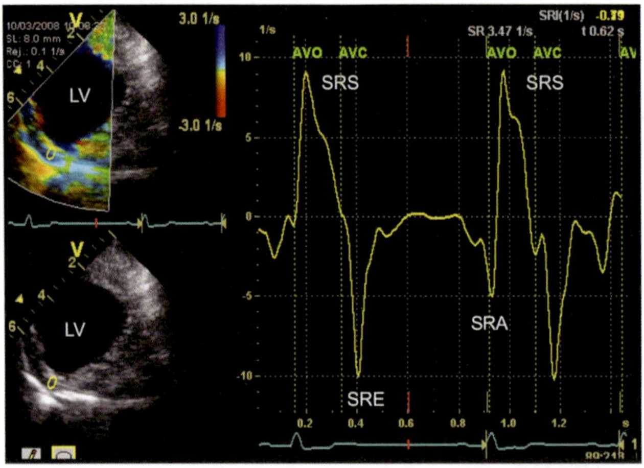

Radial hyperkinesia confirmed by regional radial strain rate recorded within the leftventricular free wall from a dog with moderate mitral valve disease. The strain rate profile is positive during systole (SRS), indicating regional thickening, and then features 2 negative diastolic peaks during early filling and atrial contraction (SRE and SRA) corresponding to a biphasic thinning phase. The SRS value is high compared to values obtained in a population of healthy dogs. The color display of strain rate is superimposed on the right parasternal trans ventricular short-axis view (left upper panel). Strain length ¼ 8 mm. Region of interest size ¼ 5/3 mm.

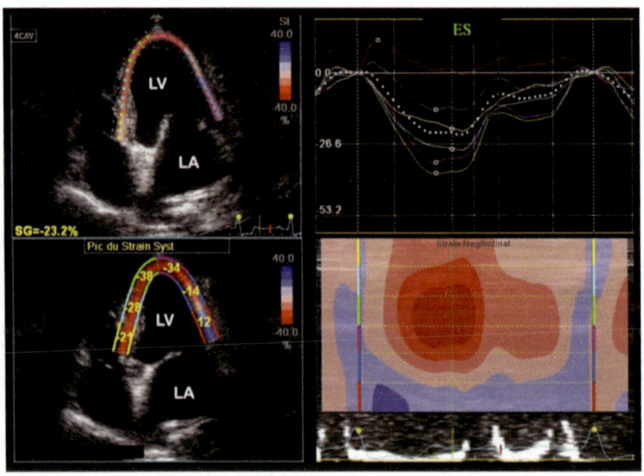

Abnormal longitudinal strain recorded in 6 myocardial segments of the left ventricle (LV)using Speckle Tracking echocardiography in a dog with mitral valve disease (left parasternal long-axis view). The software algorithm has automatically defined 6 equidistant myocardial segments within the interventricular septum and the LV free wall. The right upper panel shows the 6 corresponding LV longitudinal strain versus time curves. Five out of the 6 LV segments undergo a systolic myocardial shortening during systole (negative strain, maximal before or at end-systole (ES), which is normal). However, the values of peak systolic strain are heterogeneous, as also shown in the left lower panel. In addition, one segment (at the base of the LV free wall, red curve) undergoes an abnormal positive (instead of a negative) longitudinal systolic strain (þ12%). This dyskinesia is also apparent on the two-dimensional (left upper and lower panels) and M-curves (right lower panel) color-coded views showing the positive systolic strain in blue (instead of red). The M-curves color-coded view also shows the heterogeneous values of strain of the 5 other segments, appearing as red gradation. LA: left atrium.

References

Chetboul V. Advanced techniques in echocardiography in small animals. Vet Clin North Am Small Anim Pract 2010; 40:529e543.

Lisi M, Ballo P, Cameli M, Gandolfo F, Galderisi M,Chiavarelli M, Henein MY, Mondillo S. Mitral annular longitudinal function preservation after mitral valve repair: the MARTE study. Int J Cardiol 201.

Marciniak A, Sutherland GR, Marciniak M, Kourliouros A, Bijnens B, Jahangiri M. Prediction of postoperative left ventricular systolic function in patients with chronic mitral regurgitation undergoing valve surgery the role of *deformation imaging. E*ur J Cardiothorac Surg 2011; 40:1131e1137.

Rosenhek R, Maurer G. Management of valvular mitral regurgitation: the importance of risk stratification. J Cardiol 2010; 56:255e261.

Song JM, Kang SH, Lee EJ, Sh*in MJ, Lee JW*, Chung CH,Kim DH, Kang DH, Song JK. Echocardiographic predictors of left ventricular function and clinical outcomes after successful mitral valve repair: conventional two dimensional versus speckle-tracking parameters. Ann. Thorac. Surg 2011;91:1816e1823.

14

Theragnostic Treatment of Cancers and Electric Hyperthermia in Veterinary Practice

Domokos Máthé

Senior Lecturer and Head, In Vivo Imaging Centre, Department of Biophysics and Radiation Biology Faculty of Medicine Semmelweis University Budapest and Hungarian Centre for Excellence in Molecular Medicine – Szeged, Hungary

Precision medicine and personalised treatment of systemic or tumour diseases gain their acceptance and application in veterinary care, too. The application of personalised medical protocols and companion diagnostics is easier and ethically well reasoned within the veterinary medical field – and it can offer many advantageous lessons to human clinical transformation, too [1]. In vitro companion diagnostics for testing the applicability and sensitivity levels of certain kinase inhibitor and immunotherapeutic drugs offer a greatly increased efficiency for veterinary cancer patients, too. As the understanding of cancer biology has advanced, the field of veterinary oncology has grown significantly, paralleling developments in human oncology. Precision medicine is an innovative approach to disease treatment and prevention that considers individual variability in genes, environment, and lifestyle. In the context of veterinary medicine, precision medicine aims to provide tailored therapies that are specifically designed for the unique genetic and molecular profile of each animal's cancer. This approach moves away from the traditional "one-size-fits-all" model, instead focusing on targeted treatments that maximize efficacy while minimizing side effects. Companion diagnostics, such as molecular tests, help determine whether a dog or cat is likely to respond to a particular drug. For dogs and cats, precision medicine holds great promise in improving outcomes for cancers, which are among the leading causes of death in companion animals.

The application of precision medicine in companion diagnostics and therapies has revolutionized the way veterinarians approach cancer treatment.

Genetic profiling of the mast cell tumor can identify specific mutations or biomarkers that guide the selection of targeted therapies. The identification of KIT mutations in canine mast cell tumors can lead to the use of tyrosine kinase inhibitors like toceranib, which specifically target the abnormal proteins driving tumor growth.

This personalized approach not only improves treatment outcomes but also reduces the risk of unnecessary side effects from ineffective therapies.

Tumor Microenvironment: Where a parasite (the tumour) and its Host (the animal) Communicate and Fight

The tumor microenvironment (TME) plays a critical role in the progression, metastasis, and therapeutic resistance of cancers in dogs. Comprising a complex network of cancer cells, stromal cells, immune cells, blood vessels, and extracellular matrix, the TME influences tumor behavior and response to treatment. Understanding the TME is particularly important for developing effective therapies, such as internal radionuclide therapy (IRT), which has shown promise in treating canine cancers. IRT involves the delivery of radioactive isotopes directly to tumor cells, sparing healthy tissues and providing a targeted approach to cancer treatment.

The TME in canine cancers, such as osteosarcoma, mast cell tumors, and lymphoma, is characterized by hypoxia, acidosis, and immunosuppression, which contribute to tumor aggressiveness and resistance to conventional therapies (Khanna et al., 2006). Hypoxia, for example, is a hallmark of many solid tumors and is associated with poor prognosis due to its role in promoting angiogenesis, metastasis, and resistance to radiation therapy. IRT, however, can overcome some of these challenges by delivering radiation directly to tumor cells, regardless of the hypoxic conditions. For instance, samarium-153-EDTMP (Quadramet) and strontium-89 have been used in dogs with osteosarcoma to target bone metastases, providing pain relief and slowing disease progression (Lattimer et al., 1990). These radionuclides emit beta particles that selectively irradiate tumor cells while minimizing damage to surrounding healthy tissues.

One of the key advantages of IRT is its ability to target the TME by exploiting unique features of tumor biology. For example, radiolabeled peptides or antibodies can be designed to bind to specific receptors or antigens expressed on cancer cells or within the TME. In canine lymphoma, radiolabeled antibodies targeting CD20 or CD22 have been explored as a means of delivering radiation directly to tumor cells (Suter et al., 2004). This approach not only enhances the therapeutic efficacy but also reduces systemic toxicity compared to traditional chemotherapy. Additionally, the crossfire effect of IRT—where radiation emitted from one cell can damage neighboring cells—can help overcome the heterogeneity of the TME and target resistant cancer cell populations.

The TME also plays a role in modulating the immune response to IRT. Radiation has been shown to induce immunogenic cell death, releasing tumor antigens and stimulating an anti-tumor immune response (Golden et al., 2015). In dogs, combining IRT with immunotherapy, such as checkpoint inhibitors or cancer vaccines, could enhance the therapeutic outcome by leveraging the immune system to target residual cancer cells. For example, the combination of IRT and the ONCEPT melanoma vaccine has the potential to improve survival in dogs with advanced melanoma by addressing both local and systemic disease.

Somatostatin receptor-targeted isotope therapy (SRI therapy) is an innovative and targeted approach to treating neuroendocrine tumors (NETs) and other cancers that overexpress somatostatin receptors (SSTRs). This therapy has gained attention in both human and veterinary medicine due to its ability to deliver radiation directly to tumor cells while sparing healthy tissues. In dogs, SRI therapy holds promise for treating cancers such as pituitary tumors, insulinomas, and other SSTR-positive neoplasms, offering a novel treatment option for conditions that are often challenging to manage with conventional therapies.

Somatostatin receptors, particularly subtypes SSTR2 and SSTR5, are overexpressed in many neuroendocrine and non-neuroendocrine tumors. These receptors can be targeted using radiolabeled somatostatin analogs, such as lutetium-177 (^{177}Lu) or yttrium-90 (^{90}Y) conjugated to peptides like DOTATATE or DOTATOC. These radiopharmaceuticals bind to SSTRs on the surface of tumor cells, delivering localized radiation that induces DNA damage and cell death. In dogs, SRI therapy has been explored primarily in cases of pituitary tumors, such as corticotroph adenomas causing Cushing's disease, and insulinomas, which are common in older dogs and often metastasize, making surgical resection difficult.

For example, in dogs with insulinomas, which frequently metastasize to the liver and lymph nodes, SRI therapy can deliver radiation to both primary and metastatic lesions, providing a more comprehensive treatment approach compared to surgery or traditional chemotherapy. Studies in humans have shown that ^{177}Lu-DOTATATE (Lutathera) significantly improves progression-free survival and quality of life in patients with advanced NETs (Strosberg et al., 2017), and similar benefits are anticipated in veterinary patients.

The use of SRI therapy in dogs requires careful patient selection and diagnostic imaging to confirm SSTR expression. Techniques such as somatostatin receptor scintigraphy (SRS) or positron emission tomography (PET) using gallium-68 (^{68}Ga)-labeled somatostatin analogs (e.g., ^{68}Ga-DOTATATE) are used to identify tumors with sufficient receptor expression for effective targeting. These imaging modalities not only aid in diagnosis but also help monitor treatment response and guide therapeutic decisions.

Clinical trials and case studies in dogs have demonstrated the potential of SRI therapy. For instance, a pilot study evaluating ^{177}Lu-DOTATATE in dogs with SSTR-positive tumors reported partial or complete responses in a subset of patients, with minimal side effects (Grooters et al., 2020). The therapy was well-tolerated, with transient mild hematologic and gastrointestinal toxicity being the most common adverse effects. These findings align with human studies, where SRI therapy has shown a favorable safety profile compared to systemic chemotherapy.

In addition to its direct antitumor effects, SRI therapy may also modulate the tumor microenvironment (TME). Radiation from SRI therapy can induce immunogenic cell death, releasing tumor antigens and stimulating an immune response. This opens the possibility of combining SRI therapy with immunotherapy, such as immune checkpoint inhibitors, to enhance treatment efficacy. While this approach is still in its early stages in veterinary medicine, it holds significant promise for improving outcomes in dogs with advanced or refractory cancers.

All the above therapies are supported by a very efficient adjunct therapeutic process, namely hyperthermia and its mild, non-destructive heat version, electro-hyperthermia.

Modulated Electro-Hyperthermia in Dog and Cat Oncology

Modulated electro-hyperthermia (mEHT) is a novel, non-invasive cancer treatment that has gained attention in both human and veterinary medicine for its ability to selectively target tumor cells while sparing healthy tissues. This therapy uses electromagnetic waves to generate localized heat within tumors, inducing cancer cell death through a combination of thermal and non-thermal effects. In dog and cat oncology, mEHT offers a promising adjunct to conventional therapies such as surgery, chemotherapy, and radiation, particularly for tumors that are difficult to treat or in cases where traditional treatments are contraindicated.

Electro-Hyperthermia Applications in Dog and Cat Oncology

mEHT has been explored in veterinary medicine for the treatment of various cancers, including mast cell tumors, soft tissue sarcomas, and squamous cell carcinomas. In dogs, mast cell tumors (MCTs) are one of the most common skin cancers, and their treatment can be challenging due to their variable behavior and potential for metastasis. mEHT has been used as an adjunct to surgery and chemotherapy in dogs with MCTs, with studies reporting improved local tumor control and reduced recurrence rates (Vancsoki et al., 2013). The localized heating effect of mEHT is particularly beneficial for tumors in sensitive areas, such as the limbs or head, where surgical margins may be limited.

In cats, squamous cell carcinoma (SCC) is a common oral and skin cancer that is often aggressive and difficult to treat. mEHT has shown promise in managing feline SCC, particularly in cases where surgery or radiation therapy is not feasible. The non-invasive nature of mEHT makes it an attractive option for older or debilitated patients who may not tolerate more aggressive treatments. Case reports have documented tumor regression and improved quality of life in cats with SCC treated with mEHT, either alone or in combination with other therapies (Veterinary Cancer Society, 2020).

Synergistic Effects with Precision Therapies

One of the most compelling aspects of mEHT is its ability to enhance the effects of other cancer treatments. Hyperthermia has long been recognized as a radiosensitizer, and mEHT's selective heating can improve the efficacy of radiation therapy by increasing oxygen availability within the tumor, which is critical for radiation-induced DNA damage (Hildebrandt et al., 2002). In dogs and cats, combining mEHT with radiation therapy has been shown to improve tumor control and prolong survival in cases of soft tissue sarcomas and oral melanomas.

Similarly, mEHT can enhance the delivery and efficacy of chemotherapeutic agents. The increased blood flow and permeability of tumor vessels induced by hyperthermia improve drug penetration into the tumor, while the heat itself can sensitize cancer cells to chemotherapy. In veterinary oncology, this combination has been used successfully in dogs with hemangiosarcoma and cats with lymphoma, resulting in improved response rates and reduced side effects compared to chemotherapy alone (Veterinary Cancer Society, 2020).

Immune Modulation and Long-Term Benefits of mEHT

Beyond its direct cytotoxic effects, mEHT has been shown to modulate the tumor microenvironment (TME) and stimulate anti-tumor immune responses. The heat generated by mEHT can induce immunogenic cell death, releasing tumor antigens that activate dendritic cells and promote T-cell-mediated immunity (Frey et al., 2012). This immune activation can lead to long-term tumor control and reduce the risk of metastasis. In dogs and cats, this immunomodulatory effect is particularly valuable for cancers with a high metastatic potential, such as osteosarcoma and mammary carcinoma.

The integration of advanced therapies in veterinary oncology has opened new avenues for treating cancers in dogs and cats. Two innovative approaches—fibroblast activation protein inhibitor (FAPi) radioisotope therapy and modulated electro-hyperthermia (mEHT)—have shown significant promise individually. When used in parallel, these therapies offer a synergistic combination that targets both the tumor cells and the tumor microenvironment (TME), providing a comprehensive treatment strategy for challenging cancers. This essay explores the mechanisms, applications, and potential benefits of combining FAPi radioisotope therapy and mEHT in veterinary oncology, with implications for translational research in human medicine.

FAPi Radioisotope Therapy: Targeting the Tumor Microenvironment

Fibroblast activation protein (FAP) is a transmembrane glycoprotein expressed predominantly by cancer-associated fibroblasts (CAFs) in the TME. CAFs play a critical role in tumor progression, immune evasion, and therapy resistance by remodeling the extracellular matrix, promoting angiogenesis, and suppressing anti-tumor immune responses. FAPi radioisotope therapy involves the use of radiolabeled FAP inhibitors, such as gallium-68 (^{68}Ga) or lutetium-177 (^{177}Lu) conjugated to FAPi, to deliver targeted radiation to CAFs and other FAP-expressing cells within the TME (Lindner et al., 2018). This approach not only damages the stromal support network of the tumor but also disrupts the protective niche that shields cancer cells from immune detection and therapy.

In dogs and cats, FAPi radioisotope therapy has been explored in cancers with a dense stromal component, such as mammary carcinomas, soft tissue sarcomas, and pancreatic tumors. For example, in canine mammary tumors, which often exhibit high FAP expression, FAPi therapy has shown potential in reducing tumor growth and metastasis by targeting the stromal compartment (Veterinary Cancer Society, 2021). The ability of FAPi therapy to selectively irradiate the TME while sparing healthy tissues makes it a valuable tool for managing aggressive and metastatic cancers.

Modulated Electro-Hyperthermia: Selective Tumor Cell Killing

mEHT has been successfully used in veterinary oncology to treat a variety of cancers, including mast cell tumors, soft tissue sarcomas, and squamous cell carcinomas. In dogs with mast cell tumors, mEHT has been shown to improve local tumor control and reduce recurrence rates when used as an adjunct to surgery or chemotherapy (Vancsoki et al., 2013). Additionally, mEHT enhances the efficacy of other treatments by increasing blood flow to the tumor and improving drug delivery or radiosensitivity (Fiorentini & Szasz, 2006).

Synergistic Effects of FAPi Therapy and mEHT

The parallel use of FAPi radioisotope therapy and mEHT offers a powerful combination that targets both the tumor cells and the TME. FAPi therapy disrupts the stromal support network and sensitizes the tumor to other treatments, while mEHT selectively kills cancer cells and enhances the effects of radiation and chemotherapy. Together, these therapies create a multi-pronged attack on the tumor, addressing its structural, cellular, and microenvironmental components.

One of the key advantages of this combination is its ability to overcome therapy resistance. Many cancers develop resistance to treatment by altering the TME or upregulating protective mechanisms. FAPi therapy disrupts these protective mechanisms by targeting CAFs, while mEHT induces immunogenic cell death and stimulates anti-tumor immune responses (Frey et al., 2012). This dual approach not only improves treatment efficacy but also reduces the risk of recurrence and metastasis.

Clinical Applications in Dogs and Cats

In veterinary oncology, the combination of FAPi therapy and mEHT has the potential to revolutionize the treatment of aggressive and metastatic cancers. For example, in dogs with osteosarcoma, which is highly metastatic and resistant to conventional therapies, the combination of FAPi therapy and mEHT could target both the primary tumor and metastatic lesions while stimulating an anti-tumor immune response. Similarly, in cats with oral squamous cell carcinoma, this combination could provide a non-invasive and effective treatment option for tumors that are difficult to manage with surgery or radiation.

Case studies and preliminary trials have demonstrated the feasibility and safety of combining these therapies. For instance, a pilot study in dogs with soft tissue sarcomas reported improved tumor control and reduced side effects when FAPi therapy was combined with mEHT (Veterinary Cancer Society, 2021). These findings highlight the potential of this approach to improve outcomes in veterinary patients while providing valuable insights for human oncology.

The parallel use of FAPi radioisotope therapy and modulated electro-hyperthermia represents a groundbreaking approach in veterinary oncology. By targeting both the tumor cells and the TME, this combination offers a comprehensive and synergistic treatment strategy for challenging cancers in dogs and cats. As research continues to expand, this approach has the potential to become a standard of care in veterinary medicine while contributing to the development of similar therapies in human oncology. The integration of these advanced therapies underscores the importance of comparative oncology in advancing cancer treatment for both animals and humans.

In conclusion, the tumor microenvironment is a critical factor in the progression and treatment of canine cancers. Internal radionuclide therapy offers a targeted approach to overcoming the challenges posed by the TME, such as hypoxia and immunosuppression, while minimizing damage to healthy tissues.

By integrating IRT with other modalities, such as immunotherapy, veterinarians can provide more effective and personalized treatments for dogs with cancer. Spontaneous tumors in companion animals share many genetic, molecular, and environmental similarities with human cancers, making them valuable models for translational research.

These similarities, however, should be viewed always in a metabolism-centered concept where real life behaviour of tumours in the course of therapy is mostly defined by a complex interplay of metabolic alterations and tumour microenvironment which is entirely different in dogs and humans.

References

Andocs, G., Renner, H., Balogh, L., et al. (2009). Strong synergy of heat and modulated electromagnetic field in tumor cell killing. Strahlentherapie und Onkologie, 185(2) 120-126.

Bergman, P. J., McKnight, J., Novosad, A., et al. (2006). Long-term survival of dogs with advanced malignant melanoma after DNA vaccination with xenogeneic human tyrosinase: A phase I trial. Clinical Cancer Research, 12(10)3027-3033.

Burton, J. H., Mitchell, L., Thamm, D. H., et al. (2013). N-terminal truncation of the HER2 protein leads to increased signaling activity and induction of apoptosis in canine mammary tumor cells. Veterinary and Comparative Oncology, 11(1)1-12.

Fiorentini, G., & Szasz, A. (2006). Hyperthermia today: Electric energy, a new opportunity in cancer treatment. Journal of Cancer Research and Therapeutics, 2(2)41-46.

Frey, B., Weiss, E. M., Rubner, Y., et al. (2012). Old and new facts about hyperthermia-induced modulations of the immune system. *International Journal of Hyperthermia, 28(6)528-542.

Frey, B., Weiss, E. M., Rubner, Y., et al. (2012). Old and new facts about hyperthermia-induced modulations of the immune system. International Journal of Hyperthermia, 28(6)528-542.

Golden, E. B., Frances, D., & Pellicciotta, I. (2015). Radiation fosters dose-dependent and chemotherapy-induced immunogenic cell death. OncoImmunology, 4(9)e1049278.

Grooters, A. M., Biller, B. J., & Armbrust, L. J. (2020). Preliminary evaluation of ^{177}Lu-DOTATATE therapy in dogs with somatostatin receptor-positive tumors. Veterinary Radiology & Ultrasound, 61(3)345-352.

Khanna, C., Lindblad-Toh, K., Vail, D., et al. (2006). The dog as a cancer model. Nature Biotechnology, 24(9)1065-1066.

Lattimer, J. C., Corwin, L. A., Stapleton, J., et al. (1990). Clinical and clinicopathologic response of canine bone tumor patients to treatment with samarium-153-EDTMP. Journal of Nuclear Medicine, 31(8)1316-1325.

Lindner, T., Loktev, A., Altmann, A., et al. (2018). Development of quinoline-based theranostic ligands for the targeting of fibroblast activation protein. Journal of Nuclear Medicine, 59(9)1415-1422.

London, C. A., Malpas, P. B., Wood-Follis, S. L., et al. (2009). Multi-center, placebo-controlled, double-blind, randomized study of oral toceranib phosphate (SU11654), a receptor tyrosine kinase inhibitor, for the treatment of dogs with recurrent (either local or distant) mast cell tumor following surgical excision. Clinical Cancer Research, 15(11), 3856-3865.

Paoloni, M. C., & Khanna, C. (2008). Translation of new cancer treatments from pet dogs to humans. Nature Reviews Cancer, 8(2)147-156.

Strosberg, J., El-Haddad, G., Wolin, E., et al. (2017). Phase 3 trial of ^{177}Lu-DOTATATE for midgut neuroendocrine tumors. New England Journal of Medicine, 376(2)125-135.

Suter, S. E., Chein, M. B., von Messling, V., et al. (2004). In vitro characterization of a canine CD20-specific monoclonal antibody and in vivo activity in a severe combined immunodeficiency mouse xenograft model. *Veterinary Immunology and Immunopathology, 101(3-4)157-165.

Vancsoki, T., Vancsoki, V., & Szasz, A. (2013). Modulated electro-hyperthermia in veterinary oncology: A case report of a dog with mast cell tumor. *Conference on Advances in Veterinary Oncology, 12(3)45-50.

Veterinary Cancer Society. (2021). Fibroblast activation protein inhibitor (FAPi) therapy in companion animals: Clinical applications and outcomes. Veterinary Cancer Society Annual Conference Proceedings.

15

Recent Application of Interventional Cardiology in Cats and Dogs with Heart Diseases

Hee-Myung Park

Professor, Department of Veterinary Internal Medicine, College of Veterinary Medicine, Konkuk University, Seoul, Republic of Korea

Introduction

One of the remarkable advancements in veterinary medicine recently is the application of interventional cardiology techniques to treat various congenital heart diseases. In dogs and cats, congenital heart diseases can be treated much more easily and with fewer complications using minimally invasive interventional approaches, rather than through traditional open-heart surgery. Among congenital heart diseases, treatment options are available for conditions such as PDA (Patent Ductus Arteriosus), AS (Aortic Stenosis), PS (Pulmonic Stenosis), VSD (Ventricular Septal Defect), ASD (Atrial Septal Defect), extrahepatic shunt, and stem cell applications. These diseases often cannot be significantly improved by medical treatment alone, making the use of the aforementioned interventional techniques essential for effective management.

These congenital heart defects, especially those occurring in dogs and cats, manifest early in life and lead to various clinical signs such as growth retardation, as well as a range of cardiovascular abnormalities. Therefore, early diagnosis of these diseases through auscultation, electrocardiography (ECG), and echocardiography is crucial for prompt treatment, which is vital for the health of the pet. Among these procedures, treatments have historically involved the use of coils, vascular plugs, and ACDO (Amplatz Canine Duct Occluder). Technically, it is important to make the devices very small, ensuring biocompatibility to avoid any harm to the health of the implanted companion animals.

In congenital heart diseases such as AS (Aortic Stenosis) and PS (Pulmonic Stenosis), where stenosis occurs, balloon valvuloplasty is a technique used to expand the narrowed areas by using a balloon. This approach offers significant advantages as it allows treatment for pets with various forms of stenosis. Although these procedures often require re-intervention, in severe cases, the technique can improve the condition to a mild or moderate stage, providing an opportunity to extend the life of many pet patients. Therefore, in veterinary cardiology, this is considered a crucial therapeutic method. This technique has the advantage of being widely used in veterinary medicine to alleviate symptoms or treat chronic diseases in pets through interventional procedures, such as the implantation of stem cells. It can be applied in cases of conditions like renal failure, liver failure, and heart disease, helping to reduce disease symptoms and improve treatment outcomes.

Therefore, the purpose of this paper is to show the advantages, methods, and applicable cases of these procedures to not only general veterinarians but also veterinary specialists in internal medicine, with the aim of encouraging the broader adoption of these techniques across various fields.

Case Presentation

Case 1: ATE (Saddle embolism) in a HCM cat

Turkish Angora, 7Y 7M, CM

- Hind limb paralysis: The cat is experiencing paralysis in the hind limbs, which may indicate neurological or spinal issues.
- Cold extremities: The extremities (legs or paws) are cold to the touch, possibly suggesting poor blood circulation or shock.
- Gallop sound (Heart): An abnormal heart sound, often associated with heart failure or other cardiac conditions, where the heart rhythm resembles a galloping horse.
- Tachypnea: Rapid breathing, which may be a sign of respiratory distress or a cardiac issue.
- Harsh lung sound: Abnormal lung sounds, such as wheezing or crackles, indicating potential respiratory problems like pneumonia, fluid in the lungs, or other lung-related conditions.

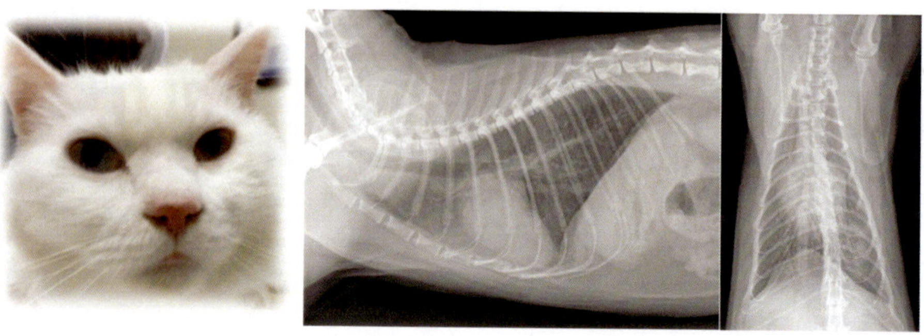

Fig. 1: There are radographic abnormalitis, such as valentine-shaped heart (LA bulging),

cardiomegaly with VHS: 9.3 (7.2-7.8), interstitial pattern and suspected pulmonary edema or hemorrhage.

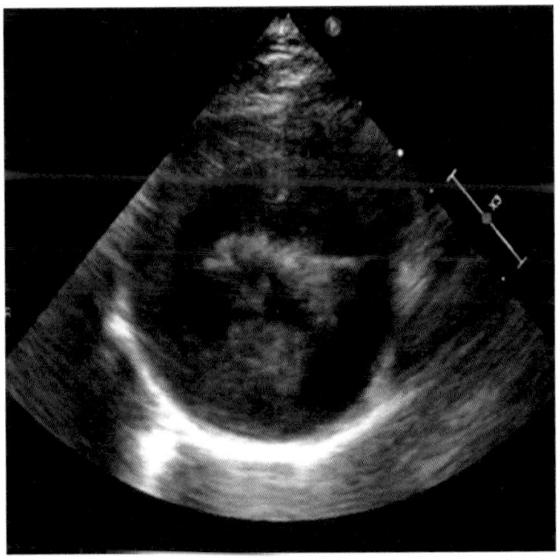

Figure 2. The echocardiographic findings show the left ventricle in a short axis view, where severe hypertrophy of the cardiac muscle is observed, resulting in a significant narrowing of the ventricular lumen. This indicates left ventricular hypertrophy, which may be associated with conditions like hypertrophic cardiomyopathy or other forms of heart disease.

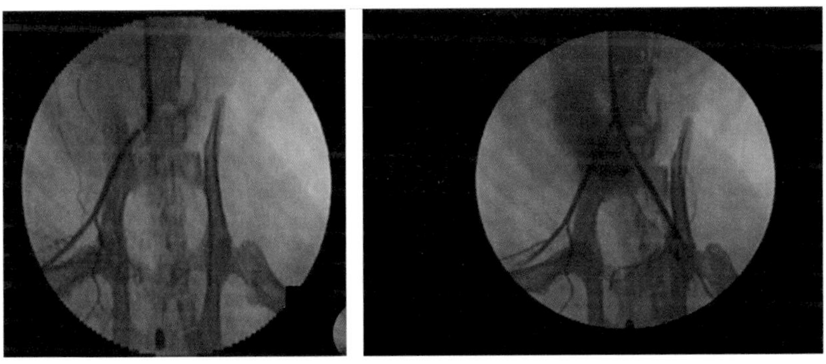

Figure 3. The following image is an angiographic view showing a saddle embolism in the left femoral artery. The right angiographic image demonstrates the post-procedural result, where blood is flowing smoothly through both femoral arteries, indicating successful restoration of circulation.

For this HCM cat with saddle embolism, the urgent thrombolysis treatment was performed using interventional angiography with the following equipment: a short introducer (4 Fr), guide wire (0.035"), angio catheter (4 Fr), and contrast media (Iohexol). Thrombolytic therapy involved the administration of Streptokinase (90,000 units infusion), and continuous cardiac medication was provided with diltiazem.

Case 2: Pulmonic stenosis in a dog

A 4.6-year-old, SF, 4.6 kg weight Poodle dog presented with symptoms of frequent coughing and shivering, especially when excited. On auscultation, a systolic murmur grade 4/6 was heard, and the point of maximum intensity (PMI) was noted in the pulmonary area

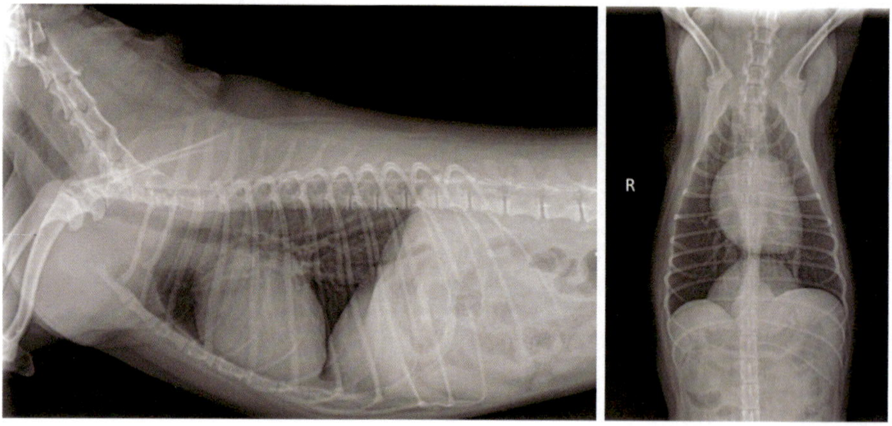

Figure 4. Radiographic findings showed a VHS of 10.6, indicating mild cardiomegaly. The right radiograph revealed increased bulging of the main pulmonary artery (MPA) at the 1-2 o'clock position in the ventrodorsal (VD) view.

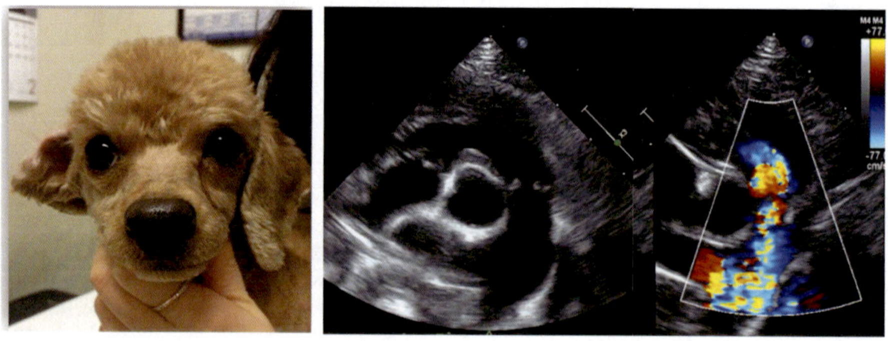

Figure 5. This echocardiogram is the result of a pulmonary flow study in a patient with pulmonary stenosis (PS). The Vmax is 8.17 m/s, and the PGmax is 267 mm Hg, indicating severe pulmonic stenosis (> 75 mm Hg) (left side). The right Doppler echocardiography findings show severe blood flow obstruction at the site of stenosis.

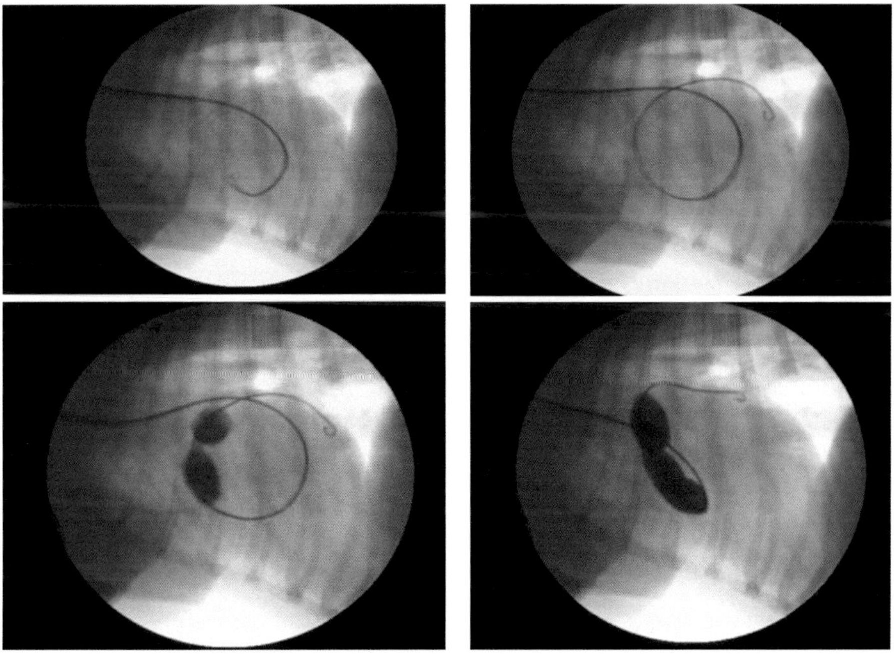

Figure 6. The top left image shows the approach of the vascular catheter through the jugular vein, demonstrating the entry of the cardiac catheter into the right atrium and right ventricle. The top right image illustrates the cardiac catheter approaching the pulmonary artery. The bottom left image shows the pulmonary artery stenosis site identified through angiography. The bottom right image describes the area where balloon valvuloplasty was successfully performed.

To treat this patient, low-dose Atenolol was administered for 2 weeks before performing balloon valvuloplasty. The dosage was up-titrated weekly as follows: 0.25 mg/kg, 0.5 mg/kg, 0.75 mg/kg, and 1 mg/kg, given twice daily (BID) orally (PO). Heart rate (HR) and blood pressure (BP) were continuously monitored. Additionally, after the balloon valvuloplasty procedure, Atenolol 1 mg/kg BID PO was continued.

Conclusions

By using interventional angiography and balloon valvuloplasty, it is suggested that if we quickly diagnose various thrombotic symptoms, such as those caused by saddle embolism due to hypertrophic cardiomyopathy in cats, including forelimb or hindlimb paralysis, these thrombotic conditions can be effectively treated. In addition, if congenital heart diseases in dogs and cats are detected early, more heart defects in companion animals can be treated through interventional cardiac procedures.

References

Bussadori, C., de Madron, E., Santilli, R. A. and Borgarelli, M. 2001. Balloon valvuloplasty in 30 dogs with pulmonic stenosis: effect of value morphology and annular size on initial and 1-year outcome. Journal of veterinary Internal Medicine, 15, 553.

Caivano, D., Birettoni, F., Fruganti, A., Rishniw, M., Knafelz, P., Moïse, N. S. and Porciello, F. 2012. Transthoracic echocardiographically-guided interventional cardiac procedures in the dog. Journal of Veterinary Cardiology Volume 14, Issue 3, 431-444

Oliveira, P., Domenech, O., Silva, J., Vannini, S., Bussadori, R. and Bussadori, C. 2011. Retrospective review of congenital heart disease in 976 dogs. Journal of veterinary internal medicine, 25:477-483.

Scansen, B. A. 2017, Interventional Cardiology: What's New?. Veterinary Clinics of North America: Small Animal Practice. Volume 47, Issue 5, 1021-1040.

16

Advanced Insights into Hemodialysis Therapy for Companion Animals Techniques, Challenges, and Outcomes

***Randhir Singh*[1], *Sachin*[2] *and S.R. Upadhayay*[3]**

[1]*Assistant Professor (Vety. Medicine), Department of TVCC, COVS, Guru Angad Dev Veterinary & Animal Sciences University, Ludhiana, Punjab*
[2]*M.V.Sc. Scholar, Department of Vety. Medicine, COVS, Guru Angad Dev Veterinary & Animal Sciences University, Ludhiana, Punjab*
[3]*Professor, Vety. Medicine & Head, VAHEE, F.V.Sc., SKUAST-Jammu Jammu and Kashmir*

Renal failure is one of the most commonly presented conditions in veterinary clinics world over. Although the potential for recovery is favorable, most animals die due to multisystemic effects induced by azotemia. Hence, extracorporeal removal of endogenous and exogenous toxins is very essential for expanding the window of recovery. Hemodialysis has been used in treatment of veterinary patients for the last 50 years and is still one of the most expensive and technically demanding treatment modalities in veterinary medicine. It is an advanced extracorporeal renal replacement therapy which has recently transitioned from a clinical curiosity to a more advanced standard for management of acute kidney injury (AKI) and chronic kidney disease (CKD) in companion animals particularly dogs and cats.

In addition to eliminating selective toxins that cause AKI, regardless of renal function, hemodialysis is also effective in the removal of pharmacokinetically active soluble uremic substances in CKD to enhance life expectancy and quality of life (Singh, 2021). Other common indications of hemodialysis in veterinary medicine include fluid overload, dysregulated body fluid composition, drug overdose or intoxications (Foster, 2020; Singh *et al.*, 2024). Medical management alone is often insufficient to control the clinical signs and metabolic abnormalities associated with uremia when AKI is severe or when there is involvement of acute on chronic kidney disease. Consequently, animals are at risk of death within a short therapeutic window, despite the potential reversibility of AKI and the improvement of life expectancy in CKD. Adjunctive hemodialysis should be introduced promptly to the conventional medical management when medical therapy alone is not anticipated to control the clinical signs and morbid clinicopathologic abnormalities associated with the disease condition, but before the animal has significantly decompensated.

Modalities for the delivery of renal replacement therapies in veterinary medicine include peritoneal dialysis (PD), intermittent hemodialysis (IHD), and continuous renal replacement therapy (CRRT). Peritoneal dialysis (PD) was one of the first renal replacement therapies introduced in veterinary therapeutics for management of uremia but it is associated with various complications including peritonitis, septicemia, abdominal pain and hernia. Due to this reason PD is now-a -days only reserved for veterinary patients where there is no facility of extracorporeal renal replacement therapies like IHD/ CRRT or where the patient size is too small to perform safe IHD/ CRRT. IHD is a type of extracorporeal renal replacement therapy which is defined by short but efficient hemodialysis sessions with the ultimate goal of removing endogenous or exogenous toxins from the bloodstream. At present, IHD remains an effective advanced treatment option for managing veterinary patients suffering from either AKI or CKD with growing acceptance. CRRT is a continuous process and once the treatment begins, therapy continues until renal function returns or the patient is transitioned to IHD. CRRT is more costly and time-consuming form of therapy as compared to IHD. Despite established integration of IHD into veterinary therapeutics for managing uremia of AKI/ CKD in the western world, in India only few teaching veterinary hospitals provide this advanced facility primarily owing to lack of technical know-how and secondarily due to financial burden and emotional drain while repeatedly dealing with clients. This paper presents recent advancements in veterinary hemodialysis, employing an evidence-based approach to techniques and technical knowledge, with a specific focus on intermittent hemodialysis (IHD).

Principles of IHD

During hemodialysis (IHD), the primary forces governing fluid and solute exchange are diffusion, convection, and adsorption. The magnitude of these exchanges is influenced by the solute's characteristics, the pore size and structural properties of the dialyzer membrane, commonly referred to as an "artificial kidney." In IHD, diffusion predominates as the primary solute and fluid exchange mechanism. Convection and adsorption generally play a secondary role. During diffusion, solutes traverse from regions of high to low concentration gradients. As they move, solutes exit the blood or dialysate fluid compartment in which they were dissolved, cross the dialysis membrane, and enter the opposing fluid compartment. Blood solutes, such as blood urea nitrogen (BUN), creatinine, and electrolytes, diffuse across the semipermeable dialyzer membrane into the dialysate, which is subsequently discarded. Conversely, solutes in high concentration in the dialysate, including bicarbonate and selected electrolytes, can diffuse across the membrane according to their concentration gradients into the blood. The rate of solute transfer via diffusion is governed by the solute concentration gradient, the kinetic energy of the solution (primarily determined by molecular weight), and membrane permeability. Diffusion is particularly effective in removing molecules with low molecular weight from the blood, such as BUN, creatinine, sodium, potassium, phosphorus, and magnesium. Convection facilitates the removal of water and dissolved solutes from the blood. Blood traveling through semipermeable dialyzer membranes encounters positive transmembrane pressure, which propels fluid (ultrafiltrate) and dissolved solutes out of the blood, across the membrane, and into the dialysate, which is subsequently discarded. The rate of fluid and solute transfer via convection is determined by the transmembrane hydrostatic pressure difference between the blood and dialysate, as well as the surface area of the dialysis membrane. Convection, although a significant force in continuous renal replacement therapy (CRRT), is not employed in IHD. It is more effective in removing molecules with low and medium molecular weights from the blood. These molecules encompass various inflammatory mediators, such as β2-microglobulin, carbamylated proteins, and parathyroid hormone, along with other uremic toxins having molecular weight of >500 Da (Yeun and Depner, 2000).

Indications of Hemodialysis

The Timing of Dialysis Initiation in Dogs and Cats with Acute Kidney Injury

Intermittent hemodialysis is an effective treatment strategy for animals with IRIS Grade IV and V AKI, removing retained uremic toxins, correcting metabolic derangements and excessive fluid overload in a short time window. However, its effectiveness decreases when applied late in the disease course or when multi-organ complications have set in. This is attributed to the fact that uremic toxins are distributed throughout body fluids, affecting almost all major body organs, making animals susceptible to multiple organ dysfunction and death if dialysis treatment is delayed (Segev *et al.*, 2008). The number of organs secondarily affected by AKI is associated with progressively increased mortality. Therefore, dialytic intervention should be proactively applied before multiorgan failure occurs, rather than as a response to it. The major indications for dialysis initiation in AKI are:

i. Serum creatinine levels >5mg/dL and exhibiting an upward trend, even after adequate hydration.

ii. Persistent anuria (>6 h) or oliguria (<0.3 mL/kg/h) unresponsive to appropriate fluid therapy and other recommended medicinal management strategies.

iii. Presence of electrolyte imbalances that cannot be effectively controlled with medical or surgical interventions (e.g., hyperkalemia, hyper and hyponatremia).

iv. Life-threatening fluid overload that is unresponsive to appropriate diuretic therapy and may lead to target organ damage.

v. For removal of toxins (sufficiently high enough to cause morbidity or life-threatening complications) when an effective antidote is unavailable or a potentially more effective therapeutic modality (e.g., hemoperfusion or therapeutic plasma exchange) is not feasible.

The Timing of Dialysis Initiation in Dogs and Cats with Chronic Kidney Disease

Intermittent hemodialysis is an effective management strategy for animals with IRIS Grade III and IV CKD with main focus on improving animal's quality of life thereby increasing life expectancy. Thus, IHD can be efficiently and safely used in patients suffering from CKD when

i. Clinical signs cannot be controlled effectively even after comprehensive medicinal therapy.

ii. All other means are not sufficient enough to normalize the animal however, before the animal has substantially decompensated (weight loss/ emaciation).

Dialysis Platform Selection

The most prevalent hemodialysis modalities in veterinary medicine are intermittent hemodialysis (IHD) and continuous renal replacement therapy (CRRT). IHD platforms are more commonly employed due to their efficiency and cost-effectiveness, while CRRT platforms are preferred for animals with critical health conditions requiring slow and continuous replacement therapy for extended periods (typically exceeding 24 hours). Although, either platform can be utilized for initial renal replacement therapy, IHD is considered more efficient and economically viable in medium to large-sized animals compared to CRRT. Prominent worldwide brands include Fresenius Medical Care (Germany), B. Braun Melungeon AG (Germany), Baxter International Inc. (USA), Medtronic plc (Ireland), DaVita Inc. (USA), and Nipro Corporation (Japan), among others. Before selecting any platform, it is crucial to ensure the availability of dialysis consumables at reasonable prices along with round the clock technical support from manufacturer.

IHD Basics

Venous Access

IHD involves removal of huge volume of patient blood out of the body by means of an extra-corporal circuit (blood tubing), its clearance through an artificial kidney (a dialyzer) followed by re-infusion of toxin free blood into animal body.

To achieve this volume, a dedicated uninterrupted venous access is a pre-requisite for performing safe and efficient IHD. In veterinary patients, this blood access is generally obtained via a dedicated double-lumen jugular catheter (DLC) having varying types and sizes. This DLC can be either temporary or permanent where temporary catheters can be kept in place for 3-4 weeks and permanent catheters can be kept in place for extended period of time usually 3-4 months. At present, most of the catheters are either made of polyurethane or silicone. Depending on individual patient size, these catheters can be of varying length (11cm to 24 cm) and diameter (7.5 Fr to 12.5 Fr). Temporary catheter is placed using a modified Seldinger technique whereas, permanent catheter is placed surgically where it is tunneled subcutaneously from insertion site. Regardless of catheter, it is mandatory to adhere to strict sterile compliance (asepsis) with provision of a dedicated sterile catheterization area/ bay, doctor(s) and technician(s) involved in catheterization must maintain proper asepsis by wearing a sterile gown, cap, mask and sterile gloves. Patient should be prepared aseptically by clipping catheterization area followed by chlorhexidine and alcohol scrub. During on-going dialysis, whole staff should adhere to strict asepsis protocol (Figure 1).

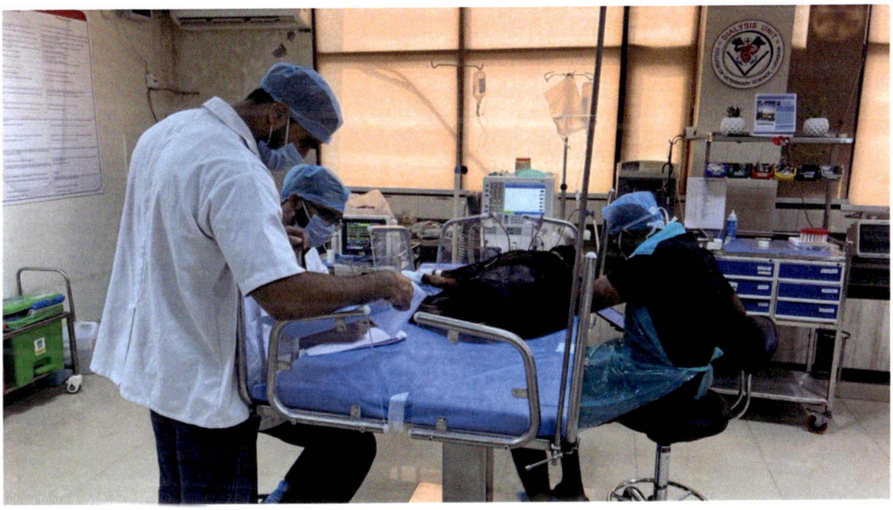

Figure 1. Patient undergoing IHD at dialysis unit, Department of TVCC, Guru Angad Dev Veterinary & Animal Sciences University. Note the strict compliance to maintain asepsis.

Selecting Dialyzer or an Artificial Kidney

The hemodialyzer is a compact, disposable extracorporeal unit containing thousands of hollow fibers that functions as an artificial kidney. It is a sealed compartment with connections on both ends to facilitate the flow of blood and dialysate through the unit. Blood circulates within the fibers, while dialysate circulates around the fibers in a countercurrent direction facilitating movement of solutes/ uremic toxins depending on concentration gradient. Selection of dialyzer is based on its surface area (Fisher *et al.,* 2004). Generally, less than 1m^2 surface area dialyzer can be used in dogs with a body weight less than 10 kg, whereas a surface area of 1-2 m^2 can be used safely in dogs with body weight up to 20kg. Dialyzers are also of two types i.e., high and low-flux dialyzers. High-flux dialyzers have a clearance of more than 20mL/min and they can remove middle sized molecules like p-Cresol and $ß_2$- microglobin whereas, low-flux dialyzers have a clearance of less than 10mL/min and they can remove small water-soluble solutes.

Blood Tubing

Blood tubing constitute the major component of extracorporeal circuit volume. Thus, before selecting a blood tubing utmost care should be given to priming/ filling volume of blood tubing according to animal body weight. Blood tubing is also available in different sizes and diameters and color coated in red (arterial line) and blue (venous line).

Dialysate Solution

The fundamental constituents of dialysate solution comprise a concentrated solute solution (part A), a concentrated bicarbonate solution (part B), and purified water. Part A may contain electrolytes such as sodium, potassium, chloride, calcium, dextrose, and magnesium in quantities that closely resemble plasma concentrations. Potassium-free, dextrose-free, and calcium-free solute solutions are also available for use in patients with hyperkalemia, diabetes, or hypercalcemia, respectively. Additionally, most contemporary IHD platforms permit sodium profiling during the session. The most commonly employed method of sodium profiling entails slightly elevating dialysate sodium relative to patient plasma (approximately 6-8 mmol/L higher) at the commencement of the session, with a gradual decline in dialysate sodium throughout the session. This elevated dialysate/plasma sodium ratio facilitates the diffusion of sodium from dialysate into patient plasma early in the dialysis session, coinciding with the most rapid diffusion of urea out of patient plasma into dialysate.

Dialysate Temperature

The dialysate temperature influences the animal's blood temperature, primarily due to the disparity between the dialysate and blood temperatures, as well as the blood and dialysate flow rates. In most instances, the dialysate temperature is calibrated to normalize or maintain the animal's body temperature. However, as all the dialysis machines are designed for human use, they may not offer a dialysate temperature setting suitable for animals. Occasionally, dialysate temperature is reduced to induce vasoconstriction as a therapeutic measure for refractory hypotension.

Ultrapure Dialysate and Water Purification System

The R.O. plant/water purification system is the foundation of hemodialysis, and its quality directly impacts dialysis outcomes. It is estimated that a 3-hour dialysis session may expose animal blood to approximately 65-70 liters of R.O. water, providing ample opportunity for impurities in R.O. water to enter the animal body. According to the Association for Advancement of Medical Instrumentation (AAMI), product water and dialysate must contain less than 100 CFU/mL of bacteria and less than 0.25 EU/mL of endotoxin. Therefore, routine R.O. plant cleaning procedures, such as backwashing, rinsing, and salt regeneration, along with periodic disinfection of the entire R.O. plant and loop, are mandatory. Commercially available dialysis R.O. plant disinfectants like Puristeril (Fresenius Medical Care) should be used for these purposes. Generally, if hemodiafiltration or high-flux dialyzers are being used, ultrapure dialysate with less than 0.1 CFU/mL of bacteria and less than 0.03 EU/mL of endotoxin should be employed (Upadhyay and Jaber, 2016).

Anti-coagulation

As blood is removed from the animal's body and circulated artificially in an extracorporeal circuit (dialyzer and blood tubing), there is a significant risk of coagulation occurring within this circuit. To mitigate this risk, anticoagulants are administered both systemically (at the commencement of dialysis) and within the extracorporeal circuit (every 30-60 minutes) during ongoing dialysis. The most commonly utilized anticoagulant is heparin sodium, administered at a dosage of 50 IU/kg body weight via intravenous (IV) infusion. Anticoagulation should be guided by hematocrit, platelet count, and activated clotting time (ACT) assessments. The standard protocol for systemic anticoagulation utilizing heparin sodium involves an initial bolus injection of 50 IU/kg body weight followed by a constant rate infusion (CRI) to prolong the baseline clotting time by 160-200% (ACT 160-200 seconds). In patients with a suspected risk of bleeding, heparin-free dialysis using repeated saline flushes is employed in human dialysis. This technique has also proven safe and effective at the author's* institutional dialysis unit for patients with bleeding tendencies, provided that the patient's fluid balance is carefully monitored. Regional citrate anticoagulation (RCA) can also be employed in high-risk patients but may require modifications in dialysate composition i.e., calcium free dialysate (Francey and Schweighauser, 2018).

IHD: Prescription and Adequacy Assessment

Priming Volume and Priming Fluids

The ideal priming/filling volume of the extracorporeal circuit should ideally be less than 10% of the animal's blood volume (BV). However, at many instances (due to low blood volume resulting from small body weight), achieving this circuit goal may not be feasible in all veterinary hemodialysis scenarios. If the circuit exceeds 15% of the animal's blood volume, consideration should be given to the composition of the priming solution to prevent hypovolemia, hypotension, and hypoxemia. If the extracorporeal circuit exceeds 20% of animal BV, there's a high risk of hypovolemia, hypotension, and hypoxemia. Therefore, the priming solution should offer effective colloidal and hemodynamic support, as well as oxygen-carrying capacity (e.g., synthetic colloid, plasma, whole blood prime). The expected hematocrit after diluting the blood with the priming solution should be ≥20%. If hematocrit is below 20%, blood transfusion before the treatment or blood priming is necessary. At author's* institutional dialysis unit, normal saline solution is the primarily used priming solution whereas, in patients where hematocrit is <18% or hemoglobin is <6g/dL, whole blood transfusion is performed before dialysis initiation. Apart from this, before initiation of dialysis if the patient's hematocrit or Hb is at borderline, simultaneous whole blood transfusion during ongoing IHD is also a common practice.

Dialysis Dose/ Intensity/ Duration

As IHD leads to the direct movement of solutes from the intravascular compartment, a concentration and osmotic gradient of uremic solutes is established between other body compartments and the vasculature. If the dialysis process is more intense, this disparity becomes more pronounced and may promote fluid shift from the intravascular space to the interstitial compartment. This fluid shift may predispose the animal to brain edema and increased intracranial pressure, leading to neurological signs such as shivering, seizures, and vocalization, collectively termed dialysis disequilibrium syndrome (DDS). Due to this reason, initial dialysis prescription is deliberately kept less efficient and azotemia, acid-base abnormalities and fluid balance is normalized slowly over a period of 24-72 hours. Estimation of urea reduction ratio (URR) is the most commonly employed ratio to assess the effectiveness of dialysis in removing waste products from the body by reducing urea levels in blood. Additionally, fractional patient urea clearance (KT/v), which normalizes the delivered urea clearance to the patient's urea distribution volume, is also utilized to evaluate dialysis efficacy. For veterinary patients the dialysis dose prescription based on URR goals as recommended by Cowgill (2011) is as under:

First treatment	
BUN <200 mg/dL	URR <0.5
200 300 mg/dL	URR 0.5-0.3
>300 mg/dL	URR <0.4
Second treatment	
BUN <200 mg/dL	URR 0.6-0.7
200-300 mg/dL	URR 0.6-0.4
>300 mg/dL	URR <0.4
Third and subsequent treatments	
BUN <200 mg/dL	URR >0.8
200-300 mg/dL	URR 0.5-0.6
>300 mg/dL	URR 0.5-0.6

Typically, the duration of the initial dialysis session is kept brief, lasting approximately 2 to 2.5 hours. Subsequent sessions are scheduled for 3 to 4 hours, with longer sessions exceeding 4 hours, depending on the patient's stability. At the author's* institutional dialysis unit, similar protocols for ultrafiltration rate (URR) are followed. Initially, the first three dialysis sessions are performed every alternate day. Subsequently, a novel approach of incremental intermittent hemodialysis (*i*-IHD) is adopted (Singh *et al.*, 2024). Following the patient's initial stabilization, which involves the first three dialysis sessions, subsequent dialysis sessions are safely performed based on the patient's residual kidney function rather than adhering to a conventional thrice-weekly regimen.

Ultrafiltration

Ultrafiltration is a process that removes excess fluid from the body through a dialysis membrane using pressure. At many instances, patients suffering from AKI and presenting for dialysis are often overhydrated, particularly when they have concurrent anuria or oliguria (D' Marco, 2022). The primary indications for ultrafiltration during IHD in companion animals include:

- Any life-threatening component of overhydration resulting in pulmonary edema, refractory hypertension, congestive heart failure, or oliguria.
- Non-life-threatening conditions such as peripheral edema, congestive neuropathy, ascites, and gut edema.

Furthermore, it is crucial to note that pleural effusions are not effectively corrected by ultrafiltration and require thoracocentesis at least two hours before dialysis heparinization to avoid potential bleeding. Ultrafiltration rates of 8-10mL/kg/hour and 5mL/kg/hour are safely tolerated in overhydrated dogs and cats, respectively.

Patient Monitoring

Patient monitoring is a vital component of safe and efficient IHD in companion animals. It is mandatory that the patient monitoring is performed by specifically trained personnel who can readily identify the complication and respond proactively. As a rule, before initiating IHD, patient should be thoroughly assessed for all baseline physiologic parameters (HR, CRT, SBP, RR, RT, hydration status), CBC, LFT, RFT, blood gas analysis, routine urine examination, urine protein creatinine ratio, urine culture, radiographic interpretation of thorax and abdomen, ultrasound, ECG and echocardiography. Blood pressure, rectal temperature, pulse rate, respiration rate and heart rate should be monitored every 15-30 minutes during an on-going IHD. At the author's[*] institutional dialysis unit, apart from mandatory pre-dialysis evaluation, continuous patient monitoring is achieved using multi-parameter monitors, doppler B.P. apparatus and bedside blood gas analysis. Pre- and post-dialysis assessments are routinely conducted to tailor post-dialysis prescriptions.

Complications

Hemodialysis is a typically safe advanced standard of care for both dogs and cats with life-threatening kidney dysfunction that cannot be effectively managed medically. However, there are numerous potential complications associated with extracorporeal procedures, which are often mitigated by experienced clinicians, appropriate equipment, and standardized procedures. The most commonly encountered complications of hemodialysis include hypotension, dialysis disequilibrium syndrome, hematoma formation at the catheter site, infection at the catheter site, and bleeding tendencies. All these complications are readily avoidable by adhering strictly to standard operating procedures (SOPs) in the dialysis unit. Therefore, clinicians and technicians must receive adequate training, and facilities must be adequately equipped prior to treating animals with extracorporeal renal replacement therapy (Bloom and Labato, 2011).

Summary

IHD is an exceptionally effective and advanced extracorporeal therapy employed primarily in veterinary medicine to manage animals with severe renal derangements when conventional medical management is inadequate or insufficient in controlling the clinical manifestations of the disease. IHD can extend the window of opportunity for recovery of uremic animals and animals exposed to selected life-threatening intoxications before the animal has decompensated substantially. Clinicians performing hemodialysis must possess a comprehensive understanding of the theoretical and technical aspects of this treatment modality, including the operation of hemodialysis equipment, appropriate and individualized treatment prescriptions, and monitoring and management of complications during and between dialysis treatments. When administered by well-trained clinicians and technicians, IHD is highly safe and effective with a low complication rate. It is strongly recommended that the clinician, technician, and other supporting staff involved in hemodialysis provide holistic and compassionate care to the patient and client, and be prepared to respond promptly to emergency situations. Authors strongly advise fellow veterinarians against performing IHD without proper training from experienced experts in the field, as it may lead to serious life-threatening consequences in an already compromised patient.

References

Bloom, C.A. and Labato, M.A. (2011). Intermittent hemodialysis for small animals. Vet Clin Small Anim. 41: 115–33.

Cowgill, L.D. 2011. Urea kinetics and intermittent dialysis prescription in small animals. Vet Clin Small Anim. 41:193–225.

D' Marco, L. (2022). Congestive nephropathy. International Journal of Environmental Research and Public Health 19: 2499.

Fischer, J.R., Pantaleo, V., Francey, T. and Cowgill, L.D. (2004). Veterinary hemodialysis: advances in management and technology. Veterinary Clinics of North America: Small Animal Practice 34: 935–67.

Foster, J.D., 2020. Extracorporeal Therapies in the emergency room and intensive care unit. Veterinary Clinics of North America: Small Animal Practice 50, 1215–36.

Francey, T. and Schweighauser, A. (2018). Regional citrate anticoagulation for intermittent hemodialysis in dogs. Journal of Veterinary Internal Medicine. 32: 147–56.

Segev, G., Kass, P.H., Francey, T. and Cowgill, L.D. (2008). A novel clinical scoring system for outcome prediction in dogs with acute kidney injury managed by hemodialysis. Journal of Veterinary Internal Medicine. 22: 301–08.

Singh, A., Singh, R., Gupta, D.K. and Singh, R.S.S. (2024). A novel study on the quality of life index in canine chronic kidney disease treated with incremental intermittent hemodialysis. Veterinary World. 17(8): 1702-14.

Singh, R. (2021). Management of Chronic Kidney Disease in a dog with Intermittent Hemodialysis. Indian Journal of Veterinary Medicine. 41(2): 58-61.

Singh, R., Sachin and Singh, R.S.S. (2024). Treatment of meloxicam induced acute kidney injury by intermittent hemodialysis. International Journal of Veterinary Sciences & Animal Husbandry. 9(4): 90-92.

Upadhyay, A. and Jaber, B.L. (2016). We use impure water to make dialysate for hemodialysis. Seminars in Dialysis. 29: 297–99.

Yeun J.Y. Depner, T.A. (2000). Principles of hemodialysis. In: Owen WF, Pereira BJG, Sayegh M, editors. Dialysis and transplantation: a companion to Brenner & Rector's the kidney. Philadelphia: WB Saunders. Pp. 1–31.

17

Novel Insight in the Treatment of Cardiac Diseases in Dogs and Cats

K. Satish Kumar

Professor and University Head, Department of Veterinary Medicine, College of Veterinary Science, Rajendranagar, PVNR Telangana Veterinary University Hyderabad, Telangana

As the heart diseases in companion animals is becoming common as in humans, the research in canine cardiac diseases is one of the most extensive studies in the present scenario. As per the available literature, the overall occurrence of various cardiac abnormalities ranges from 0.37 percent to 1.67 percent in various parts of the country. Whereas, in western parts of the globe, nearly 8 million dogs suffer from heart disease accounting 10% of all dogs in the United States. Heart diseases are common among older dogs; up to 75% of senior dogs have some type of heart condition, and unfortunately, most go undiagnosed due to varied reasons. The recognition of canine cardiac diseases has been delayed, and ignored on account of lack of awareness and knowledge by the owner and inadequate diagnostic facility in our country. Physical examination, radiography, electrocardiography and echocardiography are most useful diagnostic procedures employed in diagnosing the cardiac diseases in dogs. However, majority of the acquired cardiac diseases are being managed medically with one or a combination of drugs. Improved diet management and health care of companion animals have led to increased life expectancy, as a result, cardiac diseases have become pivotal causes of death for both dogs and cats. For such reason, a major objective has become to increase the quality of life by reducing the expansion of cardiac diseases via early detection of diseases and provision of effective treatment.

Treatment of canine cardiac disease depends on the type of the disease and the pathophysiological events. However, the following are the few goals of treatment options for heart diseases in dogs.

1. Reducing pulmonary edema as it causes diminished oxygen perfusion
2. Reducing the myocardial stretch and subsequent fibrosis.
3. Increase the cardiac output to enhance blood flow to vital organs.
4. Reduce the amount of regurgitation.

5. Regulation of heart rate and rhythm.
6. Improve blood oxygen.

The treatment protocol should be tailored in such a way that it resolves the presenting clinical signs, the respiratory and heart rates are regulated along with a good quality of life. Triple therapy is the most common and gold standard treatment prorocol followed in the management of cardiac diseases which includes diuretic, ACE inhibitor and an inotrope.

Diuretics are the most important and mainstay in the management of cardiac diseases. They are effective means to remove edema fluid from animals with heart failure and frequently is lifesaving in the short term. Among all the diuretics, furosemide is always a top priority. It acts by decreasing the resorption of sodium, chloride, and potassium in the ascending limb of the loop of Henle. It also acts as a venodilator when used IV. In refractory cases, diuresis with furosemide may be augmented by using thiazide diuretics. Thiazides suppress resorption of sodium and water at the distal renal tubules. When using a loop diuretic and a diuretic that works at the distal tubules, the ability of the kidneys to conserve water is reduced dramatically, so dehydration and hypokalemia may develop. This may be signaled by worsening azotemia, and renal values must be monitored closely in animals on multiple diuretics. Torsemide is a loop diuretic that is 10–20 times more potent than furosemide; it is typically reserved for refractory CHF or in cases of suspected diuretic resistance to furosemide. Spironolactone is a potassium-sparing diuretic that blocks the effects of aldosterone which also exerts its effect at the distal convoluted tubule. Aldactazide, a combination diuretic consisting of spironolactone and hydrochlorothiazide, may be used in cases of refractory CHF. Renal values should be monitored closely because of the risk of worsening azotemia and renal failure with aldactazide therapy.

Enalapril, benazepril, lisinopril, and ramipril are ACE inhibitors commonly used in heart failure management in dogs. They are all equally effective at blocking the conversion of angiotensin I to angiotensin II. They minimize remodelling of blood vessels and myocardium. They are part of the mainstay treatment regimen for advanced cardiac disease and heart failure. Angiotensin II receptor blockers (ARBs), formally angiotensin II receptor type 1 (AT1) antagonists, also known as angiotensin receptor blockers, angiotensin II receptor antagonists, or AT1 receptor antagonists, are a group of pharmaceuticals that bind to and inhibit the angiotensin II receptor type 1 (AT1) and thereby block the arteriolar contraction and sodium retention effects of renin–angiotensin system. Their main uses are in the treatment of hypertension, and CHF. They selectively block the activation of the AT1 receptors, preventing the binding of angiotensin II compared to ACEi.

Pimobendan, a calcium-sensitizing agent and phosphodiesterase inhibitor, is an inodilator. Pimobendan has been shown to improve the quality of life of dogs with CHF, delay the onset of CHF in preclinical dogs with degenerative mitral valve disease and improve survival in dogs with CHF. Amrinone and milrinone, analogues of theophylline that deactivate other forms of phosphodiesterase, are potent inodilators. Digitalis glycosides exert their effects by inhibiting membrane Na^+/K^+-ATPase. This increases intracellular sodium, which activates the sodium-calcium pump that increases intracellular calcium. Digoxin increases the force of myocardial contraction, slows the heart rate, and improves baroreceptor function. Sildenafil is a potent phosphodiesterase inhibitor used to treat moderate to severe pulmonary hypertension in dogs. Sildenafil has been shown to improve exercise intolerance and quality of life in people and dogs with pulmonary hypertension via pulmonary arterial vasodilation. There may also be additional beneficial effects on vascular remodeling and cardiac function. Nitroglycerin is a venodilator usually applied in a paste form to the skin inside the earflap or the mucous membranes. Sodium nitroprusside is another nitrate that is a veno- and arterial dilator. Nitroprusside can be administered IV to treat acute fulminant CHF. These two medications should never be given simultaneously or concurrently with sildenafil, because life-threatening hypotension may result.

Sotalol, amiodarone (class III antiarrhythmics) and mexiletine (IB) are among the top list antiarrhythmics used for treatment of malignant ventricular arrhythmias. Sotalol is used to treat both supraventricular and ventricular tachyarrhythmias, and it is particularly effective in treatment of Boxers with arrhythmogenic right ventricular cardiomyopathy, either alone or in combination with mexiletine. Amiodarone is useful to manage all forms of arrhythmias, including ventricular arrhythmias, and atrial fibrillation or atrial flutter. Lidocaine, a class IB antiarrhythmic, is used only IV for emergency ventricular arrhythmias such as sustained ventricular tachycardia or R-on-T morphology. Atenolol, propranolol, and metoprolol are oral beta-blockers, and esmolol is an IV beta-blocker. These drugs slow the heart rate, suppress arrhythmias, and up-regulate adrenergic receptors. Carvedilol is a beta- and alpha-adrenergic blocker that also scavenges oxygen-free radicals. Beta-blockers are often used to treat dogs with subaortic or pulmonic stenosis, and for dynamic outflow obstruction in cats with hypertrophic cardiomyopathy. Diltiazem is a calcium-channel blocker used to slow ventricular rate in animals with atrial fibrillation or supraventricular tachycardia by slowing AV nodal conduction. Atropine and glycopyrrolate are IV anticholinergic drugs that block the effects of the vagus nerve on the SA node and indicated in AV block, sick sinus syndrome.

Aspirin, clopidogrel, dalteparin, enoxaparin, and coumadin are antithrombotics that may prevent thromboembolism in cats with cardiomyopathy. Rivaroxaban and apixaban are oral factor Xa inhibitors that may prove useful for thromboprophylaxis in cats and dogs, although further studies are needed to evaluate their dosing and safety. Taurine and l-carnitine are amino acids used to prevent and treat nutritional dilated cardiomyopathy in cats and dogs with these deficiencies.

Angiotensin Receptor and Neprilysin Inhibitors (ARNi)

Previously, the inhibition of neurohormonal systems, namely the renin–angiotensin–aldosterone system (RAAS) and the sympathetic nervous system, has proven to be useful in the treatment of many cardiac diseases. Attempts have recently been made to target an additional hormonal system, that of the natriuretic peptides (NPs), which, when dysregulated, can also play a role in the development cardiac diseases. Indeed, a new class of drug, the angiotensin receptor–neprilysin inhibitors (ARNi), has the ability to counteract the effects of angiotensin II as well as to increase the activity of NPs. ARNi have already been proven to be effective in the treatment of heart failure with reduced ejection fraction. New evidence has suggested that, in the next years, the field of ARNi application will widen to include other cardiovascular diseases, such as heart failure, with preserved ejection fraction and hypertension. Eventually, it was the time for a new class of medications, known as angiotensin receptor–neprilysin inhibitors (ARNi). Indeed, ARNi combine the neutral endopeptidase inhibition, due to sacubitril, with the ATII receptor I inhibition by valsartan (an ARB), offering the benefits of this two-step approach whilst avoiding the side effects of an increase in bradykinin due to dual inhibition of its metabolism. Sacubitril/Valsartan is the most recently discovered single molecule with a dual component, which combines an ARB with the neutral endopeptidase inhibitor (NEPi) neprilysin, increasing the availability of natriuretic peptides (NPs).

The Natriuretic peptides (NPs) family includes 3 different molecules viz., atrial natriuretic peptide (ANP), brain natriuretic peptide (BNP), and C-type natriuretic peptide (CNP), that play a key role in cardiorenal homeostasis. They are mostly synthesized within the heart in response to volume overload and myocyte stress, although synthesis in response to neuroendocrine regulation has also been shown. Both ANP and BNP contribute to regulating vascular tone, mainly due to their vasodilating properties. Indeed, ANP, through the activation of the cGMP-dependent protein kinase G (PKG), leads to increased production of nitric oxide (NO) with subsequent relaxation of the vascular smooth muscle cells and a decrease in blood pressure (BP). NPs also enhance diuresis and natriuresis, leading to lower BP levels. Indeed, ANP may enhance the glomerular filtration rate (GFR) through a direct vasodilating effect on the efferent arterioles with an icrease in blood ultrafiltration. Moreover, ANP boosts natriuresis by acting directly on Na+ channels in the nephron, decreasing renin release from juxtaglomerular cells, and by inhibiting the synthesis and release of aldosterone. NPs may also influence left ventricle afterload, not only acting on vascular tone and body fluid homeostasis, but also by decreasing adverse vascular remodeling over time. Indeed, high BNP levels may reduce the expression of transforming growth factor, which is an important profibrotic molecule, and facilitate the degradation of extracellular fibrotic component. In the heart, ANP counteracts the sympathetic nerve activity and increases vagal activity, leading to a decreased heart rate and cardiac output. Moreover, NPs, by interacting with their G-coupled receptor, might antagonize pathological signaling leading to hypertrophy, such as cGMP-PKG deterioration, with titin hypophosphorylation, NO reduction with endothelial dysfunction, inflammation, and fibrosis. Due to their multiple functions, the biological signature of NPs is to reduce body fluid and maintain BP and CV homeostasis. On this basis, NPs are physiological antagonists of both SNS and RAAS, and they are fundamental actors in HF.

Sodium Glucose Co-Transportase2 Receptor Antagonist (SGLT2)

Sodium-glucose co-transporter 2 (SGLT2) inhibitors also known as gliflozins, represent one type of new-generation type 2 diabetes (T2DM) drug treatment. The mechanism of action of an SGLT2 inhibitor (SGLT2i) in treating T2DM depends on lowering blood glucose levels effectively via increasing the glomerular excretion of glucose. A good number of randomized clinical trials revealed that SGLT2is significantly prevented heart failure (HF) and cardiovascular death in T2DM patients. Despite ongoing clinical trials in HF patients without T2DM, there have been a limited number of translational studies on the cardioprotective properties of SGLT2is. As the cellular mechanism behind the cardiac benefits of SGLT2is is still to be elucidated, animal models are used to better understand the pathways behind the cardioprotective mechanism of SGLT2i.

In addition to SGLT2is' direct benefits in T2DM, studies have witnessed cardiac improvements in patients treated with gliflozins through large randomized clinical trials. These studies show the effect of SGLT2is primarily in T2DM patients at high risk of major adverse cardiovascular events (MACE) defined as cardiovascular death, myocardial infarction, or ischemic stroke which constitute as heart failure. However, the DAPA-HF trial explored the therapeutic potential of SGLT2is on HF patients, irrespective of the presence of T2DM, and found that DAPA significantly reduced cardiovascular mortality and hospitalization for HF. This suggests that the beneficial effects of SGLT2i on HF patients are not solely based on glycemic reduction and correcting metabolic disorder related to T2DM. The study highlights the following cardioprotective mechanisms that SGLT2i could be involved in decreasing blood pressure; ketone body metabolic activity; increase of red blood cells percentage and the hemoglobin level; and sympathetic nerve function and triggering of the enzyme activity of endothelial nitric oxide synthase. They also cause natriuresis, which results in modest diuresis thus reducing pulmonary congestion and edema and other signs of CHF. Other hypotheses include whether cardioprotective mechanisms are mediated by SGLT2i binding directly to SGLT2 in cardiac cells or indirectly by upregulating SGLT1 expression in cardiovascular disease. In order to better understand the main mechanism behind SGLT2i's cardioprotective properties, several animal models have been constructed.

Both diabetes and cardiology guidelines and professional societies have responded to this paradigm shift by including strong recommendations to use SGLT2i and/or GLP-1 RA, with evidence-based benefits to reduce cardiovascular risk in high-risk individuals with type 2 diabetes, independent of the need for additional glucose control. GLP-1 RA were initially developed as glucose-lowering drugs because activation of the GLP-1 receptor by these agents leads to a reduction in blood glucose and an improvement in postprandial glucose metabolism. By stimulating GLP-1R in hypothalamic neurons, GLP-1 RA additionally induce satiety and lead to weight loss. Data from cardiovascular outcome trials demonstrated a robust and consistent reduction in atherothrombotic events, particularly in patients with established atherosclerotic cardiovascular disease. Bexagliflozin (Bexacat; Elanco, elanco.com) is FDA approved for treatment of diabetes in cats, but there are no clinical reports of the use of SGLT2 inhibitors for CHF treatment in dogs or cats. No studies of SGLT2 inhibitors in dogs have been reported. In humans, SGLT2 inhibitors are strongly recommended for the treatment of heart failure with reduced ejection fraction, even in patients who are not diabetic; however, their clinical benefits at higher ejection fractions are less well established, and the mechanisms of benefit are not well understood.

A study assessed the effect of canagliflozin (CAN), an SGLT2 inhibitor, on atrial remodeling in a canine atrial fibrillation model in beagle dogs. The study which included 12 beagle dogs that received continuous rapid atrial pacing concluded that the CAN and possibly other SGLT2 inhibitors might be useful for preventing AF and suppressing the promotion of atrial remodeling in dogs. SGLT2 inhibition promotes natriuresis and osmotic diuresis, leading to plasma volume contraction and reduced preload, as well as decreases in blood pressure, arterial stiffness and afterload, thereby improving subendocardial blood flow in patients with HF. SGLT2 inhibition is also associated with preservation of renal function

Interventional Cardiac Procedures

Regenerative medicine using stem cells from various sources are emerging treatment modality in several refractory diseases in veterinary medicine. It is well-known that stem cells can differentiate into specific cell types, self-renew, and regenerate. In addition, the unique immunomodulatory effects of stem cells have made stem cell transplantation a promising option for treating a wide range of disease and injuries. Recently, the medical demands for companion animals have been rapidly increasing, and certain disease conditions require alternative treatment options. The safety of adult stem cell therapy for heart diseases has been well established in humans. The regenerative potential of CDCs has also been demonstrated in non-ischaemic cardiomyopathy and thus, it is hypothesised that the intracoronary CDC therapy can provide a safe and effective intervention for DCM; in addition, successful implementation of this intervention in a canine model of DCM will provide valuable insight in the novel approach. Cardiosphere-derived stem cells (CDCs) have been shown to reduce scar size and increase viable myocardium in human patients with mild/moderate myocardial infarction. Studies in rodent models suggest that CDC therapy may confer therapeutic benefits in patients with non-ischaemic dilated cardiomyopathy (DCM). A study to determine the safety and efficacy of allogeneic CDC in Doberman dogs with spontaneous DCM, revealed no adverse events during and after cell infusion. Histology on dog hearts (after natural death) revealed no sign of immune rejection from the transplanted cells. Canine CDCs (cCDCs) were grown from a donor dog heart. Similar to human CDCs, cCDCs express CD105 and are slightly positive for c-kit and CD90. In one study, thirty million of allogeneic cCDCs was infused into the coronary vessels of Doberman pinscher dogs with spontaneous DCM. Theoretically, autologous transplantation of cardiac stem cells (CSCs) is also possible. A previous study has demonstrated that attenuation of left ventricle remodeling causes less fibrosis in canine model of myocardial infarction after autologous CSCs intramyocardial injection. The stem cell transplantation method is also important for enhancing therapeutic efficacy and safety. Previously, stem cells were introduced into cardiomyocytes by either direct intramyocardial (subendocardial or subepicardial) injection or intracoronary injection. Direct intramyocardial injection has the advantages of providing precise targeting of cell delivery to the ischemic region and higher cell retention compared with intracoronary injection. However, direct injection may induce subsequent inflammation, which reduces the survival of engrafted cells. Intracoronary injection presents a high risk of coronary embolism and low stem cell retention.

A couple of studies have described cell-based treatment in veterinary clinical cardiac disease. One study used allogeneic cardiosphere-derived cells in 5 dilated cardiomyopathy (DCM) dogs. The beneficial effects of stem cell application were not detected in dogs with DCM during a 1-year follow-up. Another study transplanted allogeneic puppy deciduous teeth stem cells for the treatment of degenerative valvular heart disease. The efficacy of treatment was evaluated for 2 months and resulted in improved heart function with alleviated clinical signs of heart failure. Because myocardial infarction is rare in dogs and cats, all of these implications of stem cell therapy for the resolution of cardiomyocyte damage are limited by the experiments due to the use of small and no-randomized samples. Although few pilot studies provide alternative treatment options for cardiovascular disease in veterinary clinics, further research and clinical trials are needed to evaluate the short- and long-term efficacy and complications of stem-cell treatment.

18

The Canine Skin Barrier in Atopic Dermatitis: Clinical Implications and Therapeutic Approaches

Shanker K. Singh[1], Ashish Srivastava[1], S.R. Upadhyay[2]

[1]Department of Veterinary Medicine, College of Veterinary Science and Animal Husbandry, U.P. Pandit Deen Dayal Upadhyaya Pashu-Chikitsa Vigyan Vishwavidyalaya Evam Go Anusandhan Sansthan (DUVASU), Mathura Uttar Pradesh

[2]Division of Veterinary Medicine, Faculty of Veterinary Sciences and Animal Husbandry, Sher-e-Kashmir University of Agricultural Sciences and Technology (SKUAST) Jammu, R.S. Pura, Jammu, Jammu & Kashmir

Introduction

Canine atopic dermatitis (CAD) is a chronic inflammatory skin disease marked by itching (pruritus), redness (erythema), and recurrent infections. While traditionally considered an immune-mediated condition, recent studies highlight the significant role of skin barrier dysfunction in its development. A key aspect of CAD is the compromised skin barrier, which increases permeability to allergens, irritants, and microorganisms, thereby worsening the disease. The skin barrier is a complex, dynamic structure essential for protecting dogs from environmental challenges. The stratum corneum—the outermost layer of the epidermis—serves as a crucial defense against environmental insults, allergens, and pathogens. In dogs with atopic dermatitis, this barrier often becomes impaired, leading to increased transepidermal water loss (TEWL), greater allergen penetration, and secondary infections. This dysfunction both results from and contributes to the condition, creating a self-perpetuating cycle of barrier disruption, inflammation, and immune dysregulation.

Understanding the mechanisms behind skin barrier dysfunction in CAD is vital for developing effective, targeted therapeutic strategies. The "outside-in" hypothesis—which suggests that skin barrier disruption precedes immune dysregulation—has gained support in veterinary dermatology. This shift in perspective has significant implications for diagnosing, preventing, and treating CAD. This paper aims to provide a comprehensive overview of the canine skin barrier in the context of atopic dermatitis, examine its clinical implications, and discuss current and emerging therapeutic strategies.

The Canine Skin Barrier: Structure and Function

Layers of the Skin Barrier

The skin barrier, the outermost layer of the skin, is essential for maintaining homeostasis and protecting against allergens, irritants, and pathogens. It preserves the health and structural integrity of the skin in various species, including dogs. In canines, as in other mammals, the skin barrier is a complex, multilayered system comprising the stratum corneum (SC), epidermis, dermis, and associated structures such as hair follicles and sebaceous glands. The primary components of the skin barrier include corneocytes—terminally differentiated keratinocytes that provide structural support. These corneocytes are embedded in a lipid matrix composed of ceramides, cholesterol, and free fatty acids, forming a hydrophobic layer essential for barrier function. Additionally, proteins such as filaggrin, loricrin, and involucrin play critical roles in maintaining the barrier's integrity. The skin barrier consists of the following key layers:

Stratum Corneum (SC): The Primary Barrier

The SC is composed of corneocytes (terminally differentiated keratinocytes) embedded in a lipid matrix, forming a "brick-and-mortar" structure. Here, corneocytes act as bricks, while intercellular lipids—comprising ceramides, cholesterol, and free fatty acids—serve as the mortar. This unique arrangement ensures barrier integrity, hydrophobicity, and the prevention of transepidermal water loss (TEWL). The SC also provides mechanical strength and regulates skin permeability, blocking the infiltration of allergens, irritants, and microorganisms.

Epidermis: The Functional Surface

The epidermis consists of several layers—basal, spinous, granular, and the SC—predominantly formed by keratinocytes undergoing continuous turnover. Tight junctions, located in the granular layer, seal spaces between cells, forming an additional barrier that limits permeability. Langerhans cells, present within the epidermis, are crucial for immune surveillance and play a pivotal role in recognizing and responding to allergens.

Dermis: The Supportive Layer

Situated beneath the epidermis, the dermis provides structural support through a robust network of collagen and elastin fibers. Blood vessels within the dermis deliver nutrients to the skin and support immune responses. The dermis contains immune cells, including mast cells, macrophages, and dendritic cells, which are involved in inflammatory processes and hypersensitivity reactions relevant to conditions like canine atopic dermatitis (CAD).

Cutaneous Appendages

Hair follicles act as reservoirs for immune cells and allergens, contributing to the development and progression of CAD. Sebaceous glands secrete sebum, which contains antimicrobial peptides and contributes to maintaining the lipid barrier.

Functions of the Skin Barrier

The skin barrier is a multifaceted structure essential for protecting against allergens, irritants, and microorganisms, while preserving skin moisture. Disruption of this barrier elevates transepidermal water loss (TEWL), increasing the skin's susceptibility to environmental challenges. As the body's primary defense, the skin functions as a crucial immune organ, containing immune cells that detect and respond to external threats. Both innate and adaptive immune cells are integral to the skin's defense against pathogens and allergens. In canine atopic dermatitis (CAD), dysregulation of this immune barrier results in hypersensitivity reactions. A healthy skin microbiome, mainly consisting of commensal bacteria, suppresses the proliferation of pathogenic organisms. However, in CAD, microbial imbalances (dysbiosis) worsen infections, particularly those caused by *Staphylococcus pseudintermedius* and *Malassezia* species.

Clinical Implications of Skin Barrier Dysfunction

Disruption of the skin barrier has significant implications for the development of canine atopic dermatitis (CAD). A compromised barrier permits environmental allergens—such as pollen and dust mites—to penetrate deeper into the epidermis, initiating inflammatory and hypersensitivity responses. This exposure, coupled with microbial dysbiosis, results in sustained immune activation, chronic inflammation, and further degradation of the skin barrier. Consequently, the impaired barrier, along with microbial imbalances, heightens susceptibility to recurrent bacterial and fungal infections, which in turn exacerbate pruritus (itchiness) and inflammation. Additionally, increased transepidermal water loss (TEWL) leads to dry, flaky skin, intensifying discomfort and itching.

Studies indicate that dogs with CAD exhibit reduced levels of ceramides and other essential lipids in the stratum corneum (SC), contributing to weakened barrier function. These dogs also demonstrate significantly higher TEWL, reflecting severe barrier disruption that facilitates allergen penetration and triggers immune responses. The overactivation of Th2 cells and the elevated production of cytokines such as IL-4, IL-13, and IL-31 further intensify inflammation and pruritus. This creates a vicious cycle in which barrier dysfunction amplifies allergen uptake, driving ongoing inflammation and further barrier damage. Thus, skin barrier dysfunction is a hallmark of CAD and plays a pivotal role in its progression.

Therefore, disruption of the stratum corneum, abnormalities in lipid composition, microbial dysbiosis, and immune dysregulation collectively contribute to this impaired barrier. Barrier defects facilitate allergen penetration, triggering an exaggerated immune response. Common allergens include house dust mites, pollens, and molds. Sensitization is associated with elevated serum IgE levels and increased expression of pro-inflammatory cytokines such as IL-4, IL-13, and IL-31. The compromised skin barrier predisposes dogs to bacterial and fungal infections. Chronic colonization and recurrent infections further aggravate inflammation and pruritus, complicating management. The chronic nature of CAD significantly affects the well-being of affected dogs and their owners. Pruritus, sleep disturbances, and frequent veterinary visits impose a considerable emotional and financial burden.

Effective management of CAD requires addressing these underlying mechanisms through therapies that repair the skin barrier, modulate the immune response, control infections, and optimize dietary interventions. Continued research into the genetic and molecular pathways underlying barrier dysfunction will provide valuable insights for developing novel therapeutic strategies.

Therapeutic Approaches

Advancements in the treatment of Canine Atopic Dermatitis (CAD) have shifted from broad-spectrum methods to targeted, multimodal strategies. Ongoing research into CAD pathogenesis and therapeutic innovations will continue to shape veterinary dermatology, enhancing the quality of life for affected dogs and their owners. Current therapeutic objectives include reducing inflammation, controlling pruritus, repairing the skin barrier, and addressing secondary infections. Integrating conventional therapies with emerging interventions—such as cytokine inhibitors, immunomodulators, and microbiome-focused treatments—holds promise for optimizing patient outcomes.

Barrier Dysfunction and Therapeutic Approaches

The integrity of the epidermal barrier is essential for maintaining skin homeostasis. In CAD, decreased levels of ceramides and other lipids compromise the skin barrier, exacerbating transepidermal water loss (TEWL). Products enriched with ceramides, cholesterol, and fatty acids have demonstrated efficacy in restoring barrier function. Topical emulsions, such as spot-on formulations and sprays, can reduce TEWL and alleviate clinical signs. The use of colloidal oatmeal-based or humectant-containing products helps maintain hydration, enhance skin repair, and reduce irritation. Medicated shampoos formulated with ceramides or antimicrobial agents serve dual functions of barrier repair and controlling secondary infections.

Control of Inflammation and Pruritus

Glucocorticoids are synthetic derivatives of corticosteroids that mimic the effects of endogenous cortisol produced by the adrenal glands. These agents exhibit potent anti-inflammatory and immunosuppressive properties by inhibiting the arachidonic acid cascade, thereby reducing the production of pro-inflammatory mediators such as prostaglandins and leukotrienes. Glucocorticoids exert their effects primarily through binding to intracellular glucocorticoid receptors, altering gene transcription, and suppressing the activation of immune cells such as T-cells and mast cells. They also suppress the expression of cytokines like interleukin (IL)-1, IL-6, and tumor necrosis factor-alpha (TNF-α). In CAD, glucocorticoids are used to rapidly alleviate pruritus and inflammation. Short courses of systemic formulations like prednisone, prednisolone, or dexamethasone are commonly prescribed for acute flare-ups. Topical formulations, such as hydrocortisone aceponate sprays, are preferred for localized lesions to minimize systemic exposure. Prolonged use can lead to significant adverse effects, including immunosuppression, iatrogenic hyperadrenocorticism (Cushing's syndrome), polyuria, polydipsia, skin thinning, and susceptibility to infections.

Cyclosporine is a calcineurin inhibitor that selectively targets T-cell activity, reducing the immune response central to CAD pathogenesis. Cyclosporine inhibits calcineurin, a calcium-dependent phosphatase required for T-cell activation. This prevents the transcription of pro-inflammatory cytokines such as IL-2, IL-4, and interferon-gamma, which are involved in the recruitment and activation of immune cells. Cyclosporine is highly effective in managing chronic CAD, particularly in cases where glucocorticoids are contraindicated. It provides sustained anti-inflammatory effects and long-term symptom control, although the onset of action may take 2–4 weeks. Potential adverse effects include vomiting, diarrhea, gingival hyperplasia, and renal toxicity, necessitating regular monitoring. Drug interactions with P-glycoprotein substrates should also be considered.

Lokivetmab is a monoclonal antibody specifically developed for canine use, targeting interleukin-31 (IL-31), a cytokine that plays a central role in mediating pruritus and skin inflammation. Lokivetmab binds to IL-31, preventing its interaction with the IL-31 receptor complex on neurons and immune cells. By neutralizing this cytokine, the drug interrupts the signaling pathways responsible for itch perception and inflammatory responses. Lokivetmab is particularly effective for dogs with moderate to severe pruritus, providing rapid relief within 24–48 hours of administration. Its long half-life enables monthly subcutaneous injections, offering convenience and compliance. As a targeted biologic therapy, lokivetmab has minimal systemic immunosuppressive effects compared to broad-spectrum immunosuppressants. Marketed as Cytopoint (Zoetis), it is widely used in veterinary practices.

JAK inhibitors, such as oclacitinib, represent a newer class of targeted therapies for CAD, addressing both inflammation and pruritus. JAK inhibitors block the activity of Janus kinase enzymes (JAK1 and JAK3), which are integral to the signaling pathways of various cytokines involved in immune responses. These include IL-31 (pruritus), IL-4, IL-6, IL-13 (inflammation), and others. By inhibiting JAK-STAT signaling, oclacitinib disrupts cytokine-mediated activation of immune cells and itch transmission. Oclacitinib is effective in rapidly alleviating clinical signs of CAD, often within hours to days, making it suitable for acute and chronic management. It is administered orally and offers an alternative to corticosteroids and cyclosporine. Adverse effects may include gastrointestinal upset, weight gain, and rare cases of immunosuppression or neoplastic progression with long-term use. Available as Apoquel (Zoetis), it is a popular choice among veterinarians.

Expanding knowledge of cytokine involvement in CAD pathogenesis has identified additional therapeutic targets. IL-4 and IL-13 are critical in driving Type-2 inflammatory responses associated with CAD. Therapies targeting these pathways, such as monoclonal antibodies or receptor antagonists, are under investigation. IL-17 is implicated in neutrophilic inflammation and chronic skin lesions; IL-17 inhibitors may offer benefits in refractory or severe cases. Research into dual-action biologics targeting multiple cytokines simultaneously aims to improve efficacy and address heterogeneity in CAD presentations.

Immunomodulators

Allergen-specific immunotherapy (ASIT) is a cornerstone in managing canine atopic dermatitis (CAD), especially when specific allergens are identified. This approach involves gradually administering increasing doses of identified allergens to desensitize the dog's immune system and induce tolerance. ASIT shifts the immune response from a T-helper 2 (Th2)-dominated profile, characteristic of atopic reactions, to a T-helper 1 (Th1) or regulatory T cell (Treg)-dominated response. It reduces the production of allergen-specific immunoglobulin E (IgE) and enhances the production of allergen-specific immunoglobulin G (IgG), particularly IgG4, which can block allergens from binding to IgE receptors. ASIT also modulates cytokine production, reducing pro-inflammatory cytokines like IL-4, IL-5, and IL-13, while increasing anti-inflammatory cytokines such as IL-10. Subcutaneous Immunotherapy (SCIT) involves periodic injections tailored to the patient's allergen profile. Sublingual Immunotherapy (SLIT), delivered as drops under the tongue, offers a non-invasive alternative for dogs that do not tolerate injections. Allercept® Therapy Drops (Heska) is a popular SLIT option, custom-formulated based on allergen testing results. Artuvetrin® (Nextmune) is an SCIT product available in custom formulations tailored to the dog's allergen profile.

Probiotics influence gut microbiota composition, enhancing the gut-skin axis, an interconnection where gut health significantly impacts skin health. Certain strains, such as *Lactobacillus rhamnosus* and *Bifidobacterium longum*, can downregulate inflammatory pathways by modulating dendritic cell activity and promoting Treg cell differentiation. Probiotics reduce systemic inflammation and oxidative stress, both contributing factors in CAD. Studies have shown that probiotic supplementation reduces the severity of pruritus and dermatitis in atopic dogs. These effects are believed to be mediated by alterations in cytokine profiles and the gut microbiota's influence on systemic immune responses.

Dietary Interventions

Hypoallergenic diets are designed to eliminate dietary allergens that may exacerbate CAD. These diets use hydrolyzed proteins (broken into peptides too small to trigger an immune response) or novel proteins (unfamiliar to the immune system). A strict elimination diet trial is often required to diagnose and manage food-related atopic triggers. Essential Fatty Acids (EFAs) like Omega-3 fatty acids (e.g., EPA and DHA) and omega-6 fatty acids improve skin barrier function by integrating into phospholipid bilayers of epidermal cells. EFAs reduce the production of pro-inflammatory eicosanoids, such as prostaglandins and leukotrienes, thereby decreasing inflammation and pruritus. Omega-3s modulate gene expression to promote anti-inflammatory pathways. Diets enriched with zinc, biotin, vitamins E and D, and antioxidants support skin repair, reduce oxidative damage, and modulate immune responses. Hill's Prescription Diet® Derm Defense contains bioactive substances and omega-3 fatty acids to reduce inflammation. Royal Canin Skin Support features high levels of omega fatty acids and specific nutrients for barrier repair. Purina Pro Plan Veterinary Diets® HA Hydrolyzed Formula is designed for elimination diet trials.

Emerging Therapies

Biologics beyond Lokivetmab include targeted monoclonal antibodies (mAbs) that neutralize specific cytokines implicated in CAD, such as IL-4, IL-13, and IL-17. Research focusing on multi-cytokine inhibitors to simultaneously address overlapping inflammatory pathways in CAD is warranted. Gene therapy utilizes techniques such as CRISPR to correct mutations in genes associated with barrier dysfunction or immune dysregulation. While still experimental, early studies indicate potential in modifying defective filaggrin genes implicated in epidermal barrier dysfunction. Nanotechnology-based delivery systems, such as liposomes and nanoparticles, encapsulate therapeutic agents, enhancing targeted delivery to the skin and reducing systemic side effects. Examples include nanocapsules loaded with ceramides for barrier repair or anti-inflammatory agents for localized action. Phototherapy, a narrowband UVB (NB-UVB) light, modulates the immune response by reducing T-cell proliferation and inducing apoptosis of inflammatory cells in the skin. It also promotes vitamin D synthesis, which supports skin repair and immune modulation. Nanotechnology-based formulations and gene therapy products are in preclinical and clinical trial stages, representing the frontier of veterinary dermatology.

Conclusion

Canine Atopic Dermatitis (CAD) is a multifactorial disease where skin barrier dysfunction plays a pivotal role in its pathogenesis, contributing to both the clinical manifestations and the chronic nature of the disease. The impaired barrier function leads to increased allergen exposure, microbial dysbiosis, and persistent inflammation, creating a self-perpetuating cycle of damage. Recent advances in understanding the mechanisms behind this dysfunction, particularly the "outside-in" hypothesis, have shifted therapeutic approaches towards barrier repair, immune modulation, and targeted treatments. Current therapies, including topical and systemic interventions aimed at restoring barrier integrity, controlling inflammation, and managing secondary infections, offer relief to affected dogs. Emerging treatments such as biologics, gene therapy, and nanotechnology-based approaches hold promise for providing more effective and personalized treatment options. Continued research into the genetic and molecular underpinnings of barrier dysfunction will be essential in developing innovative therapies and improving the quality of life for dogs suffering from CAD.

References

Campana C, Regazzi MB, Buggia I, Molinaro M. 1996. Clinically significant drug interactions with cyclosporin. An update. Clin Pharmacokinet. 30(2):141-79.

Cosgrove SB, Wren JA, Cleaver DM, Martin DD, Walsh KF, Harfst JA, Follis SL, King VL, Boucher JF, Stegemann MR.2013. Efficacy and safety of oclacitinib for the control of pruritus and associated skin lesions in dogs with canine allergic dermatitis. Vet Dermatol24(5):479-e114.

DeBoer DJ. 2017. The future of immunotherapy for canine atopic dermatitis: a review. Vet Dermatol. 28(1):25-e6.

Dell DL, Griffin CE, Thompson LA, Griffies JD. 2012. Owner assessment of therapeutic interventions for canine atopic dermatitis: a long-term retrospective analysis. Vet Dermatol. 23(3):228-e47.

Eisenschenk MNC. 2024. The Role of Diet, Nutrition, and Supplements in Canine Atopic Dermatitis. Vet Clin North Am Small Anim Pract. S0195-5616(24)00107-4.

Fennis EEM, van Damme CMM, Schlotter YM, Sinke JD, Leistra MHG, Bartels RT, Broere F. 2022. Efficacy of subcutaneous allergen immunotherapy in atopic dogs: A retrospective study of 664 cases. Vet Dermatol. 33(4):321-e75.

Fleck TJ, Norris LR, Mahabir S, Walters RR, Martinon O, Dunham SA, Gonzales AJ. 2021. Onset and duration of action of lokivetmab in a canine model of IL-31 induced pruritus. Vet Dermatol. 32(6):681-e182.

Franco J, Rajwa B, Gomes P, HogenEsch H.2021. Local and Systemic Changes in Lipid Profile as Potential Biomarkers for Canine Atopic Dermatitis. Metabolites. 11(10):670.

Gonzales AJ, Aleo M, Mahabir S, Messamore J, Stegemann M. 2024. Oclacitinib (APOQUEL®) is a selective Janus kinase 1 inhibitor with efficacy in a canine model of flea allergic dermatitis. J Vet Pharmacol Ther. 47(6):447-453.

Lim JJ, Liu MH, Chew FT.2024. Dietary Interventions in Atopic Dermatitis: A Comprehensive Scoping Review and Analysis. Int Arch Allergy Immunol. 185(6):545-589.

Marchegiani A, Fruganti A, Spaterna A, Dalle Vedove E, Bachetti B, Massimini M, Di Pierro F, Gavazza A, Cerquetella M.2020. Impact of Nutritional Supplementation on Canine Dermatological Disorders. Vet Sci. 7(2):38.

Marsella R, Olivry T, Carlotti DN. 2011. International Task Force on Canine Atopic Dermatitis. Current evidence of skin barrier dysfunction in human and canine atopic dermatitis. Vet Dermatol. 22(3):239-48.

Marsella R, Santoro D, Ahrens K. 2012. Early exposure to probiotics in a canine model of atopic dermatitis has long-term clinical and immunological effects. Vet Immunol Immunopathol. 146(2):185-9.

Marsella R. 2013. Fixing the skin barrier: past, present and future--man and dog compared. Vet Dermatol. 24(1):73-6.e17-8.

Olivry T. 2011. Is the skin barrier abnormal in dogs with atopic dermatitis? Vet Immunol Immunopathol.144(1-2):11-6.

Outerbridge CA, Jordan TJM. 2021. Current Knowledge on Canine Atopic Dermatitis: Pathogenesis and Treatment. Adv Small Anim Care.2:101-115.

Ramió-Lluch L, Brazís P, Ferrer L, Puigdemont A. 2020. Allergen-specific immunotherapy in dogs with atopic dermatitis: is owner compliance the main success-limiting factor? Vet Rec. 187(12):493.

Santoro D, Marsella R, Pucheu-Haston CM, Eisenschenk MN, Nuttall T, Bizikova P. 2015. Review: Pathogenesis of canine atopic dermatitis: skin barrier and host-micro-organism interaction. Vet Dermatol. 26(2):84-e25.

Saridomichelakis MN, Olivry T. 2016. An update on the treatment of canine atopic dermatitis. Vet J. 2016 Jan;207:29-37.

Tamamoto-Mochizuki C, Santoro D, Saridomikelakis MN, Eisenschenk MNC, Hensel P, Pucheu-Haston C. 2024. International Committee on Allergic Diseases of Animals (ICADA). Update on the role of cytokines and chemokines in canine atopic dermatitis. Vet Dermatol. 35(1):25-39.

Tate DE, Tanprasertsuk J, Jones RB, Maughan H, Chakrabarti A, Khafipour E, Norton SA, Shmalberg J, Honaker RW. 2024. A Randomized Controlled Trial to Evaluate the Impact of a Novel Probiotic and Nutraceutical Supplement on Pruritic Dermatitis and the Gut Microbiota in Privately Owned Dogs. Animals (Basel). 14(3):453.

Wadhwa NK, Schroeder TJ, Pesce AJ, Myre SA, Clardy CW, First MR. 1987. Cyclosporine drug interactions: a review. Ther Drug Monit. 9(4):399-406.

19

Skin Lesions and Diagnostic Techniques

Anisha Tiwari and S.R. Upadhyay

Chief Vet, Suvidha Pet Care & Derma Centre AiCVD Resident (Seoul National University)

Learning objectives

1. Recognise inflammatory cell types
2. Recognise common skin pathogens
3. Diagnostic test are best for each case
4. Gain experience in interpretation
5. Recognise important artefacts

"The most crucial step towards healing is having the right diagnosis". While approaching a case, a clinician should follow appropriate steps in a systematic way for accurate diagnosis of dermatological disorders. A careful history is a first step to choose appropriate diagnostic tests.

Beginning from patient data, a detailed history, physical examination, and appropriate diagnostic tests are very much needed for a definitive diagnosis of various skin diseases of pets. Here are some of the most important diagnostic procedures for a successful dermatological practice in a sequential pattern.

1. Visual examination
2. Coat brush
3. Cytology
    a. Direct impression smear
    b. Indirect impression smear
    c. Tapestrip/impression
    d. Aspirate

4. Skin scraping
5. Woods lamp
6. Hair pluck / Trichoscopy
7. Culture (Fungal & Bacterial)
8. Biopsy

What do we want from cytology?

To establish a diagnosis, Every clinical picture can have multiple differential diagnosis and pathology can help differentiate

In house skin cytology steps

- Sampling
- Staining
- Using the microscope
- Assessing for organisms
- Assessing the cells
- Summary of findings
- Interpretation of the findings
- Using the results to formulate a next step

How to do cytology?

Cytology: Cytology can be used to obtain information on bacterial or Malassezia infection, as well as to characterize inflammatory infiltrate. Skin cytology is the most important diagnostic test for canine pyoderma.The diagnosis of superficial pyoderma needs to be supported by cytologic findings demonstrating coccoid bacteria, often associated with inflammatory cells (typically degenerate neutrophils) and, when present, bacteria phagocytosis. Cytology is also very important for identification of co-infection with other microorganisms such as Malassezia.

A. Direct impression smear: Direct impression smears may be prepared by direct impression with the glass slide pressed onto the lesion. This is a kind of superficial skin cytology. It is indicated in conditions like erosions, ulcers and/or crusting; increased secretions or exudate present in the ear canals; papules, pustules and/or epidermal collarettes, well circumscribed "moth eaten alopecia" (staphylococcal pyoderma); dry or oily scale.

Procedure: This technique involves directly pressing the slide gently on the affected skin surface. Before collecting the sample, it is best to cut the hair surrounding the lesion with clipper. A skin cytology sample can be obtained in a variety of ways, depending on the type of lesion present.

- If pustules are intact, they should be gently broken with the 25-gauge needle.
- The purulent material found is then collected by gently pressing the slide on the surface.
- Crusts must be lifted with a fine-gauge needle to expose the surface exudate.
- In the presence of erosive-ulcerative lesions, it is recommended to dry the exudative surface by rubbing it and then collect fresh exudate.

In general, apply samples to a microscope slide and stain with Diff-Quik. Then scan the sample at10X magnification for a representative area, and examine that area under 40X to 100X magnification.

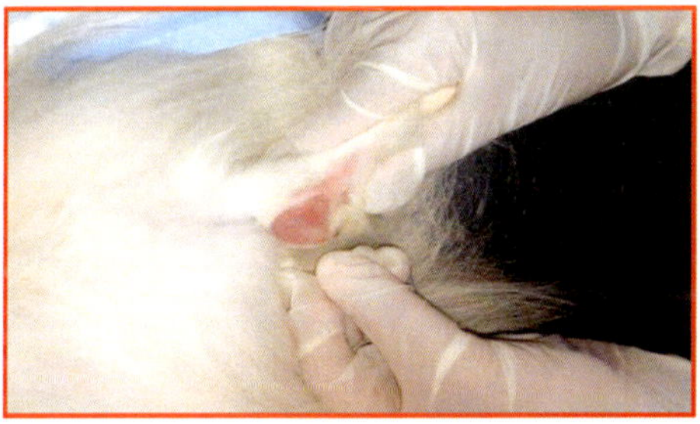

Direct Impression with the glass slide

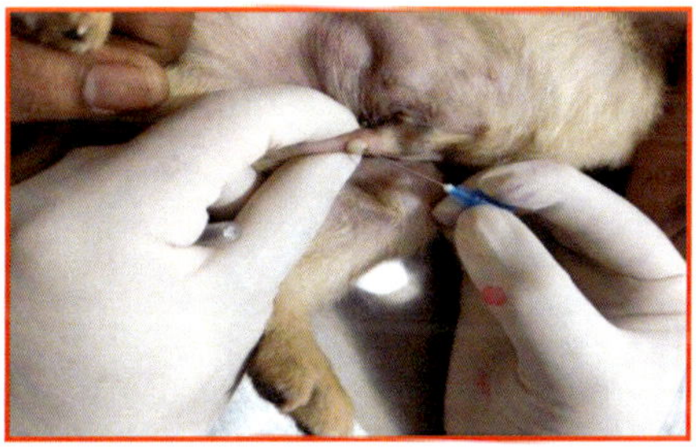

If pustules are intact then gently broken with 25 gauze needle and then collect the sample by pressing the slide onto the surface

Interpretations

- Normal findings in cytology : Keratinocytes are mostly enucleated (corneocytes) and a smaller proportion is nucleated. Frequently melanin granules are seen on the surface of epitheliated cells. A small number of cocci (<2 per immersion field [1000x]) and Malassezia (<1-2 per dry field [400x]) may be present. Absence of bacilli and inflammatory cells. Neutrophilic or pyogranulomatous inflammation can be supportive of an infectious or inflammatory process. The presence of degenerate neutrophils with intracellular cocci is diagnostic of bacterial infection.
- The presence of an elevated numbers of cocci or the presence of bacilli in the absence of inflammatory cells is diagnostic of bacterial over growth.
- The presence of non-degenerate neutrophils and numerous acantholytic keratinocytes (keratinocytes with a large nucleus and rounded hyper

basophilic cytoplasm) can suggest pemphiguscomplex (but can also be seen with chronic bacterial order matophyteinfection) and eneedforbacterialculture,biopsyandhistologicexamination.

- The presence of an elevated number of Malassezia is diagnostic of overgrowth due to Malassezia.
- The presence of eosinophils in a cytology examination of superficial skin samples in dogs is uncommon and initially suggests allergic dermatitis and ectoparasites. Eosinophils may occasionally be seen inside pustules, suggesting animmune-mediated origin of the pustule, such as pemphigus foliaceus, pemphigus erythematosus or sterile eosinophilic pustulosis.
- The presence of macrophages, lymphocytes or plasmacells together with degenerate neutrophils in a deep lesion sample (ulcers) suggests a deep pyoderma (furunculosis). In deep pyoderma there are very few bacteria and they are very difficult to identify.

B. Indirect impression smears: It is used when direct impression smear is difficult due to the location of the site by using a cotton swab to collect exudates Sampling from an exudative erosion or ulcer at skin fold or from a sinus or from the ear canal. The swab should be gently rolled along the slide, heat fixed and then stained. Examination from low to high power. Mostly taken in ear infections using ear bud/ swab.

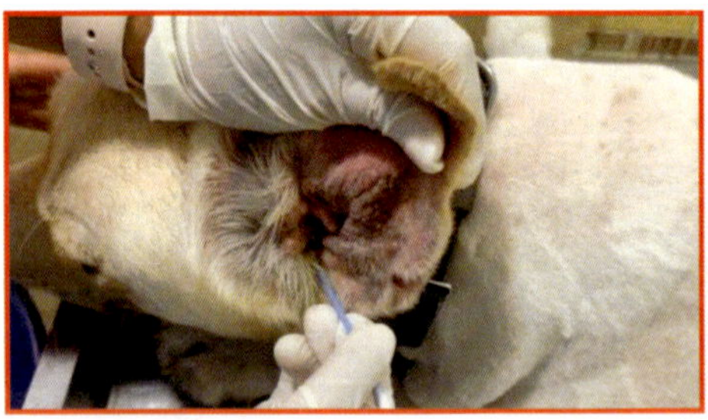

Collecting sample from ear with ear swab

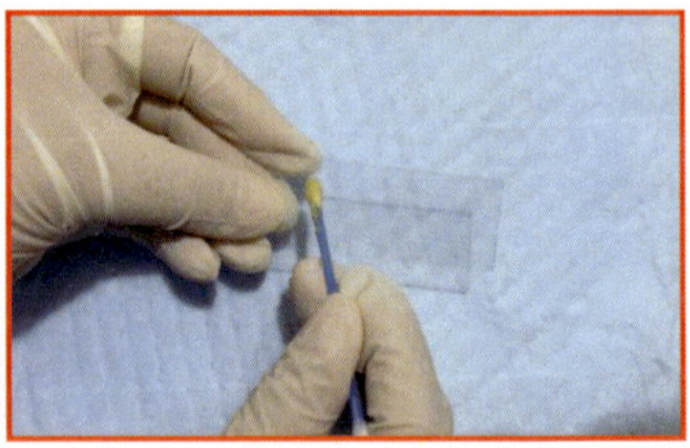

Swab should be gently rolled along the slide

C. Tape impression : Acetate tape impressions is indicated when Cheyletiella mites, Demodex mange, bacterial and Malassezia dermatitis are suspected. It also gives idea about types of epidermal cells. It can be used to sample dry, lichenified, and interdigitalareas.

- Clear, pressure-sensitive acetate tape is pressed to the skin in the affected areas.
- The tape is then stuck with pressure on a microscopic slide and examined in case of mites. Incase of Malassezia infection, a drop of Diff Quik stain is placed and then the tape is stuck with pressure on a microscopic slide.

- Attention must be paid to collect scale from the skin and not from the distal part of the hair. Superficial parasites are found very close to the skin surface.

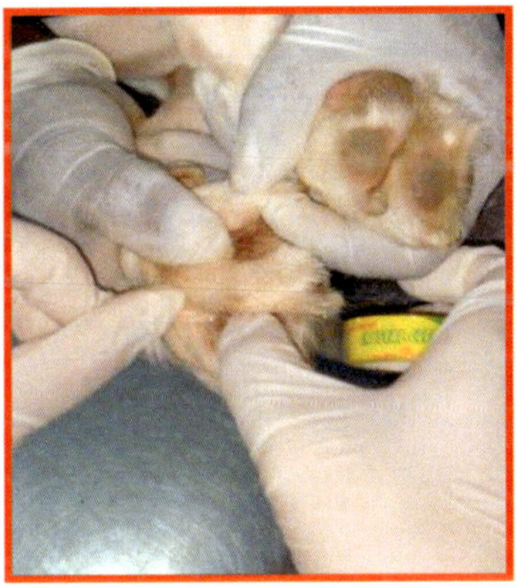

Adhesive tape strip

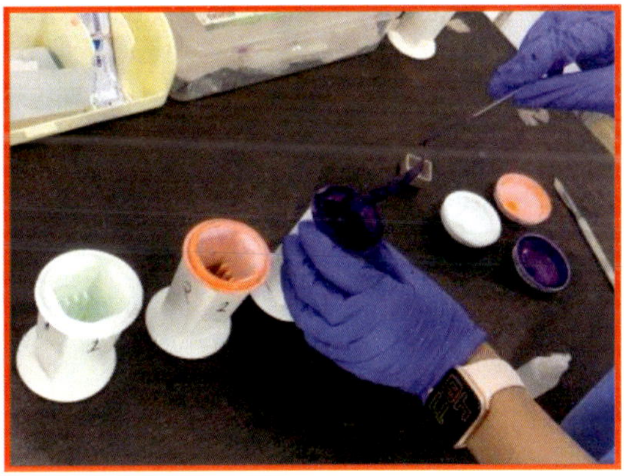

Diff quick staining

Tape strip of skin

Where to use

Dry skin, difficult sites/patients Quick

Interdigital spaces, intertriginous spaces (lips, face, tail)

What it will identify

Surface pathogens

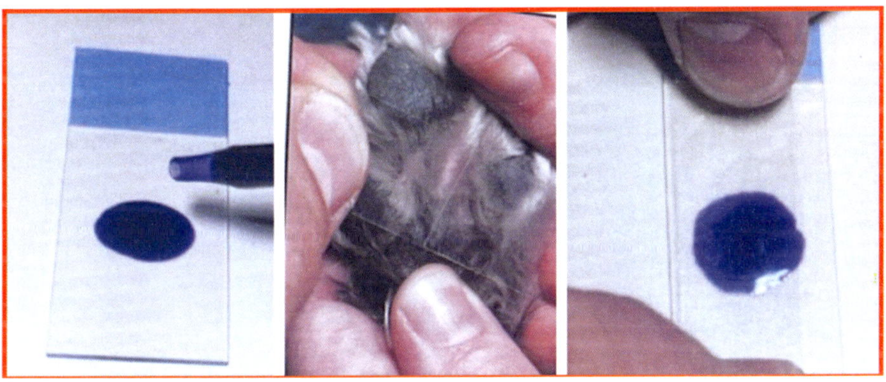

Staining of Tape Impression

Bacteria : cocci (*Staphylococcus*), rods (*Pseudomonas*), yeast (*Malssezia spp.*)
Inflammatory infiltrate

Direct impression smear

Where to use

Exudative lesions eg. erosions, ulcers, furuncles, undersides of crust- press slide onto lesions Non exudative lesions e.g. papules, pustules-pick with sterile needle, press slide onto lesion

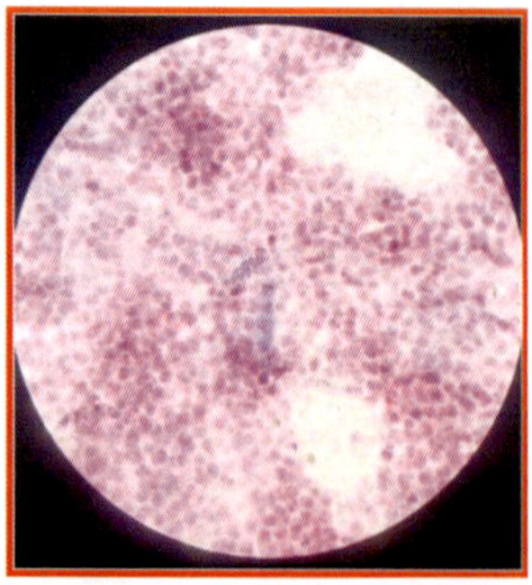

Cocci

Indirect impression smear

Where to use

Exudative and non exudative lesions inaccessible sites e.g nail beds, gums, mouth, peri ocular, ears

What it will identify

Surface pathogens

Bacteria : cocci (*Staphylococcus),* rods (*Pseudomonas*), yeast (*Malsseziaspp.*) Inflammatory infiltrate

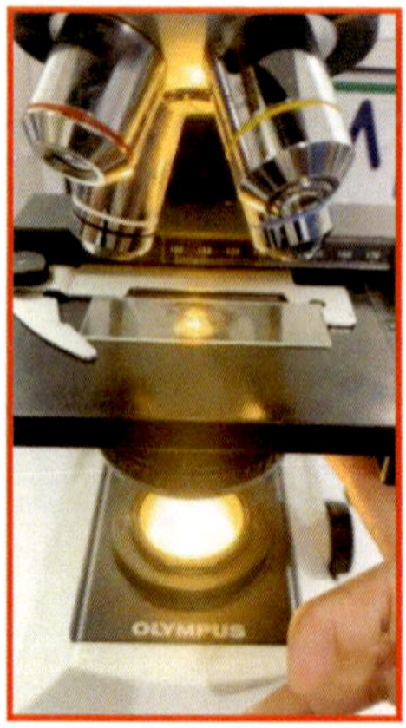

Microscope condenser up for cell detail and down for parasites

Why do Cytology?

Enables you to assess cases and decide on next steps

Are findings suggestive of inflammation, immune mediated or neoplasticdisease Are lesions infected or sterile?

What type of infection is present ? Can I treat or do I need further tests?

What do we see?

Identification of different cell types

Identification of different pathogens

Identification of artefact

Which stain?

Diff quick Gram-bacteria

New methylene blue

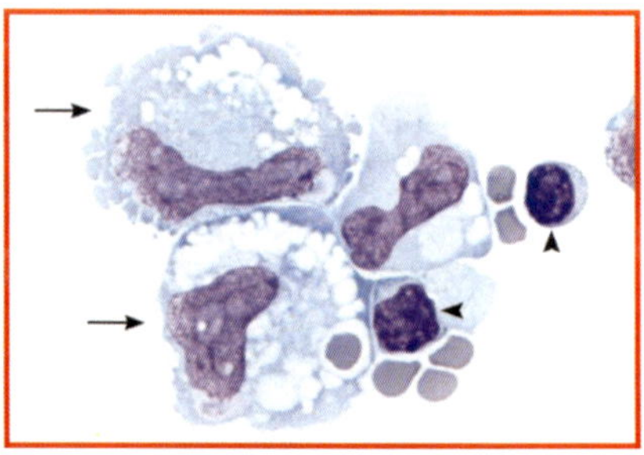

Foamy Macrophages & Lymphocytes

Keypoints to identifying inflammatory cell types Characterise the inflammation

Neutrophilic

Neutrophilic and macrophagic (pyogranulomatous)

Mixed inflammation, neutrophilic, macrophagic, lymphoplasmcytic, eosinophilic
Microscope condenser up for cell detail and down for parasites

Neutrophils

Neutrophils are important for body defence against infection First cells to arrive to fight bacteria

Distinctive multi lobed nucleus and pinkish cytoplasm

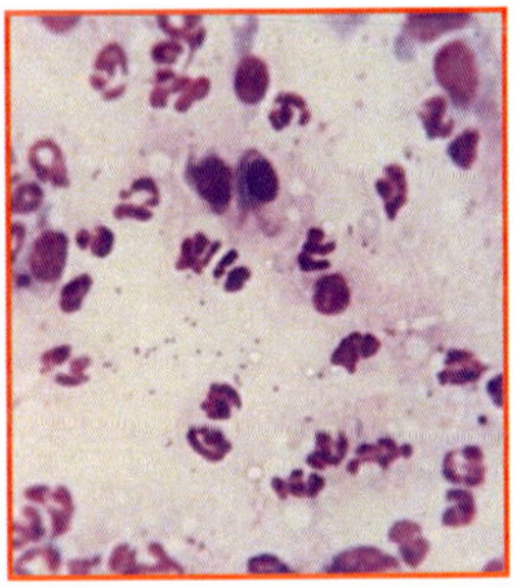

Neutrophils & Macrophages

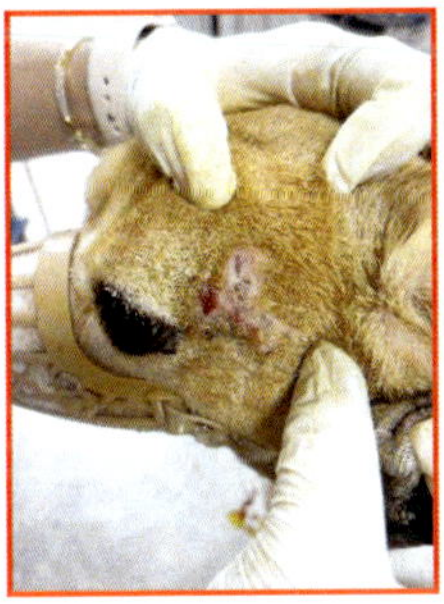

Pyogranuloma Lesion

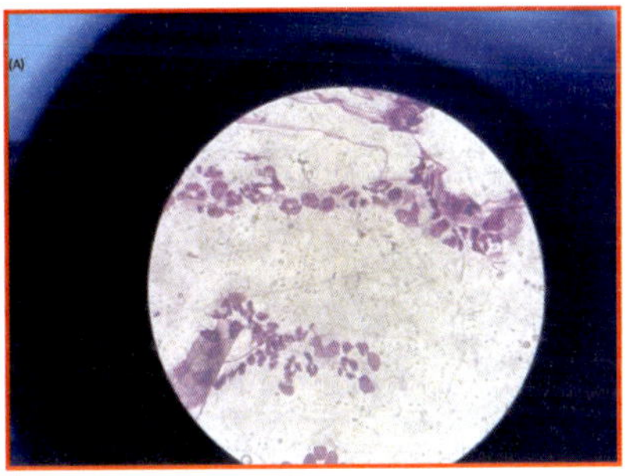

Neutrophils

Eosinophils

Eosinophils are important in parasite defence Common in feline allergy Lightly larger than neutrophil, bilobed nucleus, red cytoplasmic granules

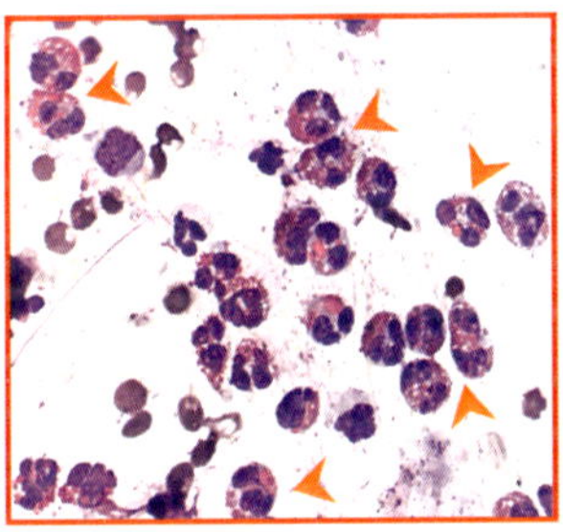

Eosinophils

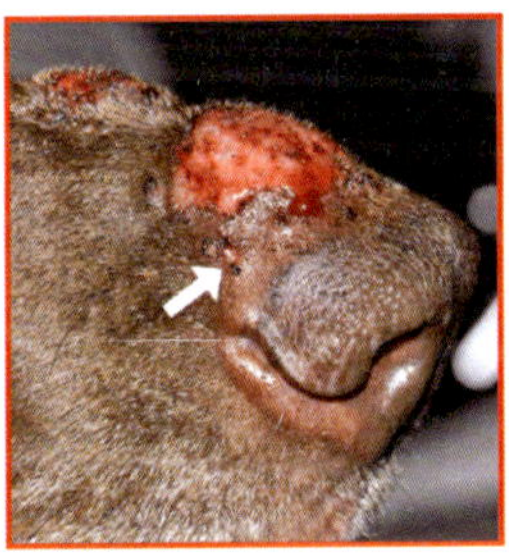

Eosinophilic

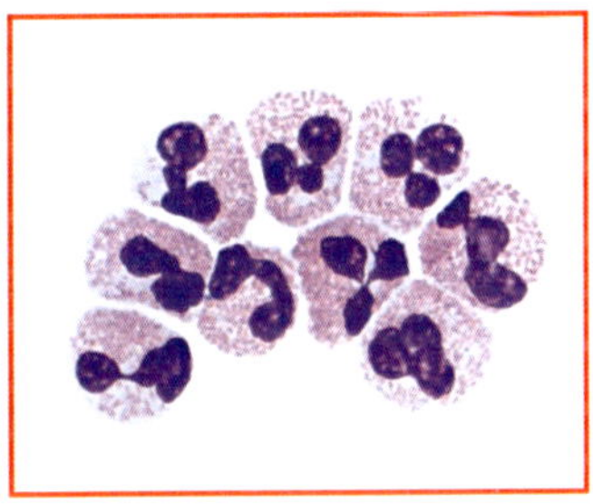

Furunculosis Eosinophils

Lymphocytes

Lymphocytes respond to exogenous antigens, seen in chronic inflammation Small cells (RBC size), nucleus round, minimal cytoplasm, smudged chromatin and no nucleoli, dark blue cytoplasm

Macrophages

Macrophages found in tissue due to chronic inflammation. Phagocytize bacteria, fungi cellular debris, foreign material Large cells, foamy vacuolated cytoplasm, nucleus oval to round

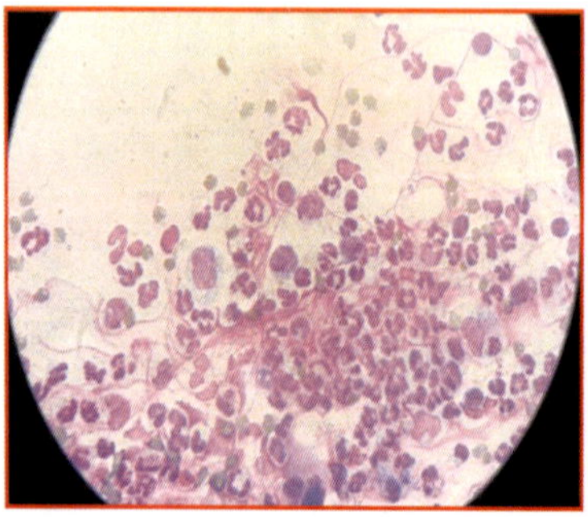

Pyogranulomatous inflammation
(Neutrophils & Macrophages)

Plasma cells

Round / oval cells, variable amounts deeply staining blue cytoplasm, occasional perinuclear clear area Round, eccentric medium sized nucleus, granular to coarse chromatin, Russel bodies can be seen in cytoplasm

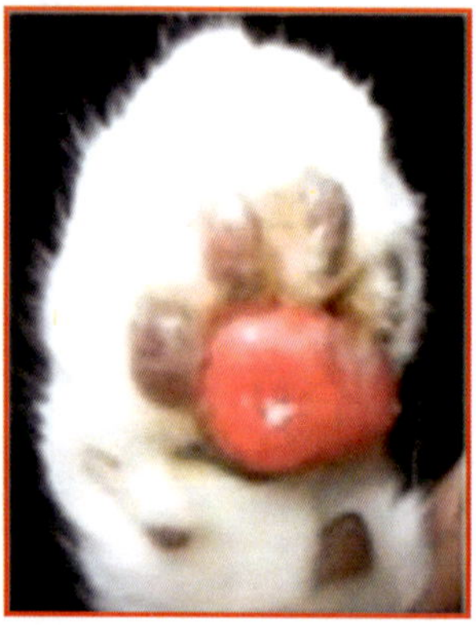

Pillow pad Plasma cell pododermatitis

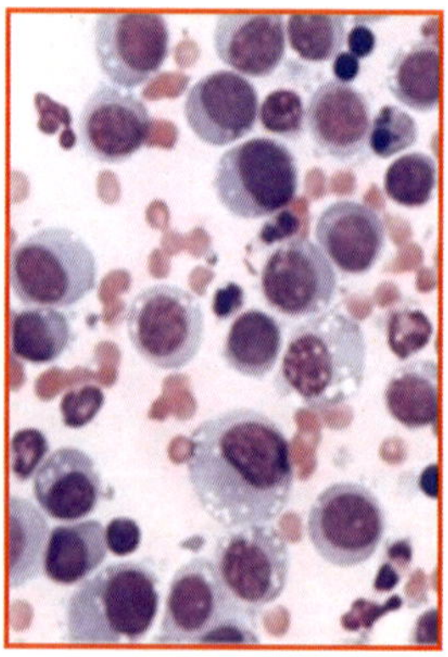

Plasma cell

Acantholytic cells

Rounded up skin cells released when cell to cell adhesion is broken Seen in pemphigus foliaceous and pyoderma Large purple blue stained nucleated cells

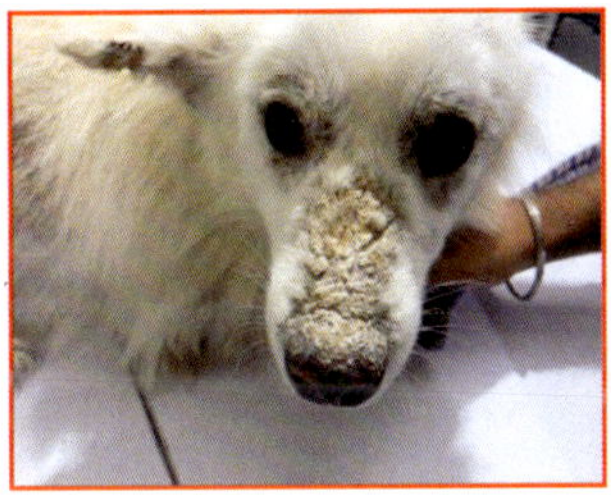
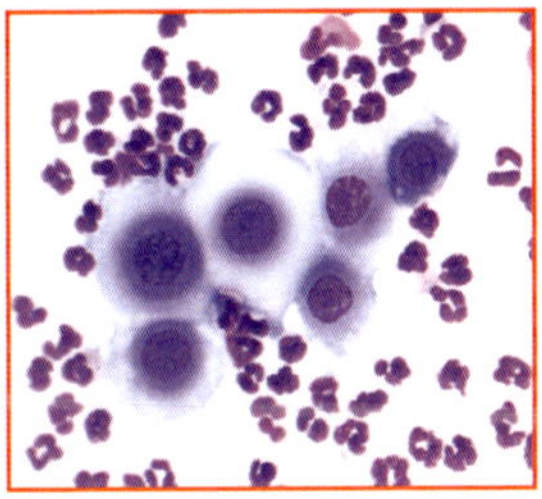
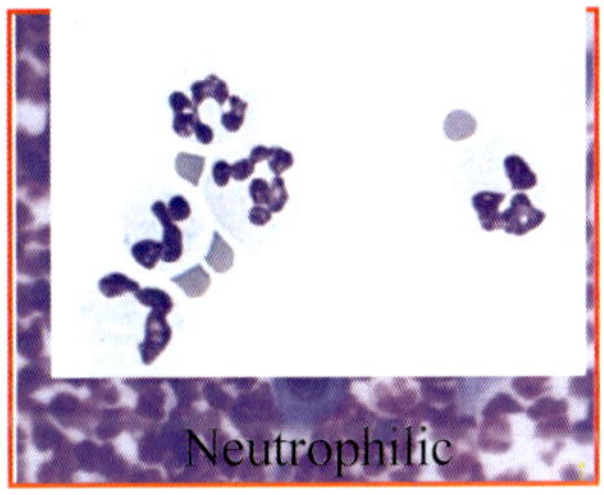

Yellow Cruston Nasal Planum

Acantholytic Cells

Pathogens

Bacteria : Cocci & rods

Yeast: Malassezia

Acantholytic Cells

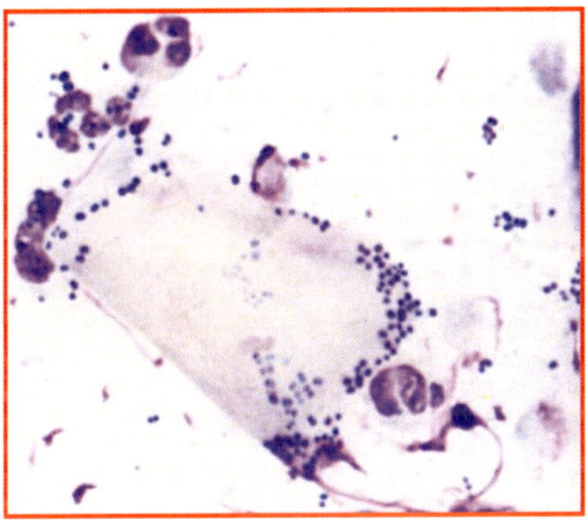

Cocci

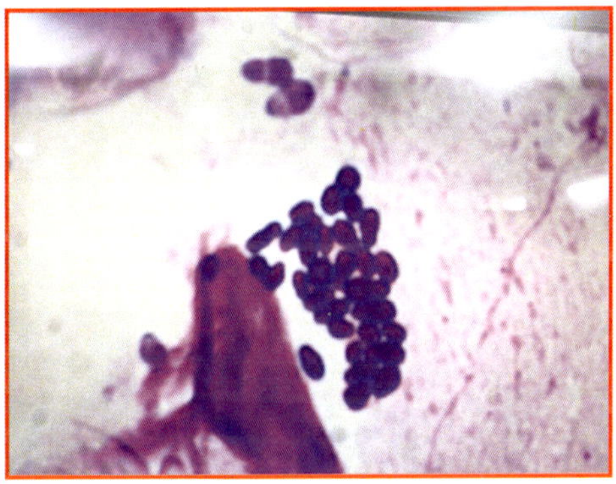

Malassezzia sp

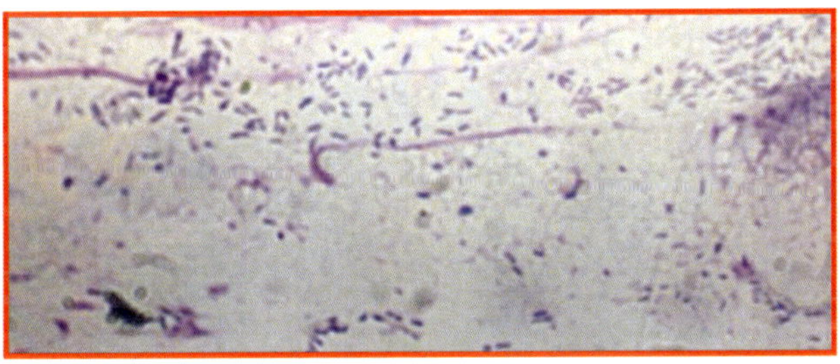

Rods

Artefacts

Excessive stain formation on the slide

Contaminants from the stain

Environmental contaminants spores, pollens

Commensal organisms

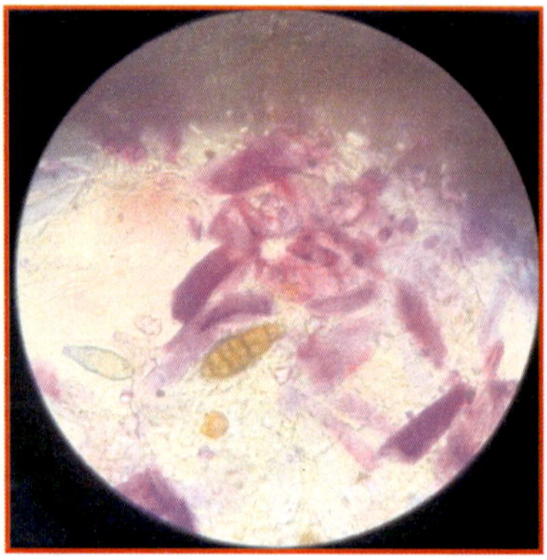

Saprophytic Spores

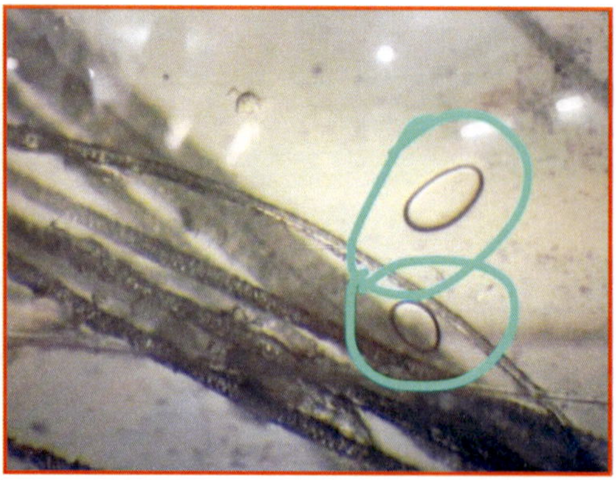

Air Bubble

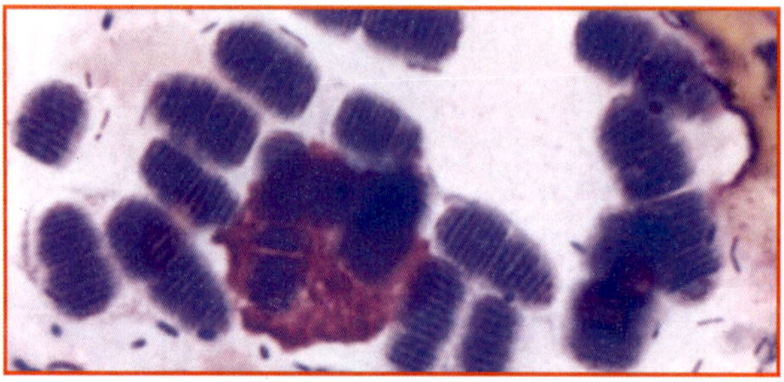

Simonsiella sp, (normal commensal)

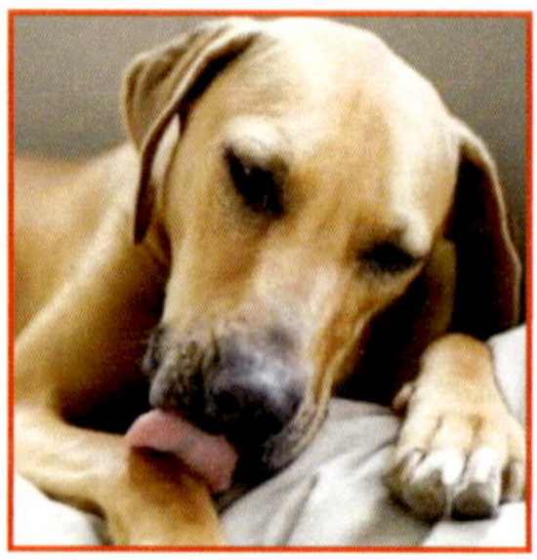

Salivary stain due to licking

Lets put our new found knowledge into practice 1)

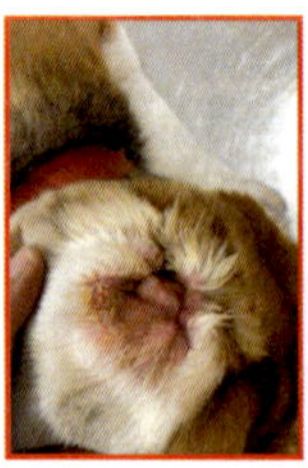

Which tests?

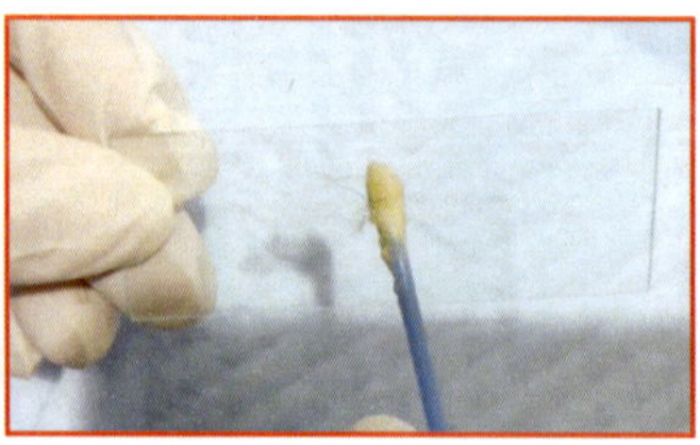

Ear swab cytology

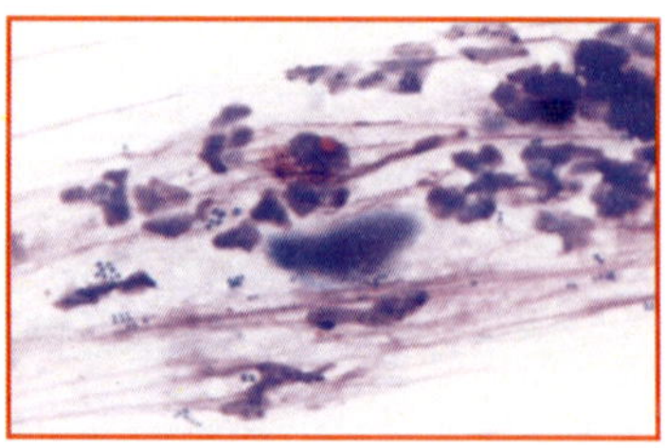

Bacteria (cocci)

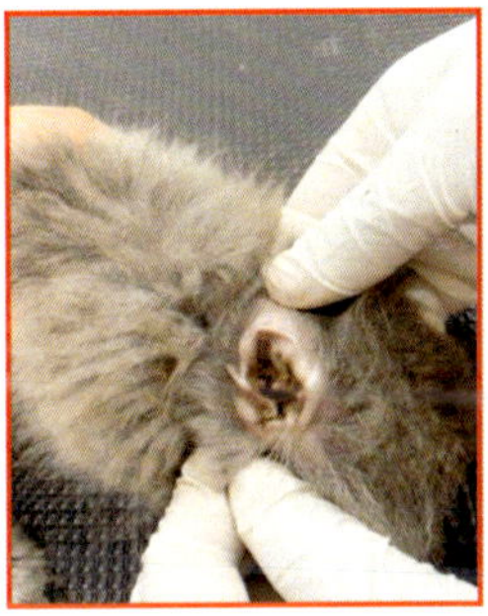

Which Tests?

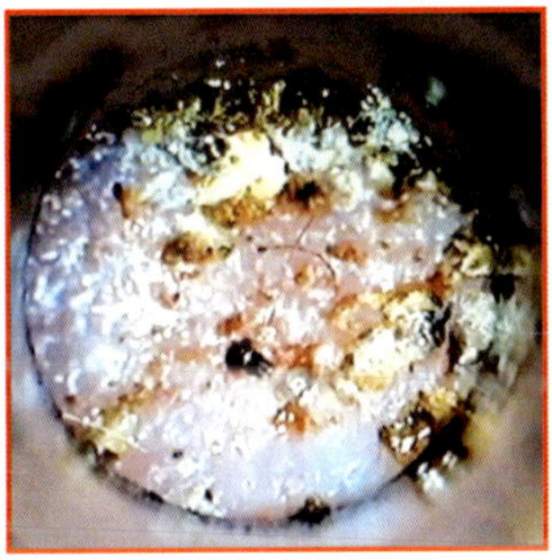

Otoscopic Examination

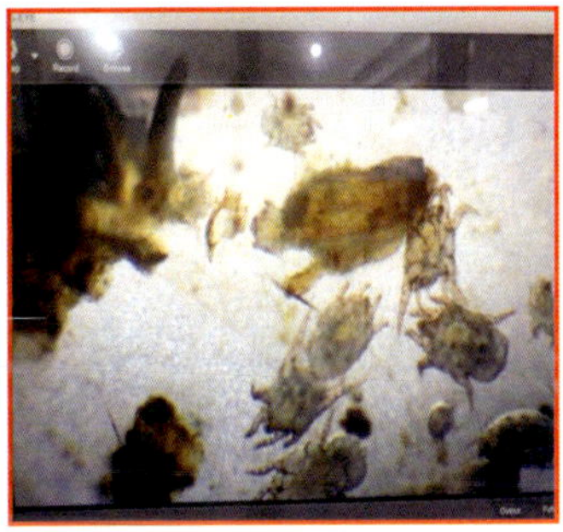

Ear Mites

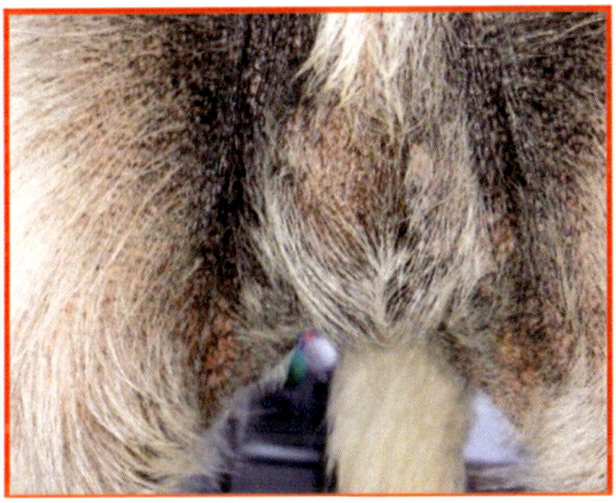

Hyper pigmentation in groin area, which tests?

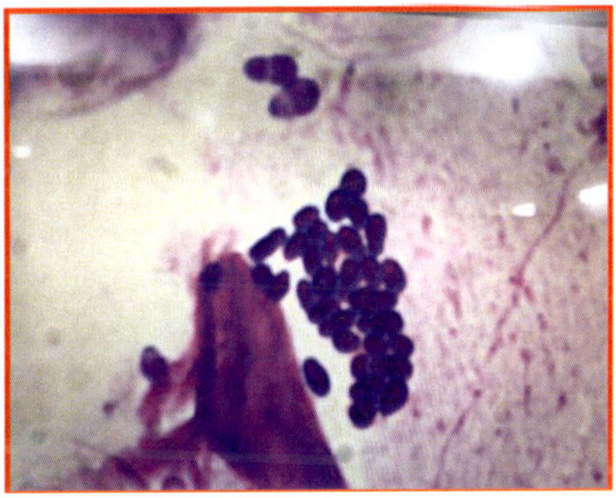

Malassezia sp.

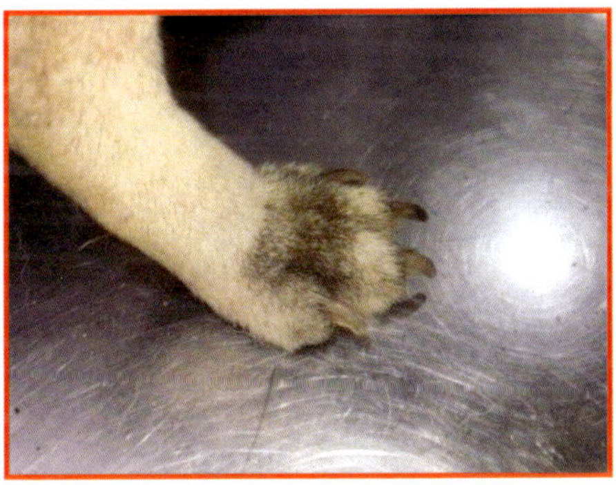

Hyperpigmentation, which tests?

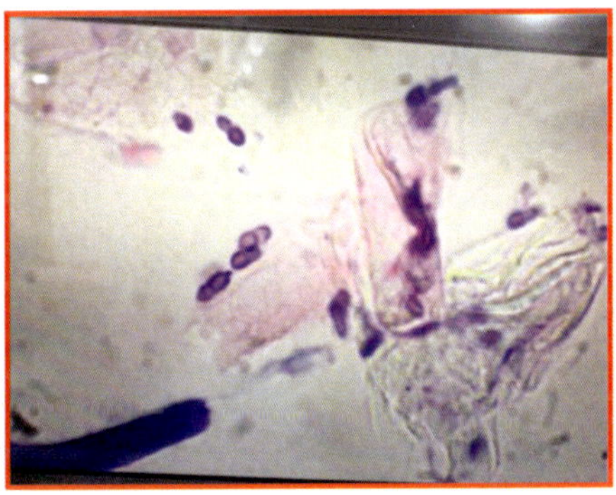

Numerous peanut shaped budding Malassezia

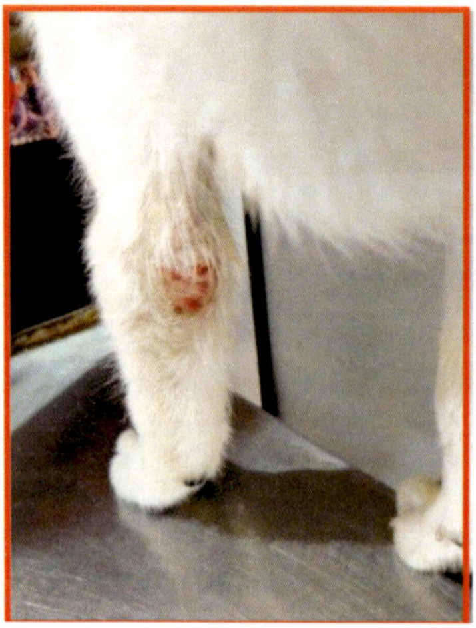

Lesion on knee, which tests?

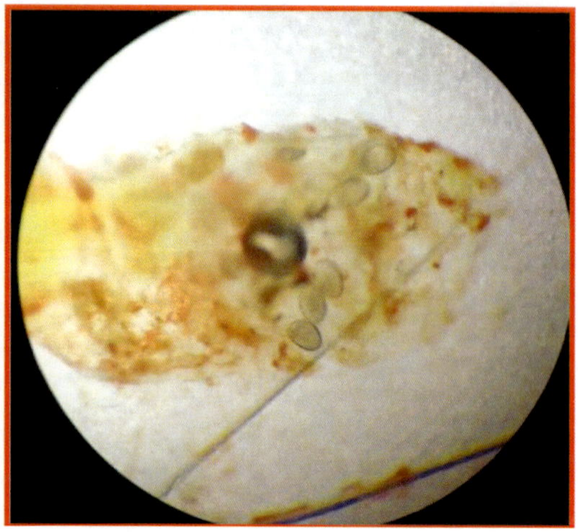

Eggs of sarcoptes

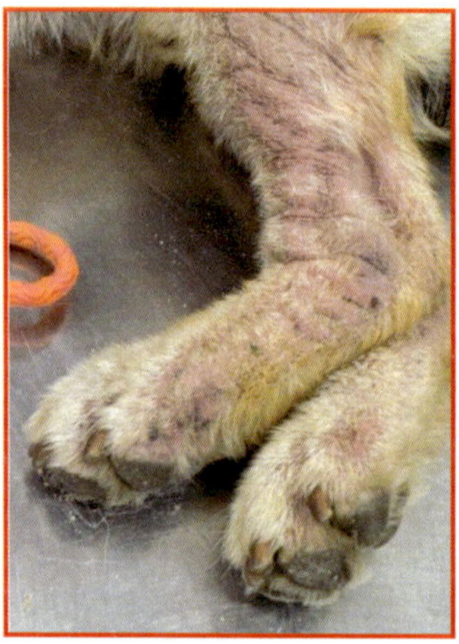

Dry erythematous lesion on dogs body, which tests?

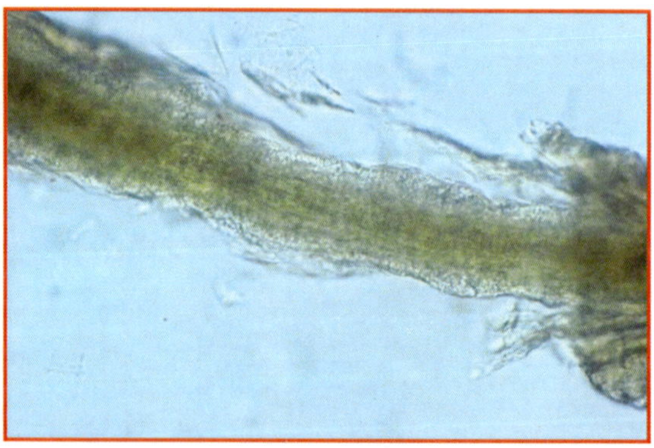

Fungal spores

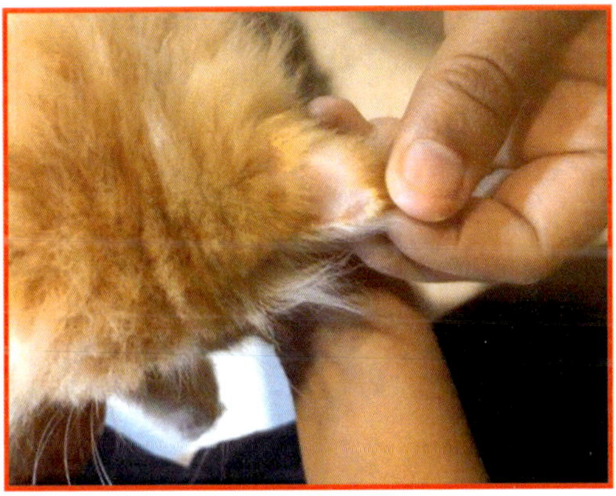

Lesion on cat pinnae, Which test?

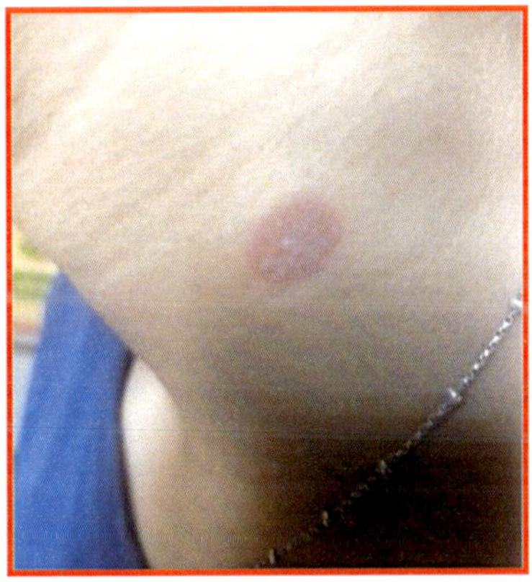

Lesion on human neck (ringworm)

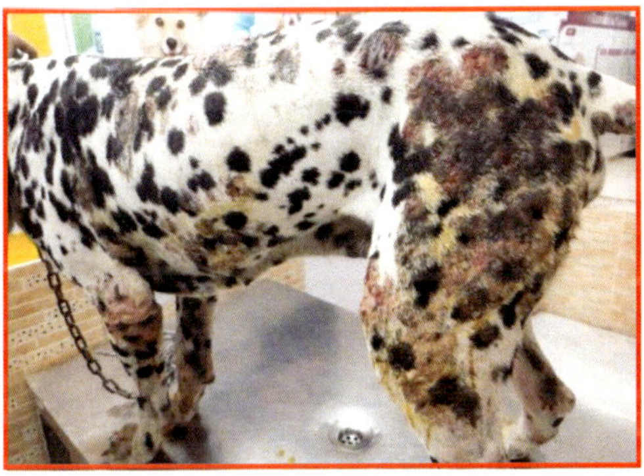

Erythematous lesion, which tests?

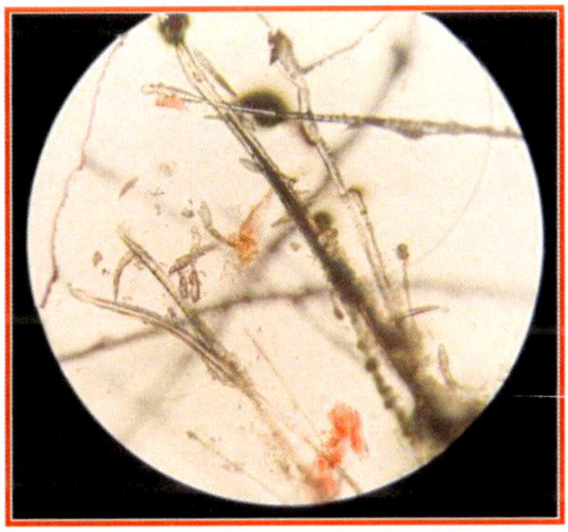

Demodex spp

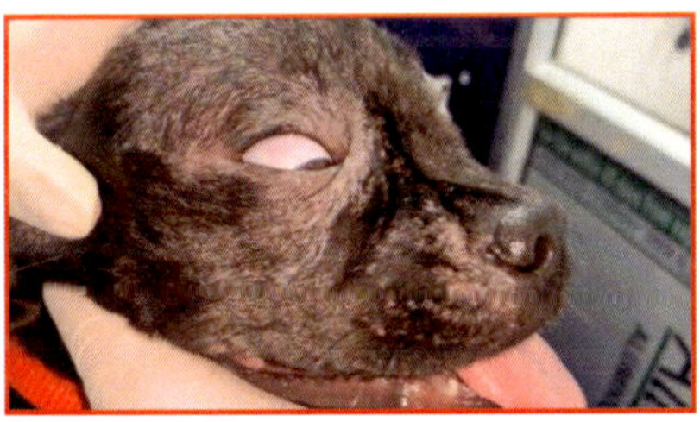

Alopeciaon face, which tests?

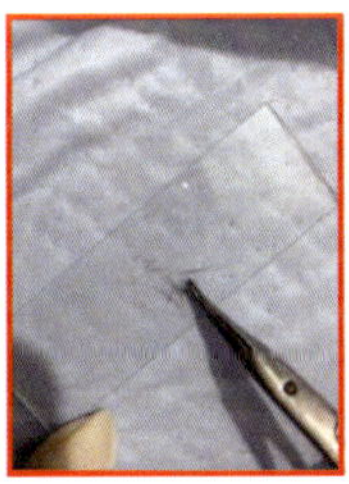

Hairpluck

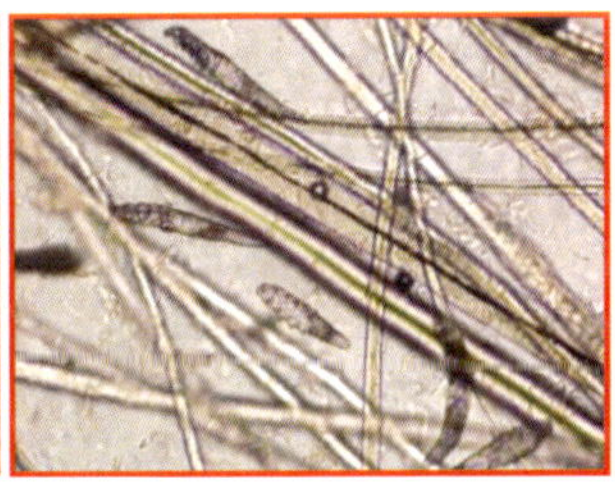

Demodex

Take Home Message

Picture correlation should never be the clinician's part of treatment protocol, since it always leads to deception. A step wise diagnostic approach must be followed. Cytology is the primary diagnostic modality, its quick, easy and low cost. It is impossible to decide on therapy or further diagnostic tests without performing cytology.

Remember

"Diagnosis is not the end, but the beginning of patient care"

20

Application of Modern Technology in Health and Well-Being of Captive and Free-Range Elephants: Space for Improvement

N. Sahoo

Professor and Head, Veterinary Medicine, Institute of Veterinary Science and Animal Husbandry, SOA Deemed University, Bhubaneswar- Odisha

Asiatic Elephant (*Elephas maximus*) is the national heritage animal of India. This particular species now exists in 13 Asian countries including India. As per 2017 census, India is home to an estimated figure of 29,964 elephants that is >60% wild population of the globe. Once distributed across the country, now they are squeezed to 14 states grouped in four regions ie., southern (14,612), north-eastern (10,139), east-central (3,128) and northern regions (2,085). There are 2675 captive elephants across different states under both private and government custody. This largest terrestrial mammal is protected under Seclude I species of Indian Wild Life Protection Act, 1972.

Both central and state Government are implementing short- and long-term programmes for health and well-being of captive as well as free-range elephants. The Central Government has established an 'Elephant Cell' at the Wildlife Institute of India (WII), Dehradun to provide technical inputs to the ministry for strengthening the efforts towards conservation of elephants. Add-on, the 'Project Elephant' was launched in 1991-92 in the Ministry of Environment, Forests and Climate Change to restore the elephant habitats and reduce their sufferings. Elephant habitats are notified as Elephant Reserves that are basic management units for elephant conservation and managements. A total of 33 Elephant Reserves has been notified in the country. A book titled, 'Caring for elephants: Managing health and welfare in captivity' is edited for field officers, veterinary professionals and elephant handlers.

Modern technologies are being applied in the different set-up to address various issues that relate to health and well-being of elephants. Diagnostic and research laboratories do exist to unfold and mitigate endemic as well as emerging health issues. Species-specific human resources such as village/local volunteers have been engaged in elephant-holding facilities. Eco-development committee members and students are being roped in for awareness campaigns. Intra- and inter-state coordination committees on elephants are framed for well fare activities. Rapid response teams and control room are actively functional. Despite aggressive actions, unusual mortality situations linked with anthropogenic activities, climate change, natural calamity, man-elephant conflict and diseases are being surfaced as breaking news. It has been recorded that half of the total deaths are due to electrocution, road and train accidents or targeted killings for tusk. Between 2019 and 2024, 483 elephants have died in Odisha and 116 in West Bengal. Of which, 208 in Odisha and 50 in Bengal. Death due to viral and bacterial pathogens have been registered in different geolocations such as elephant endotheliotropic herpes virus (EEHV), *Clostridium novyi*, *Pasteurella multocida*, *Bacillus anthracis* etc. Accidental death due to ingestion of chemicals used in the agricultural fields has been recorded in certain pockets of India.

Technologies across different sectors have been advanced tremendously during recent past. with the advent of cutting-edge technologies such as real-time polymerase chain reaction, nanopore sequencing, next generation sequencing (NGS), matrix-assisted laser desorption/ionization time—of—flight mass spectrometry (MALDI-TOF MS), Point of care tests, Artificial intelligence etc. However, the application of these modern gadgets is still young in wildlife segment. This paper throws light, as described hereunder, on the technologies currently available and/or proved beneficial in different Forest Divisions of India improving health and well-being of elephants.

Detection of antigen, antibody, nucleic acid or pathogen: There is growing demand for the technologies and methodologies that target any one of the candidates such as antigen, antibody, nucleic acid or pathogen as a whole. The following are the technologies that target one or more of the unit(s).

Targeted sequencing (amplicon sequencing): Polymerase chain reaction (PCR) amplification is performed with primer sets that individually target a taxonomically informative gene. 16S/18S/ITS sequencing targets specific regions of the microbial genome (16S rRNA for bacteria, 18S/ITS for fungi). Gene amplicon sequencing is considered the most conserved taxonomic marker as it is sequenced in considerably less time. In 16S rRNA, there are approximately 1500 base pairs (bp) in size, with nine highly conserved regions and nine variable regions (V1–V9). The conserved regions of the genes are used for primer binding during PCR amplification, whereas the hypervariable regions are used for identifying sequence diversity in prokaryotes. Hence, it is considered a gold standard for extensive phylogenetic analysis. Real time PCR and reverse transcription polymerase chain reaction (RT-PCR) using specific probes and primers are proved very sensitive in detection of targeted pathogen DNA or RNA.

Metagenomic analysis: Metagenomics is a versatile branch of science, having two basic approaches: (A) taxonomic application (B) functional application or a combination of both. It helps to identify microbial taxa and genes of interest in a subset of bio-samples, and to estimate their abundances. Further analysis of the annotation is required for in-depth analysis. Different pipelines exist with some degree of variation. It is the key that helps unlocking the mysteries of the microbial world of various environments viz., gut, soil, tissues etc. Advances in next-generation sequencing technologies have accelerated the momentum of metagenomic studies, which is in fast increasing trend.

Whole genome metagenome sequencing: Whole genome sequencing (shotgun metagenomics) method is used in characterizing the abundance of microorganisms available in a particular environment. This method not only identifies the microbial species but also can generate information about the genes (including 16S rRNA) present in the bio-sample. It is PCR independent, where there is no chance of biasing due to primer binding. This factor is helpful for finding unknown microbes in the sample, which may otherwise not be detected by targeted sequencing. This method also helps identify and discover novel viruses in the given sample. Platforms like Illumina sequencing use V3 and V4 regions to obtain the taxonomic classification by comparing these regions with those already known and available on large public databases like NCBI, SILVA, Green Gene, RDP, and 16S rRNA gene. Gene sequencing is the most widely used approach to disclose and identity pathogens as they are signature-specific sequences with higher accuracy.

Cultural examination in BSL 3/4: Around 75% of the emerging infectious diseases are zoonotic in nature and more than 70% of those zoonoses originate from wild animals with no exception to elephants. This has thus become a mandate, not only to protect laboratory workers, but also to protect the environment and community while processing bio-samples of wild animal origin. Biosafety level 3/4 (BSL-3/4) laboratories are established to tackle biosafety issues involved in handling highly pathogenic infectious disease agents or their toxins, suspected or confirmed, for basic research and diagnosis. It also supports cultural examination followed by identification employing gold standard tests.

Point of care tests (POCT): Point-of-care testing (POCT) is defined by International Standard ISO 22870 as testing that is performed near or at the site of a patient with the result leading to possible change in the care of the patient. POCT has an increasing role to play, especially in resource-limited settings. The test has a rapid turnaround time. This enables rapid decision making and faster care or treatment of the patient. In animal diagnostics, the POCT is called as pen-side, animal-side, flock-side testing. The most widely used immunoassay configuration is the enzyme-linked immunosorbent assay (ELISA) as they are easy to develop, use and validate compared to nucleic acid-based assays. However, their specificity and sensitivity are often inferior to nucleic acid-based assays. A quantitative POC - RT-PCR assay is developed by Biomeme that performs qPCR for anthrax. A point of- care tuberculosis diagnostic kit for the detection of antibodies from wild animals is developed using pathogenic mycobacteria specific recombinant antigens and purified protein derivatives of pathogenic and non-pathogenic Mycobacteria. The kit was used to determine the seroprevalence of TB in elephants. Additional tests in terms of sensitivity, specificity, turnaround time and affordability can be crafted on commonly prevalent diseases to address the situation. Multiplex POCTs that could help diagnose animal diseases with a syndromic or system-based approach with a single test would be a *win-win* for the end users and veterinarians/clinicians who treat diseases or make clinical management decisions.

Non-invasive Hormone assay

Faecal sample is considered a suitable bio-sample for the measurement of heath biomarker in the non-invasive mode. Faecal cortisol is assayed to reveal stress level in captive and wild elephants. The faecal cortisol levels between two sets of populations can be correlated to understand the managemental practices followed and in turn it will guide to extend/ implement/upgrade such facilities for better health. Reproductive management of the elephant is equally important for its conservation. To monitor its estrous cyclicity, indirect ELISA was used earlier to show that levels of fecal progesterone (P_4)-metabolite (allopregnanolone: 5α-P-3OH) in captive females sampled randomly positively correlated with serum P_4 levels. This has a potential application in the reproductive management and conservation of Asian elephants.

Thermal Drone Camera

Drone helps tracks elephants without disturbing elephant herd. Thermal drone cameras are deployed during day and night hours to curb elephant location, movement and behaviours. It helps elephant-human conflict. It scans the forest areas to monitor movements of elephants. The thermal drone hovers in a range of 2-3km, with the capacity to traverse more, if required. A single charge sustains it for around 40 minutes of continuous operation, while backup batteries extend the operational period. One can maintain a safe distance of 500 metres to 1km. Thermal drone has its limitations. During high wind pressure, it fails to work properly. It harnesses the power of AI to identify animals captured by high-resolution cameras. The drone ensures swift alerts if the herd ventures too close to human settlements. Follow up measures are planned properly.

Radio Collar with Global Positioning System

A radio collar is a thin belt equipped with global positioning system (GPS) linked with Radio Frequency Identification (RFID) technology. The device is attached to the elephant's neck. Kumki (captive and trained) elephants are usually used for the such procedure. The tool relays data in its natural habitat to a computer or a mobile app 24×7. Radio-collaring elephants is performed with loners or the herds. Real-time monitoring of the data will send early warnings if elephants are traced within human settlements. In case any elephant from the herd comes closer to the locality, follow up steps can be initiated to counter the situation. It is a fact that, once the radio collars are fixed on the elephants, the individual travel long distances. Tusker with radio collar may create panic. Each radio collar weighs around 10 kg. Indigenous radio collar is available now.

High Performance Liquid Chromatography (HPLC)/ Gas Liquid Chromatograph (GLC)

Methods such as Gas Liquid Chromatograph (GLC)/ High Performance Liquid Chromatograph (HPLC)/ UV-Visible spectrophotometer/ Fourier Transform Infra red Spectrometer/Titrimetric are useful for detection of agricultural chemicals, pesticides, insecticides, herbicides. Drugs with a narrow therapeutic index, large inter- and intraindividual variability in therapeutic response and pharmacokinetics or when the therapeutic response is difficult to monitor, above assay are helpful. These techniques proved sensitive and rapid for determining ibuprofen concentrations in elephant plasma. More than 307 pesticides registered so far can be identified applying above technologies. Poisoning due to Chlorpyrifos, a pesticide used in the agricultural filed, has been recorded in stomach content of wild elephants through GC MS.

Artificial Intelligence (AI)-Powered Camera System

Artificial Intelligence (AI) is a computer science that aims to create machines to perform tasks that typically require human intelligence. Integrating AI into healthcare holds excellent potential for improving disease differential diagnosis, treatment selection, clinical laboratory testing and management practices. AI offers increased accuracy, reduced costs, and time savings while minimizing human errors. Artificial Intelligence camera installed at the vulnerable locations along the railway tracks detects, captures and zooms the elephants approaching the line and immediately sent alerts to the control room. This early warning system allowed the Forest and Railway authorities to act swiftly in guiding the elephants away from danger. Application of this technology has proven effective during recent past and can be upscaled to different accident-prone areas. Its application has proven beneficial in elephant behavioural study.

Conclusion

It is alarming to focus on the biostatistics of the last few decades that reflects pattern of elephant mortality due to various reasons especially in some hot spots of India. The field of elephant health and wellbeing becomes undoubtedly challenging for all stakeholders. But there is tremendous space to improve quality of their life with judicious application of modern technologies. In the last few years, technology has become more affordable and accessible. Some species-specific tools have been developed and validated in elephants and are being used in some pockets. Monitoring in real time is possible through sensor technologies to record continuously and automatically the status of the elephants in their natural habitat. Assessment tool is designed and tested for routine use by elephant keepers. Cost-effective, non-invasive and validated methods are already in practice. However, there is ample scope for the application of more and more cutting-edge technologies that can be made available in each and every sector of elephant health and well-being to make our own coexistence comfortable and progressive. By protecting elephant on earth, we safeguard biodiversity and invest in a healthier, more sustainable future.

21

Clinical Appraisal of Equine Nervous System

***Umesh Maral*[1] *and S.R. Upadhyay*[2]**

[1]*Officer Commanding, 24 Dog Unit, Indian Army*
[2]*Division of Veterinary Medicine, F.V.Sc. &AH, SKUAST-Jammu Jammu and Kashmir*

Introduction

A complete neurological examination is warranted whenever an equine patient displays signs consistent with neurological disorder or to establish that the horse is neurologically normal (e.g., pre-purchase examination). Neurological examination of equine patient is challenging due to their large size, which prevents veterinarian from using many of the tests used for small animals. The key to a successful neurologic examination is to do the examination in a consistent and organized fashion. It is important to develop a routine, then do it the same way each time. This approach ensures that some parts of the examination are not forgotten and it also increases the consistency of the exam as you examine more number of equine patients. A standardized examination form is a valuable aid in this and can be concise. The goals of the neurologic examination are to determine whether disease of the nervous system exists, to localize the lesion to a particular area of the nervous system, and to describe and record the responses as a baseline for future evaluations. In this paper, a complete neurological examination is described with special emphasis on field conditions.

Method

The neurological examination can be divided into five sections: evaluation of mental status, cranial nerve examination, spinal reflexes and muscle evaluation (performed in standing position) gait and postural examination (performed while moving) and examination of recumbent patients.

Evaluation of Mental Status

Equine patient should be observed from a distance without disturbing inside stable or while grazing. Observe for encephalopathic behaviour, such as compulsive circling, head-pressing, cortical/central blindness, seizures, or significant change in mentation. If present, encephalopathic behaviour and an unknown history of vaccination should trigger an increased level of caution for rabies infection and should be handled accordingly. Subtle behaviour changes are often first noted by the handler and may or may not be indicative of neurologic disease. Normal horses are alert and responsive, although the spectrum encompasses very calm, placid horses to overly alert, anxious individuals. Hyperaesthetic horses are hyper-responsive to stimuli and often jerk or tremor when stimulated. Depressed or lethargic horses may have either mild intracranial disease, systemic disease, or pain. A thorough physical examination is necessary to tell the difference. Obtunded horses do not respond to normal stimuli (such as a stranger walking to their stable) and only respond to increased stimuli (such as loud noises, sudden movements, or firm pressure). Stuporous horses only respond to painful stimuli (such as skin being squeezed with a haemostat). Comatose horses do not respond to any stimuli.

Evaluation of Cranial Nerves

The cranial nerve examination enables evaluation of the brainstem, afferent (sensory) and efferent (motor) limbs of reflex pathways, and the responses that involve the peripheral cranial nerves. The tests listed in Table 1 are sufficient to provide a complete evaluation of the cranial nerves and can be quickly performed during a routine physical examination.

Table 1. Tests of Cranial Nerve Function

Ser No	Test	Nerve Tested	Abnormal response/ interpretation
(a)	Menace	Optic, Facial	No eye blink. Must differentiate blindness from facial nerve dysfunction
(b)	Pupillary light response (PLR)	Optic, Oculomotor	No response to bright light directed in eye
(c)	Horner's syndrome	Cervical sympathetic	Sweating around base of ear and eye, ptosis
(d)	Facial sensation	Facial (sensory)	Failure to respond to stimulation of facial skin
(e)	Facial symmetry	Facial (Motor)	Asymmetry of muzzle, +/- ear droop, food impacted in cheek
(f)	Palpebral reflex	Trigeminal, Facial (motor)	Failure to blink
(g)	Nystagmus	Oculomotor, vestibular system	Central lesions associated with positional nystagmus; peripheral lesions are non-positional
(h)	Swallow	Glossopharyngeal, Vagus	Inability to swallow as determined by observation or passing of stomach tube
(i)	Tongue tone	Hypoglossal	Failure to withdraw tongue, or tongue weak when pulled

(a) **CN I: Olfactory nerve**: This carries sensory afferents associated with smell and deficits are rarely detected. A positive response to a familiar smell such as the owner's hand or a hand containing feed, or a negative response to an unfamiliar smell such as a spirit-soaked swab can be assessed with the horse blindfolded.

(b) **CN II: Optic nerve**: Observing the animal in its normal environment may assess its function or when negotiating an obstacle course, through which the horse is encouraged to walk. Unilateral deficits can be evaluated by blindfolding one eye. Additionally, the menace response, which is absent in neonates, is evaluated by making a threatening movement towards the eye, but without touching it. Care should be taken to avoid generating air currents that may be sensed by a visually impaired horse. A normal menace response includes abrupt closure of the eyelids and occasionally moving the head away and indicates a functional pathway that includes the ipsilateral refractory media of the eyeball, the retina, the optic disc and chiasm, and primarily the contra- lateral optic tract, the lateral geniculate nucleus (thalamus), the optic radiation and the cerebral occipital cortex. Modifying pathways involve the cerebellum. The pupillary light reflexes (PLRs) are assessed by shining a bright light into each eye in turn, ideally in a darkened environment. The normal response is a reflex constriction of the ipsilateral and contralateral (consensual) pupil (CN III) – the latter being more difficult to evaluate.

(c) **CN III: Oculomotor nerve**: This is responsible for innervation of the pupillary constrictor muscles and extraocular muscles (excluding the dorsal oblique (CN IV) and lateral rectus (CN VI)). A lesion affecting this nerve will not affect vision but usually produces a dilated pupil (mydriasis). In addition, the PLR will be absent when light is directed at the eye on the affected side and the consensual PLR will be absent when light is directed at the contralateral eye. Lesions of CN III result in ventrolateral strabismus however, mild ventrolateral strabismus is seen commonly when a normal horse's head is elevated.

(d) **CN IV: Trochlear nerve**: CN IV innervates the dorsal oblique extraocular muscle. Lesions are rare, but may result in strabismus.

(e) **CN V: Trigeminal nerve**. This provides the sensory innervation for most of the head via its three divisions (mandibular, maxillary and ophthalmic). In addition, the mandibular branch provides the motor innervation for the muscles of mastication. Unilateral abnormalities of motor function may be seen as unilateral muscle wastage of the masseter and temporalis muscles. If a bilateral lesion is present, a dropped jaw and dysphagia may be evident in addition to muscle atrophy. Sensory function may be assessed by pinching the skin over the head in the regions supplied by each of the three branches of the trigeminal nerve. Gentle stimulation will usually produce local twitching of the ears, eyelids or lips, mediated via the facial nerve (CN VII). More sustained stimulation will usually induce a behavioural (withdrawal) response.

(f) **CN VI: Abducens nerve**: This is responsible for innervation of the lateral rectus extraocular and retractor bulbi muscles. Dysfunction may result in a medial strabismus together with inability to retract the globe and is assessed by placing steady digital pressure through the eyelid on the cornea (sensory CN V), and feeling for reflex retraction.

(g) **CN VII: Facial nerve**: This nerve controls movements of the eyelids, ears, lips and nostrils and is assessed during the menace response and the palpebral reflex. Facial paralysis is usually recognized by drooping of the ear and lips on the affected side with ptosis of the upper eyelid and a deviation of the muzzle and nares towards the normal side. Inability to close the eyelids, together with reduced or absent tear production, may result in corneal ulceration. If there is only weakness of the lips and a deviated muzzle, without an ear droop and ptosis, there is probably only involvement of the buccal facial nerve branches and a peripheral lesion is more likely (e.g. following trauma).

(f) **CN VIII: Vestibulocochlear nerve**: CN VIII includes the vestibular (balance) and cochlear (auditory) nerves. Hearing loss, unless bilateral and complete, is difficult to assess. Vestibular disease may present as abnormalities of balance, a head tilt or pathological nystagmus. The eyes are examined for normal vestibular nystagmus when the head is moved from side to side. Spontaneous nystagmus (horizontal, rotary or vertical) is abnormal. In general, disorders of the peripheral vestibular nerve (or inner ear) result in a head tilt (down on the affected side) and, in acute disease, the fast phase of nystagmus being directed away from the side of the lesion. Signs of vestibular disease may be exacerbated by blindfolding the animal to remove any compensatory visual input, but take care because this may result in the animal falling. Central vestibular disease can result in any form of nystagmus, or nystagmus that alters its form, and may be associated with ataxia and weakness (due to damage to the descending brainstem upper motor neuron pathways). It is important to distinguish a head tilt from a head turn: in the former, the rotation occurs around the axial plane, and the eye and ear on the affected side are lower; head turns result in the head/neck being turned away from the long axis of the horse.

(g) **CN-IX (Glossopharyngeal nerve)/ CN-X (Vagus nerve)/ CN XI (Spinal accessory nerve)**: These nerves collectively provide the sensory and motor input for normal pharyngeal and laryngeal function. Disorders of these nerves therefore result in pharyngeal and laryngeal paralysis. Normal pharyngeal and laryngeal function can be assessed by observing and listening during normal breathing and swallowing, and/or during an (un-sedated) endoscopic examination of the pharynx and larynx. Pharyngeal paralysis usually results in signs of dysphagia (nasal return of food), and laryngeal paralysis results in signs of inspiratory dyspnoea. In both cases bilateral involvement is associated with more severe clinical signs.

(h) **CN XII: Hypoglossal nerve.**This nerve provides motor function to the tongue. The tongue should therefore be evaluated for normal movement, tone and signs of atrophy.

Spinal Reflexes and Muscle Evaluation (Tone and Size)

Tendon reflexes should be performed in recumbent adult horses but may be difficult to interpret. Withdrawal reflexes should be assessed in recumbent horses. Reflexes that the practitioner should assess in the standing horse include: cervicofacial/auricular and cutaneous trunci (panniculus), tail tone, perineal reflex, and anal tone. Additionally, the clinician should carefully observe the patient for any loss of skin sensation (hypalgesia or analgesia), increased sensitivity (hyperesthesia), or abnormal sweating indicative of sympathetic denervation. All horses should be carefully inspected for any signs of muscle atrophy.

Limb Placement and Panniculus Tests

These tests can be quickly performed and have value in detecting muscular weakness and conscious proprioceptive deficits. Abnormal limb positions, particularly a base-wide stance in the front limbs, may also be associated with vestibular disease. Limb placement tests are easier to perform and interpret on the front limbs. Typically, one front hoof is lifted, then placed across the other front leg. Horses should quickly move the hoof back into normal position, or resist placement into an abnormal position. An abnormal response is to leave the hoof in this crossed position for a prolonged period (usually more than several seconds), or to attempt to move the foot back to a normal position but have difficulty in doing so. The demeanour and training of the horse must be carefully considered a slow response in a 3-year-old Thoroughbred in race training is abnormal, but a similar response in an aged gelding may be normal. Placing the foot (either front or rear) in a base-wide position can also be performed, and the expected response is for the horse to return the foot into a normal position. Limb placement tests in horses appear to have a low sensitivity for the detection of abnormalities of the CNS, and these tests should be coupled with careful observation of foot placement during dynamic manoeuvres. The panniculus response is tested by stimulating the skin over the trunk, then observing for a "skin- flick" response. Perianal skin reactions should be evaluated, for loss of this response is characteristic of herpes virus myeloencephalitis.

Gait Analysis

The gait analysis is the process of evaluating the horse in motion at a walk and possibly trot, and when the horse is asked to perform certain manoeuvres that "challenge" specific functions of the nervous system. These tests includes:

(a) Waking with the head elevated

(b) Downhill

(c) Backing

(d) Turning in tight circles.

(e) Moving over or around obstacles.

Specific neurological abnormalities that are observed during this phase of the examination include:

(a) **Ataxia:** Ataxia refers to the lack of coordination of motor movements and may be categorized as vestibular, cerebellar, or sensory in origin. Sensory ataxia seems to predominate in the horse, associated with spinal cord disease in which proprioceptive (ascending) input to the cerebellum is compromised. Ataxia is a description of clinical signs, rather than a specific diagnosis, and it may occur alone or with spasticity or paresis. Sensory ataxia is frequently associated with paresis, and it is often difficult to discriminate between the two deficits in clinical cases. Cerebellar ataxia is seen in foals with cerebellar abiotrophy, and rarely in inflammatory disease of the CNS, and is characterized by symmetric ataxia with intention tremors and retention of strength. Vestibular ataxia is usually associated with a head tilt and asymmetric ataxia. Ataxia is expressed in the horse as truncal sway, weaving during walking (i.e., placing feet out of line from one step to the next), crossing over when turning, or pivoting on the inside limb when spun. Additional signs include weaving of the affected limb during the swing phase of the stride, resulting in abnormal foot placement. Signs of ataxia are most noticeable at changes of speed and direction. Careful observation of the horse when turning in hand may reveal abducted or adducted foot placement, or pivoting. If abruptly pulled up from a trot in hand, ataxic horses will often crouch and go base wide in the rear limbs. Signs of ataxia will be exacerbated when walked on a slope or with its head elevated. These deficits are similar to those seen with proprioceptive deficits, and the two disorders often co-exist.

(b) **Paresis**: Paresis is a deficiency of voluntary movement arising from a reduction in normal muscular power. Paresis can arise from damage to upper motor neurons (UMNs), LMNs, or muscle itself. UMN weakness results from disorders that affect the UMN or their axons in the cerebral cortex, subcortical white matter, brainstem, or spinal cord. Weakness is induced by decreased activation of LMNs and may be accompanied by spasticity. Differentiation of UMN and LMN disease may help with neuroanatomic localization and understanding the distribution of the lesion resulting in the observed clinical signs (Figure 2). Table 2 describes clinical signs that can aid in the differentiation of UMN and LMN disease. Weak (paretic) horses have a low arc of foot flight, stumble, and have a poor response to the sway test. An additional sign of weakness in the horse is knuckling when going downhill, or difficulty when hopping on one thoracic limb ("hop test"). The sway test demonstrates an animal's ability to resist when being pushed off balance. When pushed at the withers, most adult horses should be able to resist, or quickly step sideways if pushed off balance. Weak horses cannot resist and recover poorly (slowly) after being pushed sideways. A similar procedure is used in the rear limbs and is referred to as the "tail-pull." In this test, the horse is pulled sideways using the tail. Most adult horses can easily resist even a strong pull. This test should also be done when the horse is walking. As the horse is walking, the tail should be strongly pulled to the side then quickly released; this should be repeated several times at different phases of the stride. Normal horses should quickly correct rear limb position with the next stride, while paretic horses are more easily pulled off balance, may take several strides to recover, or interfere while attempting to correct. Horses that demonstrate good rear limb strength standing still, but are weak when walking usually have UMN disease.

(c) **Dysmetria**: Dysmetria refers to a gait in which the limb movements are either hypermetric or hypometric. A hypermetric gait is characterized with an exaggerated range of motion and excessive joint movement and is associated with cerebellar and spinal cord (spinocerebellar) disease. Hypometria is described as limb stiffness and decreased joint flexion and gives the appearance of a "tin-soldier." It is often seen as an exaggerated flight phase in horses when going downhill, or with the head elevated. Spasticity is an increase in muscle tone that primarily affects anti-gravity muscles. Spasticity is velocity dependent and demonstrates a sudden release after reaching a maximum muscle tension (the "clasp- knife reflex"). Spasticity is generally associated with UMN disease and is due to the reduced inhibition of extensor motor neurons. Spasticity is most easily demonstrated in recumbent animals, but the "bouncing" gait seen in rear limbs of horses with cervical lesions may be an expression of spasticity and exaggerated extensor tone.

Each examiner can establish his or her own approach to performing the gait analysis. The most preferred way is to first observe the horse being led at a walk from the front, back, and side. It is helpful to walk alongside the horse, matching speed, and concentrate on detecting the various gait deficits. Each limb should be observed independently and is scored using the standardized scoring system (Table 3).

Table 2. Clinical Signs that Help to Differentiate Upper and Lower Motor Neuron Disease.

S. No.	Lower Motor Neuron (LMN) Weakness	Upper Motor Neuron (UMN) Weakness
(a)	Flaccid	Spasticity
(b)	Decreased tone	Increased tone
(c)	Diminished reflex response	Exaggerated reflex response
(d)	Profound muscle atrophy	Minimal muscle atrophy
(e)	Fasciculations present	Fasciculations absent

Table 3. Grading system for gait analysis.

S. No.	Grade	Description
(a)	0	No neurologic deficits detected
(b)	1	Neurologic deficits just detected at a normal gait but worsened by backing, turning, loin pressure, or neck extension
(c)	2	Neurologic deficits easily detected at the walk and exaggerated by backing, turning, loin pressure, or neck extension
(d)	3	Neurologic deficits prominent at the walk, with a tendency to buckle or fall with backing, turning, loin pressure, or neck extension. Postural deficits noted at rest
(e)	4	Stumbling, tripping, and falling spontaneously at a normal gait
(f)	5	Horse recumbent

Table 4. Prominent gait postural abnormalities present with neurological lesion at different locations.

S. No.	Lesion location	Postural deficit	Paresis	Ataxia	Hypometria	Hypermetria
(a)	Cerebrum	+++	0	0	0	0
(b)	Brain Stem	++	++	++	++	
(c)	Vestibular	+++	0	++	++	0
(d)	Cerebellum	++	0	+++	+	+++
(e)	Spinal cord UMN	++	++	++	++	++
(f)	Peripheral nerve/ LMN	++	+++	+	(++)*	(+++)*
(g)	Musculoskeletal	+	++	0	+	0

Grading System

(a) 0 - Not usually expected

(b) + - Mild if present

(c) ++ - Usually present

(d) +++ - Quite present (characteristically present)

(e) * - Usually only selective sensory fibre involvement

Examination of Recumbent Patients

Neurologic evaluation of the recumbent patient presents unique challenges to the clinician. The effects of recumbency may alter responses and lead to complications such as peripheral neuropathies that are not part of the primary diagnosis. In addition, fear and anxiety induced by recumbency, exhaustion from struggling, or dehydration may influence the results obtained.

(a) A general observation will reveal if the horse has normal mentation, suggesting a lesion caudal to C1.

(b) If the horse can attain a dog-sitting position, demonstrating good strength and coordination of the pectoral limbs, then the lesion is likely to be caudal to T2.

(c) Loss of pectoral limb strength, while retaining the ability to lift the head and cranial neck, suggests an extreme caudal cervical lesion, such as C6–T2.

(d) The Schiff–Sherrington phenomenon describes a condition of increased forelimb tone and flaccid paralysis of the hind limbs and has been seen in horses, associated with spinal cord lesions between T2 and L4.

(e) Specific spinal reflexes can be tested in recumbent horses. Spinal reflexes require only an intact sensory nerve, spinal cord segment(s), an intact peripheral motor nerve (LMN), and muscle. Perception of the stimulus requires intact ascending sensory pathways, and horses may have an intact reflex without perception of the stimulus. In the pectoral limbs, the flexor, triceps, and biceps reflexes can be evaluated.

(f) The flexor (withdrawal) reflex is tested by clamping the skin over the distal limb and observing for withdrawal of the limb associated with flexion of the fetlock, carpus, elbow, and shoulder. The reflex is mediated by sensory fibers in the median and ulnar nerves, spinal cord segments C6–T2, and motor fibers of the axillary, median, musculocutaneous, and ulnar nerves. Peripheral nerve trauma from recumbency can lead to sensory nerve damage, and depression and/or exhaustion can lead to a diminished response; hence this reflex must be evaluated carefully.

(g) **The biceps reflex** is tested by balloting the muscle belly of the biceps and brachialis muscles with a plexor and felling for muscle contraction. This reflex is mediated by the **musculocutaneous nerves** and spinal cord segments **C6-C7**. It is more readily detected in foals and may be difficult to detect in adult horses.

(h) **The triceps reflex** is tested by slightly flexing the limb, then balloting the distal portion of the triceps at its point of insertion. A positive reflex is the observation of triceps muscle contraction. The reflex pathway tested involves the radial nerve and spinal cord segments C7–T1.

(j) **The patellar reflex** in the rear limbs can be tested in both foals and adults. In this test, the limb is moderately flexed, and the patellar tendon balloted with a heavy plexor or the examiners hand in a "karate- chop" motion. A diminished response can be seen in horses with botulism or femoral nerve disease. Exaggerated responses to any of these segmental reflexes are associated with UMN disease cranial to the site of the spinal cord segments tested by the reflex.

Differentiating Neurogenic and Musculoskeletal Gait Abnormalities

Normal response during the nervous system examination requires a sound musculoskeletal system; hence musculoskeletal disease will lead to abnormalities of the neurologic examination. In particular, multiple limb lameness, or bilateral hind limb lameness, will cause horses to stumble, interfere, or pivot when spinning. These cases are particularly challenging because the characteristic gait abnormalities associated with a particular lameness will be altered by the presence of lameness in other limbs. Careful observation of the horse's gait and application of a few basic principles can simplify the process, however in general, the horse with a musculoskeletal problem has a gait which is regularly irregular. That is, the horse may take an abnormal step, or have abnormal placement; however, the abnormality is the same from step to step. In contrast, the gait in a horse with neurologic disease is irregularly irregular. The foot placement or step will vary from one step to the next. Furthermore, in horses with neurologic disease, the abnormality should be apparent in all phases of the gait examination, although particular manoeuvres may make the signs more obvious. If a deficit is seen only during circling, for example, yet not detected during downhill, backing, or walking in a line, then hock soreness should be investigated. Treatment of the horse with non-steroidal anti- inflammatory drugs (NSAIDs) will minimize clinical signs of musculoskeletal disease, yet will not commonly influence neurologic disorders. Hence, examination before and after treatment with NSAIDs can be a useful aid in some cases. Finally, the use of nerve blocks and joint anaesthesia, followed by a repeat nervous system examination, can be done. If local anaesthesia resolves the previously identified gait abnormality, then musculoskeletal disease must be the cause.

Neuroanatomic Localization and Case Synthesis

Once the physical examination, history, and neurologic examination are complete, neuroanatomic localization of the nervous system abnormality is determined. Differential considerations can then be constructed and evaluated. The results of the neurologic examination should allow the examiner to determine which area or areas of the nervous system are affected. Basic neuroanatomic divisions are the cerebral cortex, brain stem, vestibular system, cerebellum, spinal cord, or peripheral nerve. In general, cranial nerve signs indicate a lesion cranial to the foramen magnum. A horse with a normal sensorium and no cranial nerve deficits has a lesion(s) caudal to the foramen magnum. Gait deficits are assigned a "score" based on the criteria described in Table 3. Clinical signs associated with abnormalities of different segments of the spinal cord are presented in Table 5. In general, cervical lesions (C1–C6) result in proprioceptive deficits, weakness, and ataxia that involve all four limbs, but are one grade worse in the rear limbs than the front limbs. A gait deficit that is worse in the front limbs than the rear suggests a lesion within the region of the brachial intumescence (C7–T2). Neurologic gait deficits that involve the rear limbs with normal front limbs indicate a lesion in the thoracolumbar region. In general, the examiner should attempt to explain the neurologic deficits observed by a single lesion site; if this is not possible, multifocal disease must exist, which is important in differential diagnosis. Clinical signs associated with various parts of the nervous system are summarized in Table 6. In addition, the presence of symmetry or asymmetry must be evaluated. Some conditions, such as cervical compression, cauda equina syndrome, and EDEM, are symmetrical, while others, especially EPM, are characteristically asymmetric. The history of the neurologic disease should be considered, as some conditions have an acute onset (such as fracture), while others have a more chronic or insidious course (i.e., EPM). The presence of systemic dis- ease, fever, and anorexia is an important clue indicating the presence of an infectious disease, such as EEE, WEE, rabies, WNV, or meningitis.

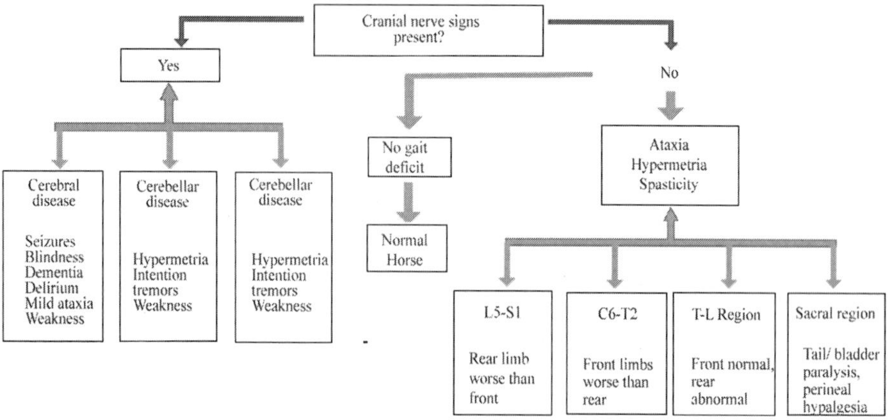

Fig. 2. A flow chart demonstrating how the results of the neurologic examination can be used to aid the clinician in neuroanatomic localization.

Table 5. Clinical abnormalities associated with different segments of the spinal cord.

S. No.	Spinal Segment	Clinical Sign
(a)	C1-C5	Spastic gait, worse in rear limbs Proprioceptive deficits Weakness +/– Horner's syndrome
(b)	C6-T2	Proprioceptive deficits, worse in front than rear Weakness Muscle atrophy, thoracic limbs +/– Horner's syndrome
(c)	T3-L3	Proprioceptive deficits, rear Normal gait, front Rear limb weakness Spasticity, pelvic limbs
(d)	S3-S5	Urinary incontinence Fecal retention Hypalgesia tail and perianal Normal thoracic and pelvic
(e)	Coccygeal	Decreased tail tone Hypalgesia caudal to lesion Normal front and rear limbs

Table 6. Clinical Signs Associated with Disease of Various Anatomic Regions of the Nervous System

Ser No	Anatomic Region	Predominant Clinical sign
(a)	Cerebral cortex	Postural deficits, seizures, altered mentation, blindness
(b)	Brain stem	Ataxia, weakness and dysmetria, mild to moderate. Dysphagia, anisocoria, or dilated pupils possible

(c)	Vestibular system	Ataxia, head tilt, postural deficits pronounced
(d)	Cerebellum	Ataxia and intention tremors
(e)	Spinal cord UMN	Paresis, ataxia, and dysmetria all present and mild to moderate. Spasticity is prominent
(f)	Peripheral nerve/ LMN	Weakness predominates

Sample Neurological Examination Form

Hops No.:	
Colour:	**Sex:**
Date:	**Age:**
History:	
Behaviour/ Mentation:	
Head/ Neck position:	

Cranial nerve examination

Reflex	Left	Right	Remarks
Vison			
Menace			
PLR			
Horner's syndrome			
Facial sensation			
Facial symmetry			
Palpebral reflex			
Nystagmus			
Swallow			
Tongue tone			

Spinal reflexes and muscle evaluation

Reflex	Left	Right
Cutaneous trunci		
Perineal reflex		
Cervicofacial / auricular		
Skin sensation		
Muscle atrophy		

Grade	Description
0	No neurologic deficits detected
1	Neurologic deficits just detected at a normal gait but worsened by backing, turning, loin pressure, or neck extension
2	Neurologic deficits easily detected at the walk and exaggerated by backing, turning, loin pressure, or neck extension
3	Neurologic deficits prominent at the walk, with a tendency to buckle or fall with backing, turning, loin pressure, or neck extension. Postural deficits noted at rest
4	Stumbling, tripping, and falling spontaneously at a normal gait
5	Horse recumbent

Gait and posture evaluation (description of stride)

Test	Description
Straight line	
Serpentine	
Head elevated	
Tail pull	
Circling	
Backing	

Grade	Description
0	No neurologic deficits detected
1	Neurologic deficits just detected at a normal gait but worsened by backing, turning, loin pressure, or neck extension
2	Neurologic deficits easily detected at the walk and exaggerated by backing, turning, loin pressure, or neck extension
3	Neurologic deficits prominent at the walk, with a tendency to buckle or fall with backing, turning, loin pressure, or neck extension. Postural deficits noted at rest
4	Stumbling, tripping, and falling spontaneously at a normal gait
5	Horse recumbent

Prominent gait postural abnormalities present with neurological lesion at different locations.

Ser No	Lesion location	Postural deficit	Paresis	Ataxia	Hypo-metria	Hyper-metria
(a)	Cerebrum	+++	0	0	0	0
(b)	Brain Stem	++	++	++	++	
(c)	Vestibular	+++	0	++	++	0
(d)	Cerebellum	++	0	+++	+	+++
(e)	Spinal cord UMN	++	++	++	++	++
(f)	Peripheral nerve/ LMN	++	+++	+	(++)*	(+++)*
(g)	Musculoskeletal	+	++	0	+	0
	Grading System (a) 0 - Not usually expected (b) + - Mild if present (c) ++ - Usually present (d) +++ - Quite present (characteristically present) (e) * - Usually only selective sensory fibre involvement					

Interpretation

Anatomic diagnosis: ______________________________

Differential diagnosis: ______________________________

Diagnostic plan: ______________________________

Therapeutic plan: ______________________________

References

Adams R, Mayhew IG. 1984. Neurological examination of newborn foals. *Equine Vet J* 16:306–12.

Chiapetta JR, Baker JC, Feeney DA. 1985. Vertebral fracture, extensor hypertonia of thoracic limbs, and paralysis of pelvic limbs (Schiff–Sherrington syndrome) in an Arabian foal. *J Am Vet Med Assoc* 186:387–8.

Greet TR, Jeffcott LB, Whitwell KE, *et al.* 1980. The slap test for laryngeal adductors function in horses with suspected cervical spinal cord damage. *Equine Vet J* 12:127–31.

Hahn CN, Mayhew IG, MacKay R. 1999. Nervous system. In *Equine Medicine and Surgery*, edited by Colahan PT, Mayhew IG, Merritt AM, Moore JN,863–996. St. Louis, MO:Mosby.

Mayhew IJ. 1989. Neurologic evaluation. In *Large Animal Neurology*, edited by Mayhew IG,15-47. Philadelphia, PA:Lea and Febinger.

Newton-Clarke MJ, Divers TJ, Delahunta A, *et al.* 1994. Evaluation of the thoraco-laryngeal reflex ("slap test") as an aid to the diagnosis of cervical spinal cord and brainstem disease in horses. *Equine Vet J* 26:358–61.

Oliver JE, Lorenz MD, Kornegay JM. 1997. Ataxia of the head and the limbs. In *Handbook of Veterinary Neurology*, edited by Oliver JE, Lorenz MD, Kornegay JM, 216–39. Philadelphia, PA:W.B. Saunders Co.

Reed SM. 1992. The neurologic examination of the horse for purchase. In *Vet Clin North Am (Equine Practice)*, edited by Beeman GM, 377–87. Philadelphia, PA:W.B. Saunders, Co.

Reed SM. 1998. Neurologic examination. In *Equine Internal Medicine*, edited by Reed SM, Bailey WM, 427–34. Philadelphia, PA:W.B. Saunders Co.

Rooney JR. 1973. Two cervical reflexes in the horse. *J Am Vet Med Assoc* 162:117–119.

Stephen M. Reed. 2008. Neurology is not a euphemism for necropsy: A review of selected neurological diseases affecting horses. AAEP Proceedings Vol 54

22

Trends of Disease Burden and Demographic Transition in Mithun *(Bos frontalis)* Populations of Northeast India

Vivek Joshi*, J.K. Chamuah, Vikram R. and P.S. Girish

ICAR-National Research Centre on Mithun, Medziphema, Nagaland
**Division of Medicine, ICAR-IVRI, Izatnagar, Uttar Pradesh*
Haryana Pashu Vigyan Kendre, Karnal, Haryana

Introduction

Mithun *(Bos frontalis),* or 'Gayal' or 'Eso' or 'Sial' or 'Sandong' or 'Wei', is a rare bovine species, exclusively found in the northeastern hill region (NEHR) of India at an altitude of 300-3000 m. It plays an important role in the socio-economic and cultural life of indigenous tribes of Arunachal Pradesh, Nagaland, Mizoram and Manipur and is aptly referred to as the 'Pride of Northeast India' (Mukherjee et al. 2019). Besides India, mithun population is distributed to China, Bangladesh, Thailand, Bhutan, Myanmar, and Malaysia. The Indian mithun is a medium- to large-sized majestic ruminant with a characteristic jet-black body, an ash-colored forehead, and 'white stockings' on all the limbs. This unique animal has a special preference for salt feeding, is a skilled browser even in steep, hilly terrain, and does not need pasture land like cattle. Mithun is primarily reared under a free-range system as an important source of lean meat, rich in amino acids, proteins, PUFA, etc. On September 1, 2023, the Food Safety and Standards Authority of India (FSSAI) officially certified the mithun as a food animal (Joshi et al., 2021; Lalchamliani et al., 2024; Ramesh et al., 2024). Compared to milk from other species, mithun milk has much larger quantities of fat, lactose, solids-not-fat (SNF), calcium, important vitamins A, D, and E, essential amino acids, and polyunsaturated fatty acids (Devi et al., 2023).

As Indian mithun inhabits remote forests with undulating topography and adverse climatic conditions, it remains one of the neglected and least studied species. The International Union for Conservation of Nature (IUCN) has classified Indian mithuns as vulnerable species. As per the 20th Livestock Census, mithun population in India currently stands at 0.39 million. However, with a constant decline in mithun population over the recent years, it is advocated to rear free-ranging mithun under semi-intensive system for its conservation (Joshi et al. 2021).

Trends of Disease Burden in Mithun

Many facets of health and diseases that affect mithun are not well understood, and research is currently ongoing, due to the species' geographic restriction to a very small part of the world and its extremely challenging hilly terrain. The clinical forms of only few diseases are prevalent, while serological investigations have documented several important diseases.

Specific Diseases	Non-specific Diseases
• Viral diseases • Bacterial diseases • Parasitic diseases • Fungal diseases • Metabolic diseases	• Inappetence/Anorexia • Diarrhea/ Constipation • Trichobezoar formation • Abscess (Facial abscess) • Conjunctivitis (Pink eye) • Cataracts • Syncope/ Sudden death

Viral Diseases

(1) Foot and Mouth Disease (FMD)

FMD has emerged as the single most economically devastating disease among mithuns in the northeastern states of India. Mithun is comparatively more susceptible to FMD than other livestock species. The morbidity of the disease is usually 60-100% with reports of high mortality. Low vaccination coverage of FMD vaccine in eligible mithuns is the commonest risk factor for outbreaks in mithun. It is primarily spread through inhalation of virus aerosols; however, airborne transmission of virus is also suspected during outbreaks. The clinical presentation in mithun is identical to FMD in cattle, including the post-mortem findings. The typical clinical sign is the development of vesicles on the muzzle, tongue, lips and in the interdigital space. Bloody nasal discharge from 3rd to 4th day is a characteristic of FMD in mithun. In contrast to cattle, lesions of the teats and mammary gland are uncommon in mithun. Maggoted wound or wound myiasis is the most serious complication of FMD in free-ranging mithuns.

In mithun, FMD is caused by serotypes O, A, and Asia-1, of which serotype O is primarily responsible for most of the outbreaks. FMD outbreaks are common in mithun during late monsoon and winter seasons. During 1974 to 2004, a total of 12 outbreaks of FMD were recorded in mithun. Over the past decade (2009-2019), there have been 120 confirmed FMD outbreaks in four mithun rearing states (Arunachal Pradesh, Nagaland, Manipur, Mizoram). The predominant serotype causing outbreaks was 'O' followed by 'Asia 1' and 'A'. These viruses isolated from mithun are genetically similar to those causing FMD in domestic cattle suggesting a situation of virus sharing between mithun and domestic cattle.

Thus, there is an urgent need to synchronously vaccinate mithuns along with cattle for the effective control and eradication of the disease (Joshi et al., 2021).

Year of outbreak	Number of outbreaks	Isolated serotype(s)
2009-10	22	O
2010-11	9	O, Asia-1
2011-12	16	O, A
2012-13	39	O, Asia-1
2013-14	12	O, A
2014-15	5	O
2015-16	10	O, Asia-1
2016-17	2	O
2017-18	4	O
2018-19	2	O

(2) Infectious Bovine Rhinotracheitis (IBR)

Red nose or IBR is a highly contagious viral disease of bovine species caused by bovine herpes virus-1 (BHV-1). It is characterized by high fever, clinical signs of upper airway and abortion. The virus is transmitted through all secretions and excretions. There is a strong possibility that IBR could also manifest in clinical or subclinical form in mithun, as a seroprevalence investigation revealed that the disease is common in this species. Arunachal Pradesh has the highest prevalence (38.46%), followed by Mizoram (18.18%) and Nagaland (15.15%). Mithuns >3 years old have the highest seroprevalence of IBR (27.03%), followed by those between 1-3 years old (18.42%) and those between 6 months-1 year (7.69%). Mithun breeding bulls have a higher seroprevalence of IBR (88.9%), which is comparable to cattle. However, unlike cattle, the overall prevalence (19%) of IBR is shown to be lower in mithun. This could be because the mithun is resistant to the illness (Rajkhowa et al., 2004).

(3) Rotavirus Diarrhea

Rotavirus was initially discovered using polymerase chain reaction (PCR) in young mithun calves that had diarrhea. Dehydration and watery diarrhea are the major clinical manifestations. According to serological research, the prevalence of antibodies was higher in free-range animals, and adult mithuns older than 3 years had higher antibody titers.

(4) Bovine Coronavirus (BCoV)

BCoV is a pneumoenteric virus that cause respiratory and enteric infections in cattle and wild ruminants. This virus is normally associated with diarrhea in neonatal calves, and winter dysentery and shipping fever in adult cattle. According to serological investigations, the overall prevalence of antibodies against coronavirus was 80%. Mithuns >3 years old had the highest seroprevalence, whereas those between 7-12 months had the lowest (Rajkhowa et al., 2007).

(5) Bluetongue

Bluetongue is an insect-borne viral disease that affects domestic and wild ruminants. It is caused by different serotypes (currently up to 26) of bluetongue virus (BTV). The disease is characterized by high fever (>105°F), reddening of the buccal and nasal mucosa, oral ulcers and inflammation of the coronary band causing lameness. Although serosurveys have indicated the presence of BTV antibodies in mithun in India, the clinical disease has not been observed. High BTV infection rate (86%) in mithun was found by serological analysis utilizing the competitive enzyme-linked immunosorbent test (cELISA). Mithun aged 1-2 years have the lowest prevalence (58%), while those aged >4 years have the highest prevalence rate (98%) (Rajkhowa et al., 2008).

(6) Bovine Viral Diarrhea (BVD)

Bovine viral diarrhea virus (BVDV) infection is a pestivirus infection affecting most even-toed ungulates. In addition to fever, decreased milk yield, abortion, diarrhea, and mortality, there can be an inapparent infection. For the first time, Singh et al. (2017) documented serological evidence of BVDV infection in mithun. The overall BVDV seroprevalence was 13.1%, which was less than the previous rates in India for cattle (37.6%) and buffaloes (30.76%). Contact with cattle during grazing is the most likely way that BVDV is contracted in mithun.

(7) Lumpy Skin Disease (LSD)

LSD is a vector-borne, notifiable disease of cattle characterised by fever (>41°C), nodules on the skin, mucous membranes and internal organs, decline in milk yield, temporary or permanent sterility in bulls and occasionally, death. It is caused by LSD virus (LSDV), belonging to the genus *Capripoxvirus* and the family Poxviridae. The first reports of LSD outbreaks in mithun were from Papum Pare (Arunachal Pradesh) and Kohima (Nagaland) in 2024. During widespread LSD outbreaks in the cattle herd, some mithuns developed signs like high fever, nasal discharge, and characteristic nodular lesions identical to those seen in LSD-affected cattle. The clinical signs in mithuns were milder than those in cattle and none of the mithuns died. Virus isolation and PCR assays that target the P32 gene were used to confirm that all mithuns exhibiting clinical signs had LSD. Mithun LSDV strains showed a 100% sequence similarity with the cattle LSDV field strain. This strongly implies that LSDV spillover from the cattle is the cause of LSD in mithun. According to serosurveys, the mithun population had a high level of LSDV exposure, with a 74.52% positive rate for anti-LSDV antibodies. Until a specific protocol is developed for mithun, the same vaccination protocol may be applied to both cattle and mithun (Reddy et al., 2024).

Bacterial Diseases

(1) Bovine Tuberculosis (bTB)

Bovine TB is a chronic infectious disease of cattle, other domesticated animals and certain wildlife populations caused by members of the *Mycobacterium tuberculosis* complex primarily by *M. Bovis*. It is a major zoonotic disease, causing tubercle formation in the lymph nodes and other tissues, fluctuating fever, intermittent hacking cough, weight loss, enlarged lymph nodes and eventual death. bTB spreads mainly through the movement of domestic animals that are infected but have not been diagnosed. bTB is recorded in mithuns by single intradermal (SID) tuberculin test and PCR. Only 1.28% of the mithuns tested positive for bTB in a PCR-based investigation, compared to 12% in the SID test. In mithuns older than six years, the SID test revealed the highest prevalence of bTB (19%) (Dubey, 2015; Rajkhowa et al., 2007).

(2) Brucellosis

Brucellosis is a contagious disease of livestock and other ruminants caused by *Brucella* bacteria. The disease is characterized by abortions or reproductive failure. Surveillance in mithuns using serological tests such as Rose Bengal plate test (RBPT), standard tube agglutination test (STAT) and avidin-biotin ELISA (A-B ELISA) revealed that mithun too suffers from brucellosis. Seroprevalence of brucellosis was recorded as 34% in A-B ELISA, 20% in STAT and 11% in RBPT. The highest seroprevalence was found in mithun cows followed by heifers and bulls (Rajkhowa et al., 2005). In a more recent investigation with a larger sample size, 8.97% of mithuns showed the prevalence of *Brucella* antibodies with RBPT (Dubey, 2015). In addition, iELISA was used to screen 160 serum samples from an organized mithun farm and the results demonstrated seronegativity for brucellosis (unpublished study).

(3) Black Quarter (BQ)

BQ is an acute, highly fatal disease caused by *Clostridium chauvoei* and is characterized by fever, inflammation with gaseous oedema of skeletal muscle and death. The clinical cases of BQ were first reported in free-ranging mithuns from Arunachal Pradesh (Heli, 1995). It occurs in mithuns aged 6 months to 2 years. Clinical signs include high fever (105-106°F) and swollen hind limb. The post-mortem reveals that the affected muscles are dark and discolored (gangrenous) with foul smelling exudate (Pradhan et al., 2023).

(4) Colibacillosis

Colibacillosis, caused by various serotypes of ENTEROTOXIGENIC *E. coli* (ETEC), is an acute disease that can cause diarrhea and SEPTICAEMIA in neonatal calves. White profuse watery diarrhea is characteristic of ETEC. Mortality rate is high and survivors are often affected by arthritis, meningitis or pneumonia. ETEC is also a leading cause of diarrhea in mithun calves. A wide range of serogroups of *E. coli* (O1, O2, O3, O4, O6, O9, O12, O15, O20, O21, O25, O26, O49, O55, O56, O68, O74, O116, O120, O141, O146, O149 O158, O161) are prevalent in mithun calves with diarrhea and can be detected through PCR. However, the frequency of ETEC in the fecal samples of mithun calves is low i.e. only very few isolates harbor ST and LT enterotoxin genes (Rajkhowa et al., 2009).

(5) Anthrax

Anthrax is an infectious disease caused by the spore-forming bacteria *Bacillus anthracis*. Antemortem clinical signs are usually absent in peracute and acute forms of the disease. Ruminants are often found dead with no indication of illness. Unclotted blood exudes from body openings and postmortem stiffening is absent. The tribal people who own mithuns have reported isolated cases with clinical signs resembling anthrax. The Monpa tribe in Arunachal Pradesh's West Kameng district is familiar with anthrax (Nivsarkar et al., 1997).

(6) Leptospirosis

Leptospirosis is caused by motile filamentous bacteria of the genus *Leptospira* and is a common cause of reproductive losses (abortion, infertility) in bovine worldwide. Recently, a total of 160 serum samples were collected from mithun and examined using microscopic agglutination test (MAT). The overall seroprevalence was 10.62%; however, additional large-scale research is necessary to have a better understanding of leptospirosis in mithun (unpublished work).

Fungal Diseases

(1) Ringworm

Ringworm is a common fungal infection of skin and hair present worldwide. In mithun, ringworm is caused by *Trichophyton verrucosum* and manifests as grey-white, slightly raised lesions with a powdery surface (2-4 cm) and alopecia (Annual Report, 2004-05).

Parasitic Diseases

(1) Nematodes

Parasitic Gastroenteritis (PGE)

PGE is a disease in ruminants caused by large numbers of gastrointestinal nematodes (roundworms) that inhabit the abomasum and intestines. The clinical disease is characterized by loss of appetite, scouring and reduced growth (up to 30%) in young calves, especially during their first grazing season. Adult animals show a decline in daily milk production. In mithun, PGE is a common condition and a major cause of morbidity and mortality in young mithun calves. The most common roundworms of mithun are *Haemonchus contortus, Oesophagostomum* spp., *Trichostrongylus* spp., *Mecistocirrus* spp., *Cooperia* spp., *Trichuris* spp., *Toxocara* spp., *Strogyloides* spp. and *Bunostomum* spp. Among these, *Toxocara vitulorum, Strongyloides papillosus, Bunostmum phlebotomum* and *Haemonchus contortus* are the major causes of anemia and mortality in mithun calves below 1 year of age (Chamuah et al., 2013).

(2) Trematodes and Cestodes

The clinical cases of fascioliosis (Fasciola gigantica) and immature amphistomosis (*Paramphistomum, Gastrothylax crumenifer, Cotylophoron cotylophorum, Fischoderius elongatus*) are occasionally observed in mithun. Among tapeworms, *Moniezia expansa* and *M. benedeni* are quite common in both adult and young mithuns. Hydatidosis is also frequently recorded during postmortem examination of mithun (Chamuah, 2005).

(3) Protozoal infection

Eimeria bovis, E. aurburnensis, E. alabamensis and *E. zurnii* are the most prevalent eimerian species in mithun (Chamuah et al., 2014). Other important protozoan parasites of mithun include *Balantidium coli, Cryptosporidium parvum* and *C. bovis* (Rajkhowa et al., 2006). Seroprevalence of *Neospora caninum* and *Toxoplasma gondii* is recorded as 10% and 42%, respectively, in free-ranging mithun. Recently, serological screening of 160 serum samples using iELISA revealed a seropositivity rate of 38.75% for trypanosomiasis in mithun.

(4) Ectoparasitic infestation (Ticks and Leeches)

Ticks (*Boophilus microplus*) and aquatic leeches (*Tyranobdella rex*) are the notable hematophagous external parasites of mithun (Joshi et al., 2022).

Metabolic Diseases

Although clinical forms of metabolic diseases are not prevalent in mithun, subclinical ketosis (SCK) and subclinical hypocalcemia (SHC) have been reported from farmed mithun population. Their prevalence rates were <20% indicating adequate health and nutritional management of farmed mithuns (unpublished work).

Demographic Shifts in Mithun Populations

Despite the promising potential of semi-intensive mithun farming, tribal farmers have not given this endeavor much thought and continue to raise mithun as a free-range animal, subjecting it to deadly diseases and unfavourable environment on a daily basis. This has led to a decrease in the number of free-ranging mithuns over the past few years. The overall number of mithun increased by 30.6%, however there were declines of 33.6% and 10.5% in Nagaland and Manipur, respectively (Livestock Census, 2019).

S. No.	Causal factors	Remedial measures
1.	Misconceptions and ignorance regarding vaccination	Routine FMD vaccination High immunization coverage of FMD vaccine in mithun populations
2.	Cross-border travel and interspecies contact (cattle, pig)	Mithun's inclusion in the National Livestock Mission (NLM) to improve vaccination rates
3.	Habitat loss due to deforestation and Jhum cultivation	Community conservation centres for mithun (1 per 3-4 villages), Longer jhoom cycles
4.	Reduction in size of the pastoral area	Fodder cultivation in nurseries that mithun relishes
5.	Absence of bankable schemes and insurance for mithun	Development of bankable schemes and insurance plans for mithun by the state govt.
6.	Predator attacks on mithun calves are common	Implementation of semi-intensive farming and the fencing of mithun raising areas
7.	Mithun is overused for table purposes	Legislative laws for the slaughter of mithun
8.	No consistent revenue from mithun	Mithun farming that is organic Alternative uses of mithun (milking, draughtability, vermicomposting, using mithun manure as FYM, etc.)
9.	Farmers' migration from rural to urban regions	Creation of village-level employment plans

References

Annual Report (2004-05) Annual Report for the year 2000–2001. National Research Centre on Mithun, Jharnapani, Nagaland, India.

Chamuah, J. K., Perumal, P., Singh, V., Mech, A., & Borkotoky, D. (2013). Helminth parasites of mithun (Bos frontalis)-An overview. The Indian Journal of Animal Sciences, 83(3).

Chamuah J K. 2005. Studies on some aspects of parasites of mithun (Bos frontalis). M.V.Sc. Thesis submitted to Assam Agricultural University, Khanapara, Guwahati-22.

Chamuah, J. K., Dutta, P. R., Borkotoky, D., Vupru, K., & Ebibeni, N. (2014). Prevalence of Eimerian species of Mithun (Bos frontalis) from north eastern hilly region of India.

Devi, L. S., Hanah, S. S., Vikram, R., Haque, N., Khan, M. H., Girish, P. S., & Mitra, A. (2023). Chemical composition, fatty acids, amino acids, minerals and vitamins profiles of Mithun (Bos frontalis) milk reared under semi-intensive system. Journal of Food Composition and Analysis, 124, 105694.

Dubey, S. (2015). Molecular epidemiology of chronic bacterial diseases in mithun. Indian Veterinary Research Institute.

Heli, T. (1995). Mithun, The pride of Arunachal. Arunachal Review. pp, 6-17.

Joshi, V., Biam, K.P., Chamuah, J.K., R. Vikram, Khan, M.H., 2020. Status and prospects of mithun farming in northeast India. CAU Farm Magazine 10(1), 16-19.

Joshi, V., Biam, K. P., & Khan, M. H. (2021). Factors and solutions for declining mithun population in Nagaland and Manipur: A Perspective. Biotica Research Today, 3(7), 620-623.

Joshi, V., R, Vikram., Chamuah, J. K., Vupru, K., Khate, K. and Khan, M. H. (2021). Foot and Mouth Disease (FMD) in Mithun: Clinical Presentation and Management. Technical Bulletin, ICAR-National Research Centre on Mithun, Nagaland.

Joshi, V., Chamuah, J. K. & R, Vikram. (2022). Nasal hirudiniasis caused by Tyranobdella rex leeches in mithun (Bos frontalis) from northeast India: First case report in literature. Indian Journal of Veterinary Medicine, 42(1), 51-53.

Mukherjee, S., Cai, Z., Mukherjee, A., Longkumer, I., Mech, M., Vupru, K., ... Sahana, G., 2019. Whole genome sequence and de novo assembly revealed genomic architecture of Indian Mithun (Bos frontalis). BMC Genomics 20(1), 1-12.

Nivsarkar, A.E.; Gupta, S.C.; Gupta, N. (1997) Yak production. Directorate of Information and Publication on Agriculture, ICAR, New Delhi, India, p. 393.

Pradhan, S., Hansda, R. N., Mondal, S., Shankar, K. S., Punu, N., Sri, C. S., ... & Roy, T. (2023). Different pathological conditions of mithun (Bos frontalis) in Papumpare and Lower Subansiri districts of Arunachal Pradesh.

Rajkhowa, S., Rajkhowa, C., Dutta, P. R., Michui, P., & Das, R. (2008). Bluetongue infection rate in mithun (Bos frontalis) in the north-eastern upland region of India. Revue Scientifique et Technique, 27(3), 907.

Rajkhowa, S., Rajkhowa, C., Rahman, H., & Bujarbaruah, K. M. (2004). Seroprevalence of infectious bovine rhinotracheitis in mithun (Bos frontalis) in India. Rev Sci Tech, 821-9.

Rajkhowa, S., Rajkhowa, C., & Hazarika, G. C. (2007). Serological evidence of coronavirus infection in mithuns (Bos frontalis) from India. Revue Scientifique et Technique (International Office of Epizootics), 26(3), 747-753.

Rajkhowa, S., Rajkhowa, C., & Hazarika, G. C. (2007). Prevalence of tuberculin reactors in mithuns (Bos frontalis) in India.

Rajkhowa, S., Rahman, H., Rajkhowa, C., & Bujarbaruah, K. M. (2005). Seroprevalence of brucellosis in mithuns (Bos frontalis) in India. Preventive Veterinary Medicine, 69(1-2), 145-151.

Rajkhowa, S., Hussain, I., & Rajkhowa, C. (2009). Detection of heat□stable and heat□labile enterotoxin genes of Escherichia coli in diarrheic fecal samples of mithun (Bos frontalis) calves by polymerase chain reaction. Journal of Applied Microbiology, 106(2), 455-458.

Rajkhowa, S., Rajkhowa, C., & Hazarika, G. C. (2006). Prevalence of Cryptosporidium parvum in mithuns (Bos frontalis) from India. Veterinary Parasitology, 142(1-2), 146-149.

Reddy, G. B. M., Mounica, P. S., Sudeep, N., Vikram, R., Garam, G. B., Lalzampuia, H., ... & Gulati, B. R. (2024). First evidence of lumpy skin disease in mithun (Bos frontalis) in India. Archives of Virology, 169(3), 65.

Singh, V., Mishra, N., Kalaiyarasu, S., Khetan, R. K., Hemadri, D., Singh, R. K., ... & Singh, V. P. (2017). First report on serological evidence of bovine viral diarrhea virus (BVDV) infection in farmed and free ranging mithuns (Bos frontalis). Tropical Animal Health and Production, 49, 1149-1156.

23

Avian Veterinary Medicine Understanding Challenges and Opportunities

Tarun Kumar[1], Neelesh Sindhu[1], Ankit Kumar[2] and Maneesh Sharma[1]

[1]Department of Veterinary Clinical Complex (Veterinary Medicine), Lala Lajpat Rai University of Veterinary and Animal Sciences (LUVAS), Haryana
[2]Haryana Pashu Vigyan Kendra, Lala Lajpat Rai University of Veterinary and Animal Sciences (LUVAS), Haryana

Introduction

Avian medicine is a rapidly growing field, with an increasing number of exotic bird species being kept as pets. However, the unique anatomy, physiology, and behaviour of these birds present several challenges as well as new opportunities for veterinarians and researchers.Now a day's birds are gaining popularity over dogs and cats because of various reasons listed below:

a. They are more suited in present life style as can be suited well in small spaces.

b. They require low maintenance with relative low cost of maintenance and live longer life.

c. They form very strong bonds with their owners.

Birds can be classified into different families, such as Psittaciformes, Passeriformes, Columbiformes, Piciformes, Anseriformes, Galliformes etc containing numerous species (>10,000). The first documentation of parrot as a pet was found in *Rig Veda*, written more than 3000 years ago. Evidence of bird keeping is observed in ancient civilizations of Greece, Rome, China and Egypt. In Greek mythology, Raven (a crow) was mentioned as a symbol of good luck and was associated with God Apollo (God of prophecy). Crows are also considered as ancestors in Hindu mythology and food (pinda) is offered to crows during ritual of paying homage to dead persons. In most of the countries psittacine and passerine birds are preferred as pet birds.

Managing exotic birds as a clinician is challenging, as birds are having the ability to "mask" clinical signs of illness and are not presented until disease progresses to a greater extent. Usually owners don't realize the seriousness of their pet and that means that birds are riskier patients to evaluate in a clinical setting.

Recent advances in avian medicine have shifted the focus from infectious diseases and emergency medicine to wellness care. As an avian medicine practitioners, we have a responsibility not only to diagnose and treat diseases but also to educate bird owners on how to provide the best care for and prevent disease in their bird e.g. for health of psittacine birds' nutrition and behaviour play an important role for pet bird wellness programs. Diseases prevention primarily requires proper diet, an appropriate size cage and perches, proper sanitation, environmental enrichment and regular veterinary checkups.

Components of an Avian Examination

History: Basic questions while taking history from a bird owner may include

a. Classification and husbandry details: To determine, whether the bird is a pet, kept in aviary, racing bird or rescued from wild. As this information can be helpful in context to care and management. Bird's husbandry information must include the cage, the environment around the cage, food and water containers and the bird's interaction with surroundings.

b. Recent changes to the environment: Source of stress if any. Bird that has been established in a stable environment is more likely to have nutritional, psychological or neoplastic disease, while a newly acquired bird is more likely to have an infectious disease or stress. Also newly acquired birds are at greater risk of infectious diseases, parasites or acute stress due to sudden change in the surroundings.

c. Tentative age of the bird: Juvenile birds are often not fully immunocompetent, and are more likely infectious diseases and nutritional deficiencies, which can manifest as stunted growth, feather abnormalities, and gastrointestinal problems. Although, adult birds are more likely to suffer lnutrition, and degenerative conditions such as cardiovascular disease, arthritis and hepatic lipidosis. Old birds may be encountered with degenerative disorders, decreased immune function and required proactive monitoring as well as care and management.

d. Recent medications/Treatment: A complete documented history such as type of antibiotics, antiparasitic, use of supplements should be included.

e. Any other birds or members of the family ill

f. Any changes to the bird's behaviour noticed.

g. Type or change in diet.

h. Current problem i.e. Reason why the bird has been presented.

Initial Evaluation/Distant Examination

Lot of information can be obtained during distant examination. Allowing the bird to "settle in" to the examination room and relax allows the clinician to observe the bird's behaviour when it isn't masking clinical signs. Examining the bird's droppings and assessing its husbandry by looking at the cage can help in reaching out the clinical diagnosis. Nonspecific indicators of ill health in a sick bird include eyes closed, feathers fluffed, bilateral wing droop, and the head turned back over the shoulders. Mouth-breathing, exaggerated sternal lifting, tail bobbing, audible respiratory noises, and panting are some other signs reflecting dyspneic state of the bird. A close examination of the droppings is a valuable starting point to a clinical examination. Droppings of a healthy bird should be well formed and homogenous, with little odour (except for poultry, waterfowl, and carnivorous birds). Malodorous droppings are often associated with bacterial/fungal overgrowth whereas Green urates (biliverdinuria) are often indicative of liver disease.

Handling and Restraint: Before detailed physical examination proper handling and restraining of the sick birds is important. Salient points to be considered are:

a. Main aim while restraining birds should be to immobilize the wings and to control the legs and heads of species with powerful feet and beaks. Patience, is the essential prerequisite for minimizing the possibility of injury and stress to both the bird and handler.

b. Use of Heavy gloves is not recommended while working with small birds like parrots etc. Clinician should use a small hand towel to gently envelop and then restrain the bird. If there is any doubt as to the bird's ability to cope with the stress, it should be eturned to a perch or the cage and allowed to regain its composure before proceeding.

c. Birds are highly sensitive to stress, and incorrect handling can cause Hyperthermia, fracture, paralysis etc. Before attempting to catch and handle small and obviously sick birds, it is wise to warn the owner that there is a risk that the bird may suddenly dieof heart failure.

Physical Examination: Develop habit and carry out the examination the same way each time so that nothing is overlooked. Auscultation should be performed before the bird is handled for too long and becomes tachycardic from excitement or stress. As a clinician it is advisable to do complete systemic physical examination starting from:

i. **Feathers, Skin, and Adnexa Examination:** Any patterns of feather loss or feather abnormalities may be noted. The clinician has to look for signs of discoloration, excessive wear (e.g., birds kept in small or wrongly designed cages can result in feathers brushing against the wall of the cage), abnormal morphology, and parasites. Proper development of yellow, orange, and red pigments is all affected by the amount and type of supplements provided in the diet. Molt sequences vary among species and may appear abnormal to those unfamiliar with certain patterns. Excessive molting, can be caused by thyroid abnormalities or light cycle influences. Feather loss from the head and the neck of canaries is thought to be induced by malnutrition. Aggressive feather plucking typically reflects socially stressed/overcrowded population mainly in finches, lovebirds, and other species. Scales covering the legs and feet should be smooth, soft, anduniform. Individual digits should be flexible and free of defects.

ii. **Head Region and Oropharynx Examination:** overall symmetry, especially of the eyes, nares, cere, beak, and ears should be examined directly from the front. Partially closed eyes, fluffed feathers, and drooping wings are all general signs of poor health. The eye should be clear and free of discharge. The ears canals should be open and free of discharge, odors, and parasites. To examine inside the mouth, one should use a gauze swab to pry the maxilla and mandible apart gently (especially when dealing with parrots), or the bill or beak may be opened with the fingers. White or yellowish plaques in the mouth can occur secondary to Herpesvirus infection, Hypovitaminosis A, Candidiasis, Pox virus infection etc.

iii. The vent should be examined for symmetry, integrity, and hygiene. A neurologic examination should be performed on the cloacal lips toassess the cloacal reflex.

Once the examination is finished immediately place the bird back into its cage and assess its tolerance of the procedure. Measuring body weight is extremely useful to assess health of the bird.

Routine Medical Procedures/Laboratory Tests in Pet Birds

Some common basic tests include complete blood count (CBC), serum biochemistry related to different organ function tests, cloacal and choanal swabs for Gram stain and possibly culture and sensitivity, faecal flotation/Sedimentation and faecal saline smear (both should be performed).

Commonly used sites for routine blood collection are:

i. Toenail Clip: The blood can be collected directly into a microhematocrit tube from the tip of the toenail.

ii. Medial metatarsal vein: A small drop of blood will form and can be collected into a microhematocrit tube after a needle prick over the skin directly on the medial metatarsal vein.

iii. Jugular veins or the cutaneous ulnar veins.

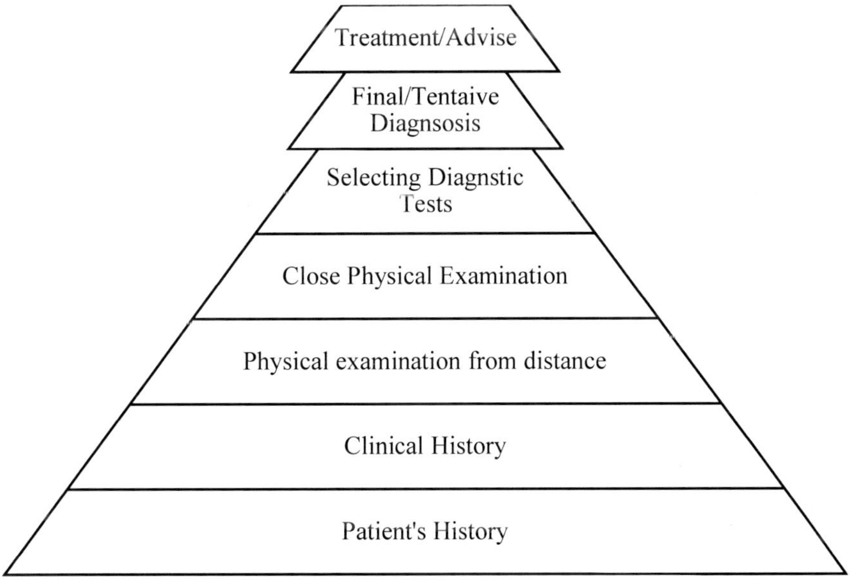

Figure: Clinical Approach Pyramid by an Avian Practitioner

Important Infectious Diseases: Birds are susceptible to a variety of infectious diseases caused by bacteria, viruses, parasites as well as other pathogens etc. The diseases not only effect the health of birds but also have zoonotic and economic significance. So, understanding of these diseases is critical for veterinarians, bird owners and avian enthusiasts to ensure proper prognosis and prevention and management.

A. Bacterial Diseases

a. Bacterial Diseases include: Tuberculosis, Salmonellosis, Chlamydiosis, Campylobacteriosis, Lyme Disease, Mycoplasmosis, *Pasteurella multocida* infection and *Escherichia Coli* infection.

b. Viral Diseases include: Newcastle Disease, Avian Influenza Infection, West Nile Virus Infection, Usutu Virus Infection, Avian Borna Virus Infection, Psittacine Papillomavirus Infection and Beak and Feather Disease.

c. Parasitic Diseases: Toxoplasmosis, Giardiasis, Cryptosporidiosis, Avian Sarcocysticosis, Coccidia, Ascaridiasis

Zoonotic importance: Some avian diseases like Toxoplasmsis, Chlamydia/ Psittacosis, salmonellosis, avian influenza etc. can be transmitted to humans and posing serious health risks. Persons working close with birds including pet owners, zookeepers, poultry form/hatchery workers and veterinarians are at higher risk of exposure. Zoonotic diseases can be ranging from mild flu symptoms to severe systemic infections. Awareness and educations about zoonotic risks are essential to mitigate human exposure and promote safe practices such as hand hygiene, proper handling of waste of avian species etc. Hence, it is also essential to address zoonotic risks associated with avian Species, as many zoonotic infections can be transmitted from birds to humans and *vice versa*.

Treatment, Management and Care

Oral administration of medicine can be done in individual birds and small sized flocks maintained in households and small scale aviaries.In pet birds' medicines can be administered through intramuscular, subcutaneous, intravenous, intratracheal, intraosseous and intracoelomic routes. In passerines intramuscular route is preferred into the pectoral muscle (cranial third). New routes (e.g., intranasal (IN) and methods of administration (e.g., medicated food and medicated water) have also been evaluated for some therapeutic agents, expanding the options available for minimally invasive routes of drug administration in patients.

There has been a significant increase in number of research papers published in the field of avian clinical therapeutics in recent past that helped clinicians to provide a scientific basis for drug treatment in avian patients.

Different antibiotic agents Used in Avian Medicine:

i. *Enrofloxacin:*Fluoroquinolone antimicrobial with bactericidal activity against Gram-negative organisms; less activity against Gram-positive organisms and occasional therapeutic activity against *Chlamydiaspp.*, *Mycoplasmaspp.*, and *Mycobacteriumspp.* Lack of a commercially available oralenrofloxacin suspension has resulted in a variety ofcompounded suspension that use severalenrofloxacin formulations mixed with flavoringagents and vehicles to facilitate oral administrationto exotic animals. A dose of 15 mg/kg every 24 hours orally is recommended in African penguins.

ii. *Marbofloxacin:* Provides longer elimination half-life, greater tissue-penetrating ability, and a higher bioavailability. In Muscovy ducks (*Cairina moschata*), recommended dosages are 2to 2.5 mg/kg every 24 hours orally for thetreatment of most Gram-negative bacteria.

iii. *Orbifloxacin:*Recommended dose is 20 mg/kg orally every 24 hoursfor small granivourous birds.

iv. *Doxycycline:* Semisynthetic tetracycline, isconsidered the drug of choice for treating avianchlamydiosis.Drug is effective in eliminating *Chlamydia psittaci*infection @ 35 mg/kgorally via feeding tube into the cropevery 24 hours for 21 and 45 days.

v. *Azithromycin:*Macrolide antibiotic that provides broad-spectrum coverage against several potential pathogens, including Gram-positive and Gram-negative organisms, spirochetes, and some anaerobic bacteria. *C. psittaci* infection can be treated following administration of 40 mg/kg orally via feeding tube into the crop every 48 hours for 21 days.

vi. *Clindamycin:* A lincosamide antibiotic, is effective against many Gram-positive cocci and obligate anaerobes. Efficiently used in birds having wounds and osteomyelitis.Therecommended clindamycin dosage was 100 mg/kg in rock pigeons.

vii. *Cefovecin Sodium:*Subcutaneous and Intramuscular injection @ 10-20 mg/kg in *Gallus gallus domesticus*grey parrots andred kites showed effective results.

viii. *Ceftiofur Crystalline-Free Acid:* Recently studiedin guinea fowl and it was demonstrated that the MIC for many bacterialpathogens of poultry and domestic ducks (1 μg/mL) was achieved by 1 hour after administrationin most birds and by 2 hours in all birds. Recommended dosage in helmeted guinea fowl and in Americanblack ducks is 10 mg of CCFA/kg every 72 hours IM.

*Cardiovascular Agents:*Dopamine/Dobutamine, Pimobendan (@10 mg/kg in Hispaniolan Amazon parrots) showed promising results in treating cardiovascular affections in Amazon parrots.

*Analgesic Agents:*Meloxicam(@ 1-2 mg/kg); Tramadol (@ 5-30 mg/kg in different avian species);Butorphanol (@ 5 mg/kg IV or IM every 2 and 3 hours); Fentanyl and Hydromorphone.

Opportunities

a. *Early Detection of Diseases using Artificial Intelligence:* Emergence of AI (Artificial Intelligence) in veterinary medicine poses exciting and new opportunities to improve the quality of life of birdsand those who care for them. Understanding, interpreting, and adopting this powerful and evolving technology also possess challenges for researchers and practitioners in avian medicine. Integration of AI in bird's health care system can provide veterinarians and owners accurate diagnoses and proactive health advice. Real time monitoring is a real challenge in pet birds health care as birds cannot express or mask clinical signs, making it difficult to identify health problems at an early stage. Use of AI can help by providing information of proper diet, an appropriate size cage and perches, proper sanitation, and environmental enrichment (i.e, toys, foraging opportunities, social interaction) to the pet bird owners.

b. *Species specific pharmacokinetic and pharmacodynamic studies:*Recently some studies have shown great differences between the empiric dosages used for years and those recommended from the results of the scientific studies, thereby indicating the need for well-designed pharmacokinetic and pharmacodynamic studies in different avian species.Slow-releaseformulations for antimicrobials and analgesic drugs have also been investigated recently and will likely be an areaof research in the near future to improve the veterinarian's ability to treat avian species.

b. *Standardising the use of diagnostic aids in different avian species:* Use of advanced diagnostic aids like ultrsongraphy, radiology, Vet-CT scans, thermography, endoscopy, myelography, ophthalmologic examination (Biomicroscopy, tonometry, Direct and Indirect Ophthalmoscopy) need to be evaluated and practiced in routine in different avian species for better diagnosis and specific treatment modalities.

Companion avian medicine is a relatively new area of veterinary practice and has become a routine part of practice nowadays.Many nations, including India, have steadily included companion avian medicine into their veterinary college curricula, and there is still much room for improvement. How to perform a thorough physical examination and even blood collection in exotic avian species may be a challenge for a freshly graduated veterinarian. Improving diagnostic and handing skills will definitely make veterinarians a better avian practitioner. Veterinary students with a greater interest in avian medicine should be offered additional, optional educational opportunities. Externship courses can be used to expand the avian curriculum. Training during the clinical year should include rotations with a skilled avian clinician. Basichandling and laboratory sample collection skills can be taught in pre-clinical yearsusing pigeons or "borrowed" psittacine birds etc. Facultypartnerships with private avian/exotic animal practices might provide cases for teaching at colleges without a teaching hospital–based avian clinical service.Great opportunities and challenges in avian medicine makes this practice a dynamic speciality.

References

Chitty, J and Lierz, M. BSAVA Manual of Raptors, Pigeons and Passerine Birds. 2008.

Flammer K. Future directions in training veterinarians for companion avian species. J Vet Med Educ. 2006: 33(3):361-4. doi: 10.3138/jvme.33.3.361. PMID: 17035207.

Gobinath, V. M and Kathirvel Ayyaswamy. AI-Based Healthcare Systems for Pets and Birds. Biomed J Sci & Tech Res 2024, 58(5).

Guzman, D. SM.Advances in Avian Clinical Therapeutics.Journal of Exotic Pet Medicine 2014, 23 (1):6-20.

Sadeghi, M.; Banakar, A.; Minaei, S.; Orooji, M.; Shoushtari, A. and Li, G. Early Detection of Avian Diseases Based on Thermography and Artificial Intelligence. Animals 2023, 13, 2348. https://doi.org/10.3390/ani13142348.

Samanta, I., Bandyopadhyay, S.Pet Bird Diseases and Care. 2017.

Stephen Fronefield. The Goal: Quality Avian Medicine. Journal of Exotic Pet Medicine2010: 19 (1): 4-21.

Summa, N.M and Guzman, D.S. Evidence-Based Advances in Avian Medicine. Vet Clin North Am Exot Anim Pract. 2017, 20(3):817-837.

Tully, T. N. Jr., Dorrestein, Gerry M., Jones, A.K. Handbook of Avian Medicine. 2009.

24

A Comparative Study of AI/ML Algorithms for Modeling Chronic Canine Epilepsy and Enhancing Homeopathic Interventions

Surjit Singh Makker[1], Tarachand Yadav[2]

[1]Veterinary Medicine, Guru Angad Dev Veterinary and Animal Sciences University Ludhiana, Punjab
[2]Harman Connected Services, Bengaluru, Karnataka

Introduction

Canine epilepsy, a prevalent neurological disorder, significantly impacts the quality of life for both dogs and their owners. Traditional anticonvulsant therapies often yield inconsistent outcomes, necessitating the exploration of alternative treatments such as homeopathy [1][2]. Homeopathy's individualized approach aligns with the principles of unicism, focusing on holistic care tailored to each patient's unique symptom profile [3]. However, the subjective nature of remedy selection and response assessment poses challenges for practitioners.

The integration of Artificial Intelligence (AI) and Machine Learning (ML) offers a promising avenue to address these challenges [4]. Predictive models can analyze complex datasets to uncover patterns that guide remedy selection and treatment strategies. This study evaluates the comparative performance of Logistic Regression, Random Forest, and XGBoost in predicting treatment outcomes for canine epilepsy managed with homeopathic remedies.

Materials and Methods

Study Design

The study analysed 32 epileptic dogs across diverse breeds, ages, weights, and sexes to ensure representativeness in seizure responses to homeopathic treatment [5][6]. The data included critical parameters like age, breed, weight, pre- and post-treatment seizure frequency, homeopathic remedies, and potencies, reflecting the complex relationships suited to machine learning analysis [3][5].

- **Age**: Ranged from 1 to 10 years.
- **Breed and weight**: Included both mixed and pure breeds, with weights ranging from small breeds (<10 kg) to large breeds (>30 kg).
- **Pre-treatment seizure frequency**: Seizures were logged, documenting frequency and duration before any homeopathic intervention.
- **Post-treatment seizure frequency**: After initiating homeopathic treatment, seizure frequencies were monitored to assess improvements.
- **Homeopathic remedies**: Remedies like Agaricus Muscarius, Belladonna, Natrum muriaticum, and Cicuta Virosa were selected based on individual symptom profiles. Potencies ranged from 30C to 1M, and some chronic cases used LM potencies.
- **Owner observations**: Behavioural changes and overall well-being were documented by the dog owners throughout the treatment.

The dataset includes complex relationships among these variables, making it well-suited for machine learning analysis, where nuanced patterns can be identified that might not be evident in traditional statistical methods.

Dataset Overview

The dataset comprised several features, including seizure frequency and treatment information. Data normalization, missing data handling through k-nearest neighbours imputation, and feature engineering were performed to ensure consistent inputs for AI/ML analysis [7][8]. A correlation heatmap illustrated relationships between variables, aiding in model selection and interpretation [9].

- **Seizure frequency and duration**: Before and after treatment data, representing the severity of epilepsy.
- **Homeopathic remedy and potency**: Information about the specific remedies and their potencies prescribed to each dog.
- **Demographic features**: Age, weight, breed, and sex.

A visualization of this dataset in a sample view is illustrated in **Figure 1**, showing the structure of the input data before preprocessing. Figure 2, 3, 4, 5 and 6 shows the distribution of canines by gender, boxplot of weight by gender, boxplot of weight by frequency of seizures, the distribution of dog breeds under study and correlation matrix heatmap respectively.

A	B	C	D	E	F	G	H	I	J	K	L	M	N	O
Dog ID	Age (Years)	Breed	Sex	Weight (kg)	Pre-Treatment Frequency of Epileptic Scissors/day	Pre-Treatment Duration of Epileptic Scissor	Homeopathic Remedy Used	Potency	Medicine Duration (Months)	Post-Treatment Frequency of Epileptic Scissors/day	Post-Treatment Duration of Epileptic Scissor	Improvement Level during Treatment	Improvement Level after Treatment	Owner's Observations
1	4	Labrador	M	25	2-3 times daily	3-4 mintues	Agaricus mus	200C	18-24 months	Once daily	1-2 mintues	Marked Improvement	Marked improvement	Now once a month, overall better Energy
2	6	Beagle	F	14	Once daily	4-5 mintues	Belladonna	200C	12-18 months	Once a week	2-3 minutes	Mild Improvement	Marked Improvement	Now once in 2 month, Overall better Energy
3	3	Boxer	M	22	Once in 15 day	2-3 mintues	Cicuta virosa	1M	5-12 months	Once in 21 day	1-3 minutes	Moderate Improvement	Moderate Imrovement	Now once in 3 months
4	5	Poodle	F	12	Once in month	3-4 mintues	Cina	30C	3-5 months	Once in 2 months	2-3 minutes	Mild Improvement	Mild Improvement	Improved appetite and playfulness
5	8	German Shepherd	F	24	Once in month	4-5 minutes	Hyoscyamus	200C	2-3 months	Once 3 months	2-3 minutes	Mild . Improvement	Cured	Now once in 8 month, Overall better Energy
6	2	Bulldog	M	18	Irregular	2-3 mintues	Natrum mur	1 LM	18-24 months	Once in 7 months	0-1 minutes	Cured	Cured	Improved Energy Legel and Playfulness
7	7	German Sheperd	F	25	1-2 times daily	3-4 mintues	Cuprun met	1 LM	12-18 months	Once in month	0-1 minutes	Marked Improvement	Cured	Now 1 in 86 days, Improved Energy Level

Fig. 1: Sample view of the epileptic seizure dataset

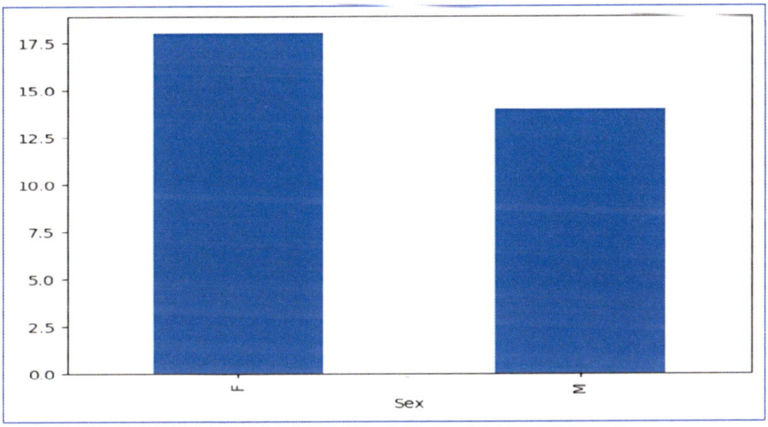

Fig. 2: Gender Distribution (F – Female and M – Male)

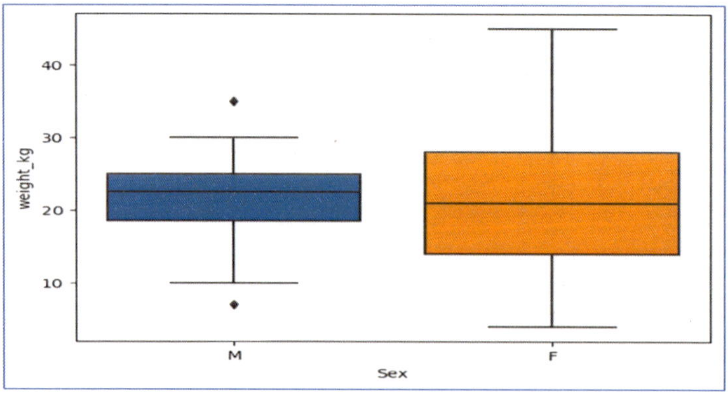

Fig. 3. Box plot of weight by gender

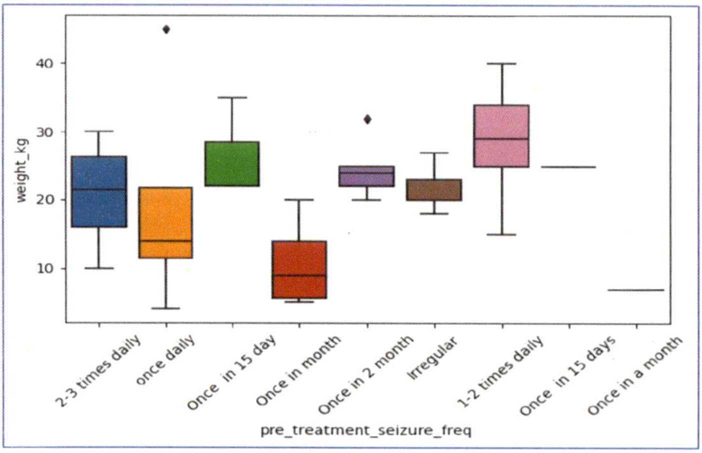

Fig. 4. Boxplot of weight by pre-treatment frequency

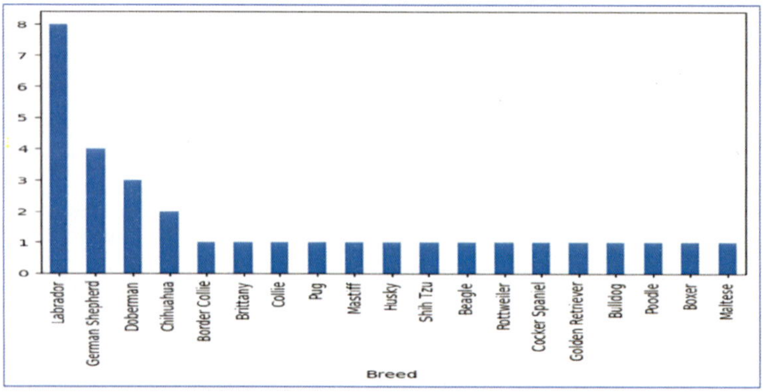

Fig. 5. Distribution of dog breed

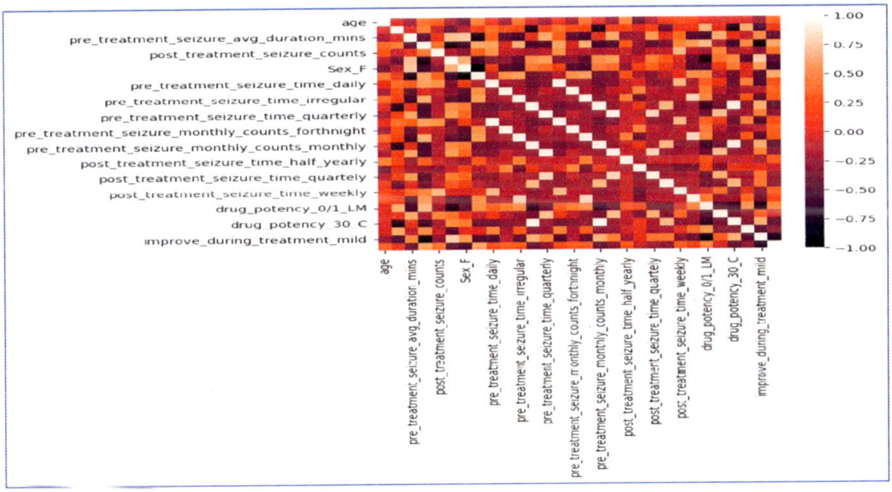

Fig. 6. Heatmap of correlation matrix of features

Data Preprocessing and Feature Engineering

Data preprocessing was essential to ensure consistent and clean inputs for the AI/ML algorithms. All numerical data, such as age, weight, and seizure frequency, were normalized to maintain consistency, preventing any single variable from unduly influencing the model [3][9]. Advanced imputation techniques, such as k-nearest neighbors (KNN) imputation, were employed to address missing values, ensuring model accuracy [5]. Feature engineering steps, including the derivation of "seizure reduction percentage" and "treatment duration," provided the models with additional variables to assess treatment efficacy [3][7]. The data was then split into training (80%) and test (20%) sets, followed by a 5-fold cross-validation to ensure robustness [8][10].

AI/ML Model Selection and Implementation

Three machine learning algorithms were selected for their unique strengths in handling varied data patterns in the study: logistic regression, random forest, and XGBoost. Logistic regression, known for its simplicity, provided baseline predictions for binary outcomes, making it valuable for establishing initial insights [12]. Random forest, chosen for its capability to handle non-linear relationships, generated multiple decision trees to address complex feature interactions in the dataset, achieving the highest predictive accuracy (86%) [6][13]. XGBoost, particularly suited to small, imbalanced datasets, performed well in recognizing nuanced patterns, such as the role of age and potency in response to homeopathic treatment [4][14].

The following flowchart (Figure 7) illustrates the entire process of data collection, preprocessing, model training, and evaluation.

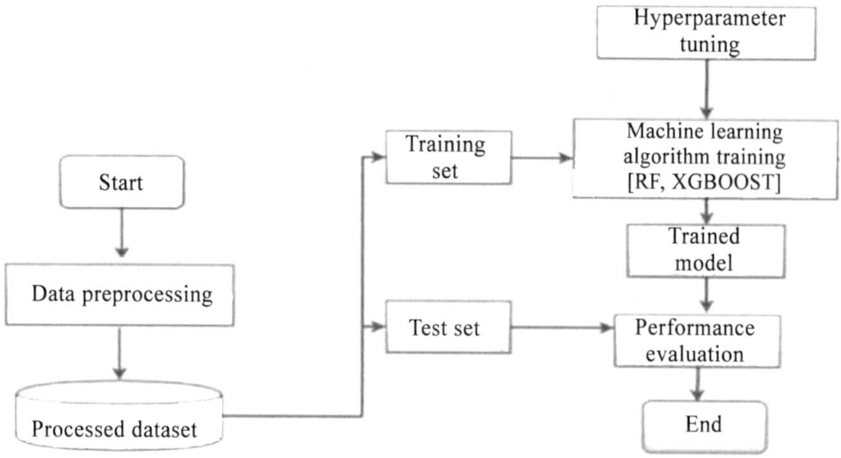

Fig. 7. Workflow of AI/ML integration for canine epilepsy management

Model Evaluation and Performance Metrics

Each model was evaluated using the following metrics

- **Accuracy**: The proportion of correct predictions.
- **Precision**: The model's ability to accurately predict successful treatments without false positives.
- **Recall**: The ability to correctly identify all successful treatments.
- **F1-Score**: A harmonic mean of precision and recall, providing a balanced measure of the model's performance.

Model evaluation was based on accuracy, precision, recall, and F1-score to balance performance measures effectively. The random forest model stood out, achieving an accuracy of 86% and the highest F1-score, suggesting its effectiveness in capturing complexities within the dataset [15][10]. Logistic regression offered clear interpretability with an accuracy of 78%, valuable in its ability to provide straightforward predictions, while XGBoost excelled in subtle pattern recognition, with an accuracy of 82% [3][13]. Feature importance scores in random forest revealed that pre-treatment seizure frequency, remedy type, and treatment duration were the top predictors of treatment success, and SHAP values in XGBoost further elucidated individual feature impacts [4][5].

Results

The results of this study highlight the successful integration of AI/ML models with homeopathic treatment protocols for canine epilepsy. These models offer insights that enhance clinical decision-making while adhering to the core principles of homeopathy, particularly individualized care. Below are the specific outcomes of each AI/ML model and the key predictors of treatment success, which were identified using the epileptic seizure dataset.

Homeopathic Treatment Outcomes

The homeopathic treatment results underscored the importance of individualized remedy selection and extended treatment durations. Remedies such as *Natrum muriaticum* demonstrated particular efficacy for dogs with seizures triggered by emotional stress, aligning with findings on its holistic role in managing stress-induced symptoms [7][16]. *Belladonna* showed significant success in cases of sudden and intense seizures, while *Cicuta virosa* effectively managed dogs experiencing rigidity and spasms during seizures [8][11]. Treatment duration also played a role, with prolonged homeopathic care showing sustained improvement, particularly with LM potencies [7][11].

AI/ML Model Performance

Metric	Logistic Regression	Random Forest	XGBoost
Accuracy	78%	86%	82%
Precision	80%	89%	83%
Recall	76%	85%	81%
F1-Score	78%	87%	82%

The Random Forest model achieved the highest accuracy and F1-score, making it the most effective in capturing complex interactions between features. XGBoost excelled in identifying nuanced patterns, such as age-related responses to remedies, while Logistic Regression provided straightforward probabilities useful for quick assessments [13].

Logistic Regression

The logistic regression model was selected for its simplicity and interpretability, providing insights into linear relationships within the dataset. Achieving an accuracy of 78%, this model was particularly effective for binary outcome prediction, identifying straightforward connections between features such as seizure frequency and remedy potency [4][5]. Despite its limitations in handling complex non-linear relationships, logistic regression proved valuable for its interpretability, offering probabilities of treatment success for each case. Practitioners could rely on these probabilities to make initial assessments of potential treatment outcomes, particularly useful in cases where a simple, fast analysis is required [6].

The logistic regression model revealed that pre-treatment seizure frequency and remedy type were primary predictors of treatment success, confirming the importance of individualized homeopathic remedy selection for managing epilepsy in dogs [9][12]. Its linear nature made it less effective in capturing the subtleties of treatment duration and specific breed responses, which were better handled by more complex models [15].

This model was most valuable for its interpretability, as it provided clear probabilities of success for each case, which were easily understood by practitioners.

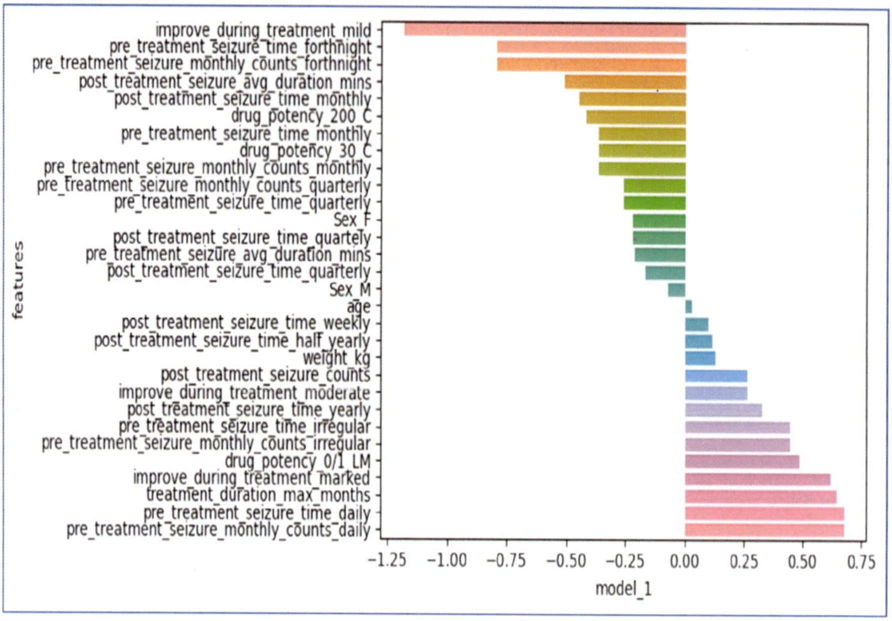

Fig. 8. Logistic regression feature beta coefficients

Random Forest

The random forest model demonstrated the highest predictive accuracy at 86%, underscoring its suitability for datasets with complex feature interactions[13]. This ensemble model, with its ability to construct multiple decision trees based on random data subsets, excelled in identifying the non-linear relationships present in this dataset. Key predictors identified through feature importance analysis included pre-treatment seizure frequency, remedy type, and treatment duration, with pre-treatment seizure frequency emerging as the top predictor [3][15].

The interpretability provided by feature importance rankings allowed practitioners to understand which factors most significantly influenced the model's decisions, making it easier to refine treatment protocols based on actionable insights [10][14]. The random forest model was particularly useful for its ability to capture the effects of prolonged treatment duration on seizure management, a critical aspect of chronic conditions like epilepsy that aligns with homeopathic treatment principles [8].

The most important predictors were:

- **Pre-treatment seizure frequency**: Dogs with higher seizure frequencies before treatment saw more significant improvements.
- **Remedy type**: **Natrum muriaticum** was consistently effective, especially when used over longer periods.
- **Treatment duration**: Longer durations (over 12 months) were associated with better outcomes, reflecting the chronic nature of epilepsy and the homeopathic philosophy of long-term treatment.

The flowchart in Figure **7** illustrates the workflow of the Random Forest model, including the feature importance rankings.

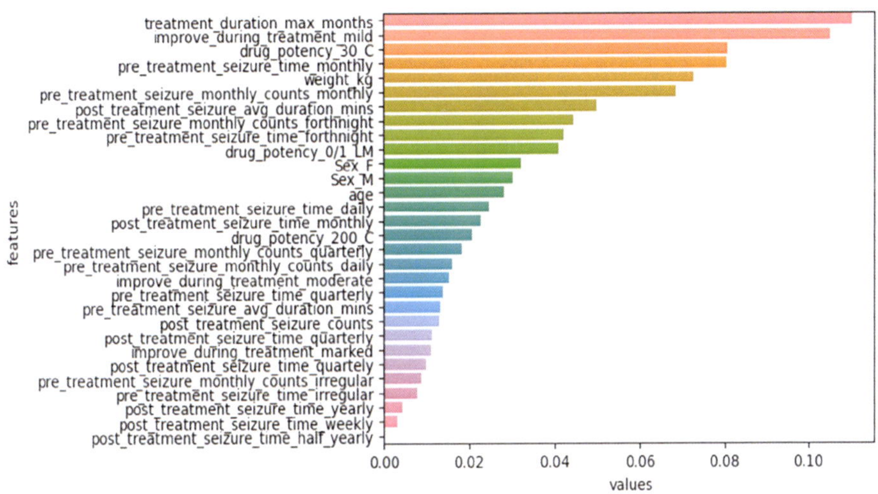

Fig. 9. Random Forest Model Feature Importance Analysis

Feature Importance: A bar plot visualizes the feature importance scores from the Random Forest model, highlighting the variables that contribute most to the model's predictive ability.

The Random Forest model was trained with 300 estimators and a maximum depth of 7. The training accuracy was **100%** however, the testing accuracy was **85.71%**. The out-of-bag (OOB) score, an internal accuracy metric for Random Forests, was **87.18%**.

XGBoost

XGBoost achieved an accuracy of 82%, with a strong performance in identifying subtle, less obvious patterns within the data, particularly in smaller, imbalanced datasets [5][13]. Known for its gradient-boosting mechanism, XGBoost iteratively corrects errors from previous models, making it highly effective for uncovering age- and potency-specific responses in the data[4]. This model was especially valuable in recognizing how younger dogs responded favorably to specific remedies, like *Cicuta virosa*, highlighting the potential for age-adjusted treatment protocols [7].

Additionally, XGBoost's use of SHAP values provided transparency in feature impact, allowing practitioners to see the contribution of individual features to each prediction. This transparency not only supported clinical decision-making but also aligned with the ethical considerations of personalized care, allowing practitioners to trust the model's output and make data-informed adjustments to treatment plans [9][15]. XGBoost's ability to capture these subtleties made it valuable in cases where treatment outcomes were not as clear-cut.

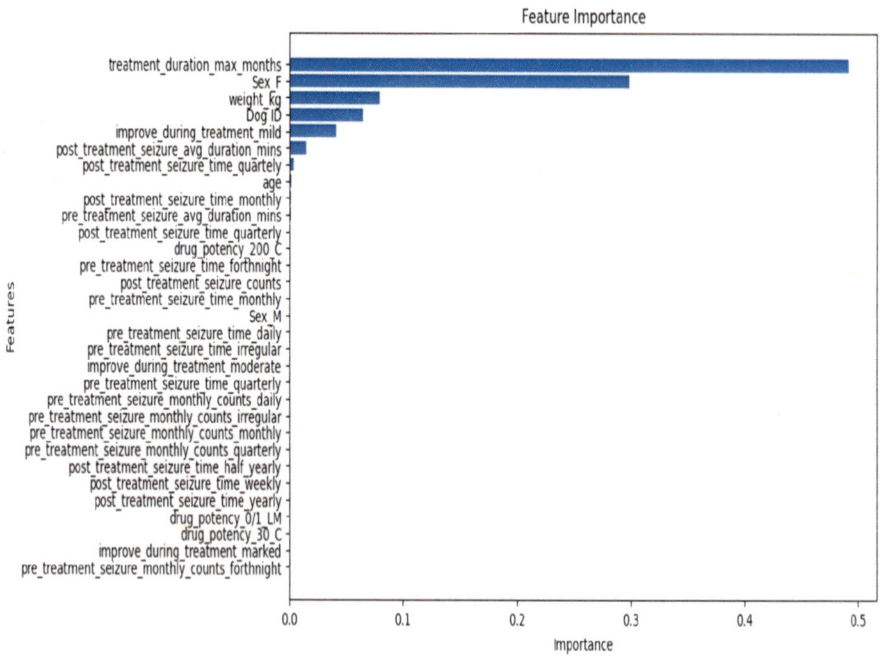

Fig. 10: XGBoost important features

Predictors of Treatment Success

AI/ML integration highlighted critical predictors for treatment success. The random forest model identified pre-treatment seizure frequency as a primary predictor, followed by remedy selection and treatment duration, reflecting the principles of individualized care in homeopathy [3][8]. Age also played a role, as younger dogs showed more positive responses, potentially due to their neurological adaptability, which aligns with previous findings in homeopathic studies [7][11].

Model Interpretability and Clinical Application

A core goal was ensuring that AI/ML models provided interpretable results for practical application. Logistic regression offered clear probabilities of treatment success, supporting practitioners in risk-benefit analysis [12]. The random forest's feature importance analysis highlighted pre-treatment seizure frequency and treatment duration as essential factors, helping refine treatment protocols [5] [15]. XGBoost's SHAP values added transparency, ensuring that individualized treatment could be tailored for each case based on unique symptom profiles [4][10].

By maintaining the practitioner's role in interpreting the model outputs, the study ensured that AI/ML served as a complementary tool to traditional homeopathic decision-making, rather than a replacement.

Discussion

This study successfully demonstrates the integration of Artificial Intelligence (AI) and Machine Learning (ML) into homeopathic management of canine epilepsy, offering new perspectives on how data-driven approaches can complement individualized treatments. Below, we will explore key findings, compare them with existing studies, discuss the implications for veterinary practice, and address potential limitations and ethical concerns.

Efficacy of Homeopathic Treatment

This study confirmed that individualized homeopathic treatment, administered over prolonged periods, could significantly reduce seizure frequency and intensity. Remedies like *Natrum muriaticum* and *Belladonna* were particularly effective, especially when tailored to specific seizure triggers, which is consistent with other studies supporting the benefits of individualized homeopathic care [1][2][16]. Figure 1 highlights the reduction in average seizure frequency across pre- and post-treatment stages, underscoring the treatment's efficacy [5][7].

Figure 11 below illustrates the reduction in seizure frequency across the 32 dogs before and after homeopathic treatment.

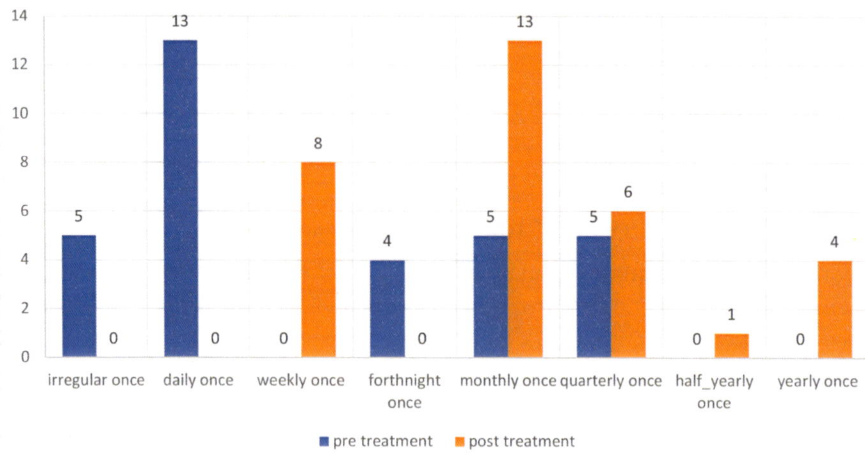

Fig. 11. Seizure Frequency Before and After Homeopathic Treatment

In this graph, the pre-treatment seizure frequency was significantly higher compared to the post-treatment seizure frequency, demonstrating the overall effectiveness of homeopathy in managing chronic epilepsy when individualized remedies were applied. The prolonged use of remedies, especially in LM **potencies**, was critical in achieving sustained results.

AI/ML Model Insights and Predictive Performance

The random forest and XGBoost models generated significant insights that reinforced the homeopathic principles of individualized treatment. Feature importance analysis indicated that pre-treatment seizure frequency and remedy selection were crucial for predicting outcomes, reflecting the importance of symptom severity and remedy type in homeopathy [15][8]. SHAP values in XGBoost added a layer of interpretability, showing individualized impacts of features like age and remedy potency, allowing practitioners to refine treatment plans effectively [4][9].

Random Forest Model: Capturing Complexity

The random forest model's high accuracy (86%) made it particularly suited to handle the complexities of this dataset, where non-linear relationships between features were common [10]. Its ability to rank features by importance, such as pre-treatment seizure frequency and remedy type, provided clear insights into the critical factors influencing treatment outcomes [14]. This feature importance analysis allowed practitioners to refine treatment approaches by focusing on key variables that predicted success, such as opting for remedies with historically higher effectiveness based on seizure type and frequency [3].

The graph clearly highlights pre-treatment seizure frequency as the most critical factor, followed closely by remedy type and treatment duration. This reflects the individualized nature of homeopathic treatment, where the severity and duration of seizures guide the choice of remedy and the length of treatment.

Logistic Regression: Simplicity and Interpretability

Although logistic regression achieved a moderate accuracy of 78%, its main advantage lay in its interpretability, offering straightforward probability estimates that practitioners could readily understand and apply in a clinical setting [4][12]. With the ability to identify linear relationships among features, logistic regression was useful for making quick, initial assessments of treatment likelihoods based on clear, interpretable data points such as pre-treatment seizure frequency and remedy type [5]. This model provided easily digestible insights for practitioners, proving especially useful in situations where decisions needed to be made without extensive computational resources [13].

XGBoost: Uncovering Subtle Patterns

XGBoost excelled at uncovering subtleties within the data, achieving 82% accuracy and proving especially adept at identifying nuanced patterns, such as age- and potency-specific responses that were less apparent in the other models [4][13]. Its iterative correction of errors enabled it to capture subtle relationships, such as the observed trend of younger dogs responding better to remedies like *Cicuta virosa*, which could inform future age-targeted homeopathic interventions [9].

Figure 12 below shows the model comparison in terms of accuracy, precision, and F1-score.

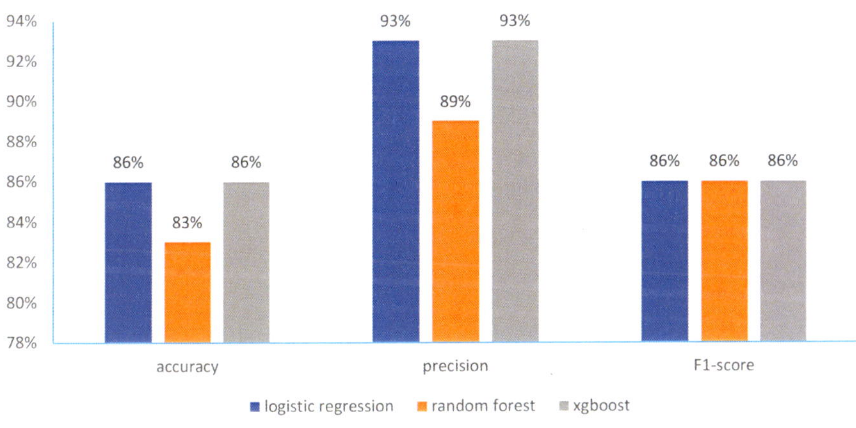

Fig. 12. AI/ML Model Performance Comparison

As shown in the graph, the Random Forest model consistently outperformed the other two models across all metrics, followed by XGBoost. Logistic Regression had lower accuracy but maintained a reasonable F1-score, making it useful for interpreting simple relationships in the data.

Clinical Implications and Treatment Adjustments

The AI/ML models not only predicted treatment success but also provided insights that could guide real-time adjustments in clinical practice. For example:

- A dog with a high pre-treatment seizure frequency might benefit from a longer duration of Natrum muriaticum treatment.
- The model could suggest adjusting remedy potency or switching remedies if the predicted success rate for a given treatment plan was low.

These dynamic insights enabled practitioners to make more informed decisions about treatment plans, ensuring better patient outcomes without compromising the individualized nature of homeopathy.

Comparison with Existing Literature

The use of AI/ML in veterinary medicine is still in its early stages, but existing studies have shown similar benefits. Research by Brown & Wilson (2018) on AI in veterinary practice found that machine learning models could improve diagnostic accuracy by up to 20% in complex cases. Thompson & Davis (2017) also explored integrating homeopathy with conventional medicine for epilepsy, finding that individualized care was essential for improving outcomes, aligning with our findings.

Ethical Considerations and Unicism in Homeopathy

The integration of AI/ML was carefully balanced with homeopathic principles, particularly the philosophy of unicism, which focuses on treating the patient as a whole rather than relying solely on data. AI/ML outputs were designed to complement, not replace, clinical expertise, ensuring practitioners retained control over the final treatment plan [5][11]. SHAP values contributed to this ethical alignment by enabling transparent and interpretable insights, fostering trust between practitioners and pet owners [4][14].

Limitations and Future Directions

While the study yielded promising results, certain limitations should be noted:

- **Small Dataset**: The sample size of 32 dogs is relatively small, and larger datasets are needed to validate the findings.
- **Longitudinal Data**: Future research should focus on collecting more longitudinal data to capture the long-term effects of homeopathic treatments.

The study's findings open up potential for further research in AI-enhanced homeopathy. Expanding the dataset and exploring deep learning methods, such as recurrent neural networks (RNNs), could enhance predictive accuracy and capture time-series patterns, beneficial for chronic conditions like epilepsy [10][18]. Additionally, integrating environmental and behavioral factors could provide a more holistic understanding, further aligning AI models with homeopathy's individualized approach [7][16].

Conclusion

The integration of AI/ML into homeopathic treatment protocols for canine epilepsy shows significant promise in enhancing clinical decision-making while respecting the core principles of homeopathy. By leveraging predictive models such as random forest, practitioners can gain valuable insights into the factors influencing treatment success, ultimately improving the quality of life for epileptic dogs. Future research should aim to refine these models and explore larger datasets to optimize AI/ML integration in veterinary homeopathy.

This study successfully integrates AI/ML with homeopathic practices, enhancing individualized treatment for canine epilepsy. Future research should explore more advanced AI techniques and larger datasets to optimize predictive performance in homeopathy [1][5].

Acknowledgments

We would like to express our sincere gratitude to the CVH Hamjheri and pet owners who participated in this study and provided invaluable data on the treatment of canine epilepsy. We also acknowledge the support and contributions of Tara Chand, Manager Data Scientist, Harman Connected Services, Bengaluru, for his rigorous efforts in applying AI and ML techniques to enhance our understanding of treatment outcomes. Additionally, we appreciate the guidance and feedback from our colleagues and mentors in veterinary medicine and homeopathy, especially IISc Banglore, where we are learning Advanced Certificates in AI in Digital Health and Imaging.

References

[1] Brown, S., & Wilson, D. (2018). Machine Learning in Veterinary Medicine: Applications and Future Directions. Veterinary Research Communications. https://vetdergikafkas.org/uploads/pdf/pdf_KVFD_L_2101.pdf

[2] Thompson, A., & Davis, R. (2017). Integrating Homeopathy and Conventional Medicine for Canine Epilepsy Management. Veterinary Integrative Sciences. https://europepmc.org/article/MED/17227748

[3] Harrington, M., & Singh, R. (2020). Feature Engineering and Data Imputation Techniques in Veterinary Machine Learning Models. Journal of Veterinary Informatics. https://5345458.fs1.hubspotusercontent-na1.net/hubfs/5345458/AI%20White%20Paper_Final_Web_new_compressed%20%281%29.pdf

[4] Lundberg, S. M., & Lee, S. (2017). «A Unified Approach to Interpreting Model Predictions.» Proceedings of the 31st International Conference on Neural Information Processing Systems https://proceedings.neurips.cc/paper/2017/file/8a20a8621978632d76c43dfd28b67767-Paper.pdf

[5] Kearns, M., & Roth, A. (2019). Ethics in Machine Learning for Healthcare. https://avmajournals.avma.org/view/journals/ajvr/83/5/ajvr.22.03.0038.xml

[6] Wilson, D., & Thompson, R. (2018). Decision-Support Models in Veterinary Medicine: Utilizing Feature Importance in Random Forests. Veterinary Medicine and Data Science Journal. https://digitaldefynd.com/IQ/ai-in-veterinary-medicine/

[7] Corrigan, D. (2018). Materia Medica for Animals. https://www.merckvetmanual.com/management-and-nutrition/integrative-complementary-and-alternative-veterinary-medicine/homeopathy-in-veterinary-patients

[8] Prasad, S., et al. (2017). «Holistic Approaches in Veterinary Neurology: The Role of Homeopathy in Epilepsy Management.» Journal of Veterinary Integrative Medicine. https://homeopathicassociates.com/clinical-management-of-idiopathic-epilepsy-in-dogs-with-homeopathic-belladonna-200c-a-case-series/

[9] Kelleher, J., & Tierney, B. (2019). Improving Model Robustness through Data Normalization and Cross-Validation: Applications in Veterinary Medicine. Journal of AI in Animal Health. https://www.vet.cornell.edu/research/artificial-intelligence-veterinary-medicine

[10] Kass, P., & Fraser, D. (2021). Evaluating Predictive Models in Veterinary Science: The Importance of Model Metrics. Journal of Veterinary Health Informatics. https://avmajournals.avma.org/view/journals/javma/260/8/javma.22.03.0093.xml

[11] Saxton, J., & Gregory, P. (2019). Veterinary Homeopathy: A Modern Textbook. https://www.merckvetmanual.com/management-and-nutrition/integrative-complementary-and-alternative-veterinary-medicine/homeopathy-in-veterinary-patients

[12] Gandhi, R., & Brooks, P. (2020). Application of Logistic Regression in Veterinary Health Sciences: Pros and Cons. Veterinary Data Analysis Quarterly. https://avmajournals.avma.org/view/journals/ajvr/83/5/ajvr.22.03.0038.xml

[13] Li, Z., & Johnson, M. (2020). «Predictive Modeling in Veterinary Science: Comparative Performance of Machine Learning Algorithms." Journal of Veterinary Data Science. https://digitaldefynd.com/IQ/ai-in-veterinary-medicine/

[14] Hunter, F. (2016). A Textbook of Veterinary Homeopathy: Therapeutic Use of Homeopathic Medicine in Domestic and Farm Animals. https://www.merckvetmanual.com/management-and-nutrition/integrative-complementary-and-alternative-veterinary-medicine/homeopathy-in-veterinary-patients

[15] Sarkar, S., & Mukherjee, P. (2019). Visualizing Model Performance for Improved Interpretability in Veterinary AI. Journal of AI Applications in Veterinary Medicine. https://avmajournals.avma.org/view/journals/javma/260/8/javma.22.03.0093.xml

[16] Liu, F., & Jones, S. (2022). «Improving Predictive Accuracy with Feature Engineering in Animal Health.» Journal of Computational Veterinary Medicine. https://digitaldefynd.com/IQ/ai-in-veterinary-medicine/

[17] Bohlouli, M., & Das, S. (2020). Feature Importance and Interpretability in Veterinary Predictive Models. Veterinary Informatics and Data Analysis. https://avmajournals.avma.org/view/journals/ajvr/83/5/ajvr.22.03.0038.xml

[18] Jones, D., & Miller, T. (2020). «Cross-Validation in Small Sample Veterinary Datasets.» Journal of Veterinary Data Science. https://digitaldefynd.com/IQ/ai-in-veterinary-medicine/

25

Herbal Plant Extracts and Wound Healing: Potential Epigenetic Pathway

***Gunjan Das*[1] *and S.R. Upadhyay*[2]**

Department of Veterinary Medicine, CoVSc & AH, CAU, (I), Jalukie Peren District Nagaland

Division of VMD, FVSc & AH, SKUAST-J, Jammu and Kashmir

Introduction

Wound is a disruption to the epithelial integrity of the skin, extended in-depth to subcutaneous tissue and other body parts such as ligaments, muscles, blood vessels, nerves, and bone (Robson et al. 2001). An appropriate wound healing is essential for the restoration of disrupted anatomical continuity (Begum, 2000). We have observed increasing interest in research based on traditional medicines of the world in the recent era (Medina-Franco et al. 2013). Traditional and complementary medicine regains popularity not only in developing countries but also in developed countries. Common and known practices across the globe of traditional medicines include Herbal, Ayurveda, Siddha, Unani, Iranian, Islamic, Vietnamese, Chinese, Acupuncture, African and other pseudo-medical knowledge (Dorai 2012). According to World Health Organization (WHO), traditional medicine 'the health practices, approaches, knowledge and beliefs incorporating plant, animal and mineral-based medicines, spiritual therapies, manual techniques and exercises, applied singularly or in combination to treat, diagnose and prevent illnesses or maintain well-being'. Saxena et al. (2013) reported that phytochemicals present in plants are liable for preventing disease and promoting health. Antibiotics used in the treatment of wound infections are now proved to have adverse effects in the human body and in pathogens where resistance is emerging. Attention has, therefore, turned towards extracting biologically active compounds from plant species having wound healing property (Pattanayak and Sunita, 2008).

Process of Wounds Healing

The mechanism and stages of the wound healing process will start with hemostasis where aggregated platelet is trapped and form the bulk of the clot to prevent blood loss. Activated platelets release growth factors to promote adhesion and aggression, thereby a provisional matrix is formed. Then during inflammation, different immune cells release pro-inflammatory cytokines for cleaning the wound infection by removing bacteria and denatured matrix components. They also release some growth factors FGF to recruit and activate the fibroblasts and epithelial cells to initiate subsequent phases of proliferation and synthesis of new ECM. After migration, fibroblast alters their morphology, settling down and replacing the provisional fibrin matrix with a new matrix. In the new matrix, epithelial cells detach and change their internal structure, then migrate, proliferate and differentiate over the granulation tissue to close the wound surface. Matrix remodelling is the final phase of the healing process where granulation tissue matures into the scar and the density of fibroblast and capillary decreases. Finally, the scar is replaced by ECM, similar to normal skin.

Herbs and Wound Healing

Wound contraction with polyherbal formulation containing *Utleria solicifolia curcas*, *Clerodendrum infortunatu* and *Centella asiatica* has (Pushpangandan et al. 2008). Traditional practices for the treatment of burn wounds, soft tissue wounds, ulcerated wounds, postnatal wounds, treatment of leech bites and skin infection with fresh leave decoction of *Chromolaena odorata* (Das et al. 2022). The ethnic Naga tribes use the mashed leaves of *Ageratum conyzoides* to apply on cuts and injuries (Das et al. 2020). Healing of the chronic ulcers with *Centella asiatica* has been reported (Kishore et al. 2011). Local tribes use *Aloe vera* succulent stem juice taken as raw for gastritis (Bharali et al. 2017). The ethnic tribes of Nagaland use mashed leaves of *Mikania micrantha* to apply in fresh cuts, injuries and wounds to stop bleeding (Das et al. 20220). The leaf juice is used to remove warts, treat wounds and eczema; leaves are crushed and used to wash latex or sap stains from hands (Nelia and Limasenla 2020). Methanolic extract of *Mimosa pudica* shoot and root showed very good wound healing activity of (Kannan et al. 2009). *Psidium guajava* leaves paste by grinding with little water or oil have been traditionally used for healing various wounds (Lam et al. 2016). *Lantana camara* is used in herbal medicine for the treatment of skin itches, as an antiseptic for wounds, and externally for leprosy and scabies (Nayak et al. 2009). According to Azarkan et al. (2003), *Carica papaya* fruits possess wound healing properties and its latex is used to apply on burnt wound using hydrogel. *Calendula officinalis* flowers' infusion is used to treat antifungal and antiseptic in wounds, marks, sprain, and freckles (Rehecho et al. 2011). *Curcuma longa* is mashed, warmed, and applied on wounds, skin problems, scabies and cuts an antiseptic (Velayudhan et al. 2012). Topical herbal oil formulation with *Heterophragma roxburghii* bark extract is an important natural curing therapy for different medical conditions like burn wounds, diabetic foot ulcer, untreated open wounds, snakebite wound (Sharma et al. 2021). *Rubia cordifolia* root is used by Indian folklore for treatment of cuts, wounds, burns and also uses in skin diseases like eczema, dermatitis, skin ulcers, etc. (Karodi et al. 2009).

Molecular Mechanism of Wound Healing

The wound healing response has long been recognized as a complex process requiring the dynamic interaction of cellular and blood-borne elements. Many cellular, extracellular, vascular, and cytokine-related components interact with one another during the three major phases of wound healing; the inflammatory response, proliferative phase and remodeling phase. During the early phase of cutaneous wound repair, new stroma, often called granulation tissue, begins to form approximately 4 d after injury (Tonnesen et al 2000). Macrophages, fibroblasts, and blood vessels move into the wound space as a unit, which correlates well with the proposed biologic interdependence of these cells during tissue repair. Macrophages provide a continuing source of cytokines necessary to invite myofibroblast and angiogenesis. Fibroblasts construct new extracellular matrix (ECM) necessary to support cell in growth, and blood vessels carry oxygen and nutrients necessary to sustain cell metabolism. Angiogenesis, formation of new blood vessel is a critical component of wound healing. Endothelial cells digest and penetrate the underlying vascular basement membrane, invade the ECM stroma and form tube-like structures that continue to extend. These events require a dynamic temporally and spatially regulated interaction between endothelial cells, angiogenesis factors, and surrounding ECM proteins (Madri et al. 1996). Injuries could induce transient TGF-β signaling as observed during wound healing and this stimulation subsequently increases the level of β-catenin in desmoids cells and has been shown in wound healing. In the case of chronic injuries, this would reoccur and the cells would have repeated periods of β-catenin accumulation due to activation of TGF-β pathway. TGF-β exerts its biological effects through TGF-βI and TGF-βII receptors, which form a heteromeric complex to facilitate signaling (Zhang et al 2009). The activated type 1 TGF-β receptor phosphorylates Smads-2 and -3, which in turn interact with Smad-4, resulting in nuclear translocation and activation of target gene transcription. Further, macrophages (via IL-1 and TNF-α) and fibroblasts via (fibroblast growth factor-2), KGF-2 and TGF-β mediate angiogenesis through keratinocyte-stimulated release of vascular endothelial growth factor (VEGF), which is a significant promoter of endothelial proliferation and angiogenesis (Zhang et al 2009). β-Catenin has long been established as a component of adherens junctions in association with cadherins. Adhesion proteins include epithelial cadherin (E-cadherin), neural cadherin (N-cadherin), placental cadherin (P-cadherin), muscle cadherin (M-cadherin), and vascular endothelial cadherin (VE-cadherin or CDH5).

Epigenetic Regulation of Wound Healing

Epigenetic regulatory mechanisms are essential for epidermal homeostasis. However, while the epigenetic regulation of epidermal homeostasis is now becoming active area of research, the epigenetic mechanisms controlling the wound healing response remain relatively untouched (Christopher et al.,

2014). Epigenetics is heritable changes in gene function without altering the nucleotide sequence. Epigenetics mainly includes three main mechanisms, DNA modification, histone modification, and regulation of non-coding RNAs (ncRNAs) (Zeybel et al., 2013). Precise epigenetic regulation is crucial for maintaining skin homeostasis and shaping the processes of wound healing. The epigenetic mechanism in the wound healing process is still not well understood. Considerable progress is witnessed within the last decades in understanding epigenetic mechanisms controlling gene expression including noncoding RNA and microRNA-dependent regulation. Epigenetic regulators intrinsically involved in the processes of wound repair and are able to dynamically regulate keratinocyte proliferation, differentiation, migration, dermal regeneration and angiogenesis. A series of complex regulatory mechanisms are involved to achieve this goal. This paper summarized to understand the epigenetic modification functioned during wound healing course, mainly including DNA methylation, histone modification, and regulation of siRNA interference. Regulating the wound healing process through precise epigenetic regulation might bring novel insights to accelerated wound healing.

Plant Extracts Enhancing Wound Healing Through Activation of Cell Signalling Pathway

We evaluated the wound healing effects of extract of *MM* using in vitro studies and in vivo studies. The modulation of cell signalling molecules after the treatment of the excision wound was evaluated to characterize signalling pathways involved in the healing process. Various in vitro studies, such as proliferation and migration in HDFa cells, invasion studies in HUVECs, and protein expression in HDFa cells using Western blot, were conducted. Gel zymography was conducted to determine the level of enzymatic activity of MMP-2 and MMP-9 in order to determine the extent of the degradation of ECM. Immunohistochemistry and other staining techniques were used to confirm the presence of the protein marker CD31 and cytokeratin for assessing angiogenesis and remodelling quality. In vivo studies like western blot assays for expression of FAK, Akt, mTOR, MMP-2, and MMP-9; immunohistochemistry for CD31 to confirm angiogenesis and assess the quality of wound healing. Use of *MM* increases HDFa cell migration and proliferation at a concentration. *MM* treatment of HUVECs and cutaneous wounds in rats also showed improvement in angiogenesis. The results of a western blot study revealed the activation of the FAK/Akt/mTOR cell signalling pathway in the healing tissue after the topical treatment of the cutaneous wound with the extract of *MM.* This signalling pathway is known to play a crucial role in the development, proliferation, and migration of different types of cells as well as the modulation of MMPs. The treatment showed upregulation of MMP-2 and MMP-9 expressions as well as an increase in their activities in both in vitro and in vivo studies. Our study demonstrated that use of the cold methanolic extract of *MM* accelerated wound healing in both in vitro and in vivo studies.

Conclusion

Traditional knowledge blended with advanced research may contribute immensely as many medicinal plants gifted by nature are yet to be explored and might have potential wound healing properties. The knowledge of various indigenous medicinal plants from village elderly and ethnic groups can be of immense significance to the researchers of alternative medicine. Further, better understanding of the underlying causes of cellular malfunction in chronic wounds, as well as the epigenetic targets of healing interventions, is essential for future development of herbal medicine for proper wound healing. Plant extract *MM* modulates fibroblast proliferation, migration, and invasiveness, angiogenesis, and MMP-2 and MMP-9 expressions and activities via activation of the FAK/Akt/mTOR cell signaling pathway.

References

Aggarwal BB, Sundaram C, Malani N, Ichikawa H. 2007. Curcumin: The Indian solid gold. The molecular targets and therapeutic uses of curcumin in health and disease, 1-75.

Ahmad W, Aquil Z, Alam SS. 2020. Historical background of wound care. Hamdan Med J;13:189-95. DOI: 10.4103/HMJ.HMJ_37_20.

Azarkan M, El Moussaoui A, Van Wuytswinkel D. 2003. Fractionation and purification of the enzymes stored in the latex of Carica papaya. J Chromatogr B Anal Technol Biomed Life Sci; 790: 229–238. DOI:10.1016/S1570-0232(03)00084-9.

Begum D, Nath SC. 2000. Ethnobotanical review of medicinal plants used for skin diseases and related problems in Northeastern India, Journal of Herbs. Spices and Medicinal Plants 7: 55–93.

Bharali R, Bharali L, Borkotoky D, Singh RK. 2017. Ethno medicinal plants used in traditional health care by Chakhesang tribe of Phek district. Bull. Env. Pharmacol. Life Sci., Vol 6 Special issue 1: 46-49.

Broughton G, Janis JE, Attinger CE. 2006. The basic science of wound healing. Plast Reconstr Surg; 117(7suppl): 12S – 34S. DOI: 10.1097/01.prs.0000225430.42531.c2.

Christopher, J. L. , Andrei., N. M. , Andrey, A S., Michael Y F., and Vladimir, A B.. (2014). The Epigenetic Regulation of Wound Healing, Adv Wound Care (New Rochelle).,3(7):468–475.

Das G, Thou K Mondal P, Meeran SM 2022. Review: Ethnomedicinal plants used for wound healing and dermatological problem in the North-Eastern Hill Region of India. Asian J Ethnobiol 5: 102-119.

Debbarma M, Nazir A Pala, Munesh K, Rainer W Bussmann. 2017. Traditional knowledge of medicinal plants in tribes of Tripura in northeast, India. Debberma et al., Afr J Tradit Complement Altern Med., 14 (4): 156-168. DOI: 10.21010/ajtcam.v14i4.19.

Dorai AA. 2012. Wound care with traditional, complementary and alternative medicine. Indian Journal of Plastic Surgery: Official Publication of the Association of Plastic Surgeons of India, 45(2), 418-424. DOI:10.4103/0970-0358.101331.

Kannan S, Aravinth S, Aravinth J, Sam E, Kumar J, Kayarohanam S, Suthakaran R, Ravi M, Devi BP. 2009. Wound healing activity o*f Mimosa pudi*ca Linn. formulation. IJPR; 1(4):1554-58.

Karodi R, Jadhav M, Rub R, Bafna A. 2009. Evaluation of the wound healing activity of a crude extract o*f Rubia cordifol*ia L. (Indian madder) in mice. International Journal of Applied Research in Natural Products.Vol. 2(2), pp. 12-18. http://www.healthy-synergies.com.

Khare CP. 2004. Encyclopedia of Indian Medicinal Plants, Springer, Germany, 405-406.

Kishore B, Siva Prasad M, Murthy GK. 2011. Comparison of the dermal wound healing of *Centella asiatica* extract impregnated collagen and cross linked collagen scaffolds. J Chem Pharm Res 3(3):353–362.

Lam KY, Ling APK, Koh RY, Wong YP, Say YH. 2016. A review on medicinal properties of orientin. Advances in Pharmacological Sciences. DOI: 10.1155/2016/4104595.

Madri, JA, Sankar, S & Romanic, AM: Angiogenesis. In: RAF Clark, ed. The Molecular and Cellular Biology of Wound Repair New York, Plenum Press, pp. 355–372, 1996.

Medina-Franco JL, Giulianotti MA, Welmaker GS, Houghten RA. Shifting from the single to the multi target paradigm in drug discovery. Drug Discov Today. 2013 May; 18 (9-10):495-501. DOI: 10.1016/j.drudis.2013.01.008. Epub 2013 Jan 20. PMID: 23340113; PMCID: PMC3642214.

Mordeniz, C. 2019. Integration of Traditional and Complementary Medicine into Evidence-Based Clinical Practice. In (Ed.), Traditional and Complementary Medicine. IntechOpen. DOI:10.5772/intechopen.87061.

Mordeniz, C. 2019. Introductory Chapter: Traditional and Complementary Medicine. In (Ed.), Traditional and Complementary Medicine. IntechOpen. DOI:10.5772/intechopen.86373.

Nair RV and Sala A V. 1995. Indian medicinal plants-a compendium of 500 species. Hyd: Ori Long Pvt Ltd, 4, 15-17.

Nayak BS, Raju SS, Eversley M, Ramsubhag A. 2009. Evaluation of wound healing activity of *Lantana camar*a L.- a preclinical study. DOI:10.1002/ptr.2599.

Nelia L, Limasenla. 2020. Traditional knowledge of medicinal plants used by the Chakhesang Naga tribe in Phek District of Nagaland, India. Pleione. 14. 237-247. DOI:10.26679/Pleione.14.2.2020.237-247.

O'Toole EA. 2001. Extracellular matrix and keratinocyte migration. Clin Exp Dermatol; 26 (6):525–30. DOI: 10.1046/j.1365-2230.2001.00891.x.

Panyaphu K, On TV, Sirisa-Ard P, Srisa-Nga P, ChansaKaow S, Nathakarnkitkul S 2011: Medicinal plants of the Mien (Yao) in Northern Thailand and their potential value in the primary healthcare of postpartum women. J Ethnopharmacol. 135, 226–237. DOI: 10.1016/j.jep.2011.03.050.

Pattanayak, S.P and Sunita, P. (2008). Wound healing, anti-microbial and antioxidant potential of Dendrophthoe falcata (L.f) Ettingsh., J Ethnopharmacol, 120(2):241-7.

Pushpangadan P, Mehrotra S, Rawat AKS, Rao CV, Ojha SK, Aziz I. 2008. Herbal composition for cuts, burns and wounds. US 7344737. http://www.freepatentsonline.com/7344737.html.

Rafique Khan SM, Akhter T, Hussain M. 2021. Ethno-veterinary practice for the treatment of animal diseases in Neelum Valley, Kashmir Himalaya, Pakistan.PloS ONE 16(4):e0250114. DOI: 10.1371/journal.pone.0250114.

Rahman IU, Afzal A, Iqbal Z, Ijaz F, Ali N, Shah M, Ullah S, Bussmann RW. 2019. Historical perspectives of ethnobotany. Clinics in Dermatology, 37(4), 382-388. DOI: 10.1016/j.clindermatol.2018.03.018.

Rehecho S, Uriarte-Pueyo I, Calvo J, Vivas LA, Calvo MI. 2011. Ethnopharmacological survey of medicinal plants in Nor-Yauyos, a part of the Landscape Reserve Nor-Yauyos-Cochas, Peru. J Ethnopharmacol;133:75-8. DOI:10.1016/j.jep.2010.09.006.

Rehman S, Iqbal Z, Qureshi R, Rahman IU, Sakhi S, Khan I, Hashem A, Al-Arjani A-BF, Almutairi KF, Abd_Allah EF, Ali N, Khan MA and Ijaz F. 2022. Ethnoveterinary Practices of Medicinal Plants Among Tribes of Tribal District of North Waziristan, Khyber Pakhtunkhwa, Pakistan. Front. Vet. Sci. 9:815294. DOI: 10.3389/fvets.2022.815294.

Robson MC, Steed DL, Franz MG. 2001. Wound healing: Biologic features and approaches to maximize healing trajectories. Curr Probl Surg 38: 72-140. DOI:10.1067/msg.2001.111167.

Santhosh AM, Shravanthi V, Jhansi SU. 2015. An Overview of herbs possessing wound healing activity. Eur J Pharm Med Res; 2(7): 329–332.

Saxena M, Saxena J, Nema R, Singh D, Gupta A. 2013. Phytochemistry of Medicinal Plants. Journal of Pharmacognosy and Phytochemistry 1 (6):168-182.

Sharma A, Khanna S, Kaur G. 2021. Medicinal plants and their components for wound healing applications. Futur J Pharm Sci **7**, 53. DOI:10.1186/s43094-021-00202-w.

Tonnesen MG, Feng X, Clark RA. Angiogenesis in wound healing. J Investig Dermatol Symp Proc. 2000. 5(1):40-6.

Velayudhan KC, Dikshit N, Abdul Nizar M. 2012. Ethnobotany of turmeric (Curcuma longa L.). Indian Journal of Traditional Knowledge. 11(4), 607–614.

Velnar T, Bailey T, Smrkolj V. 2009. The Wound Healing Process: an Overview of the Cellular and Molecular Mechanisms: The Journal of Intern*ational Medic*al Research; 37: 1528 – 1542. DOI: 10.1177/147323000903700531.

Verma RK, Verma SK. 2006. Phytochemical and termiticidal studies of Lantana camara var aculeata leaves. Fitoterapia 77: 466-468. DOI: 10.1016/j.fitote.2006.05.014.

WHO Traditional Medicine Strategy: 2014–2023, ISBN: 9789241506090, http://www.who.int/traditional-complementary-integrative-medicine/en/.

Zeybel M., Mann D. A., Mann J. (2013). Epigenetic modifications as new targets for liver disease therapies. *J. Hepatol.* 59 (6), 1349–1353.

Zhasa NN, Hazarika P, Tripathi YC. 2015. Indigenous knowledge on utilization of plant biodiversity for treatment and cure of diseases of human beings in Nagaland, India: a case study. Intl Res J Biol. Sci 4 (4): 89–106.

26

Fostering Antibiotics Stewardship in Farming Communities: An Extension Approach

***Pranav Kumar*[1], *Veerta Bhagat*[2] *and S.R. Upadhyay*[3]**

[1]*Division of Veterinary & A.H. Extension Education, Faculty of Veterinary Sciences & Animal Husbandry (VAHEE), SKUAST-Jammu, Jammu and Kashmir*
[2]*Division of VAHEE, Faculty of Veterinary Sciences & Animal Husbandry, SKUAST-Jammu, Jammu and Kashmir*
[3]*Veterinary and Animal Husbandry Extension Education, Faculty of Veterinary Sciences & Animal Husbandry, SKUAST-Jammu, Jammu and Kashmir*

Introduction

As India is the leading global economy with livestock contributing 4.66% in total GVA to Indian Economy (PIB, 2024) and ranks 1st in Milk Production, 2nd in Egg production, 5th in meat production (BAHS, 2024). Being the largest exporter of milk and meat in the world , this has led to the intensification of animal production due to the increasing demand of major livestock products (MLPs), which has led to an increasing overall use of antimicrobials. Antimicrobials are invariably used to preserve animal and public health, but also as growth promoters at a sub-therapeutic level. The overuse and misuse of antibiotics can contribute to antimicrobial resistance. The growing resistance to antimicrobial drugs could reverse the therapeutic benefits; animals' resistance to antimicrobial drugs, reduces productivity and leads to economic losses. Unwanted antimicrobials residues may be present in products of animal origins, in animal waste contaminating soil and water and the environment. Seventy-five to ninety percent of antimicrobials used in livestock are excreted, mostly unmetabolized. AMR poses a serious threat to the safety and quality of animal origin food, food security and livelihoods. Unhealthy and unproductive animals are no longer able to generate food products of acceptable safety and quality for human consumption and can no longer contribute to income generation. Insufficient standards for residues in animal food products, reduces the livestock sectors potential of access to trade and increases public health risks (https://www.fao.org/antimicrobial-resistance/key-sectors/animal-production/en/). This emergence of antibiotic-resistant bacteria has become a global concern, threatening the effectiveness of antibiotics in treating human and animal diseases. Farming communities, particularly those involved in livestock production, play a critical role in addressing this issue. This write-up explores the importance of fostering antibiotic stewardship in farming communities and proposes an extension approach to promote responsible antibiotic use.

The Problem of Antibiotic Resistance

Antibiotic resistance occurs when bacteria develop mechanisms to resist the effects of antibiotics. The overuse and misuse of antibiotics in livestock accelerate the development of antibiotic-resistant bacteria. Unwanted antimicrobials residues may be present in products of animal origins, in animal waste contaminating soil and water and the environment. These resistant bacteria can spread to humans through the food chain, contaminated water, and direct contact with infected animals. The consequences of antibiotic resistance are severe. In humans, antibiotic-resistant infections can lead to increased morbidity, mortality, and healthcare costs. In animals, antibiotic resistance can result in reduced treatment options, increased disease transmission, and economic losses.

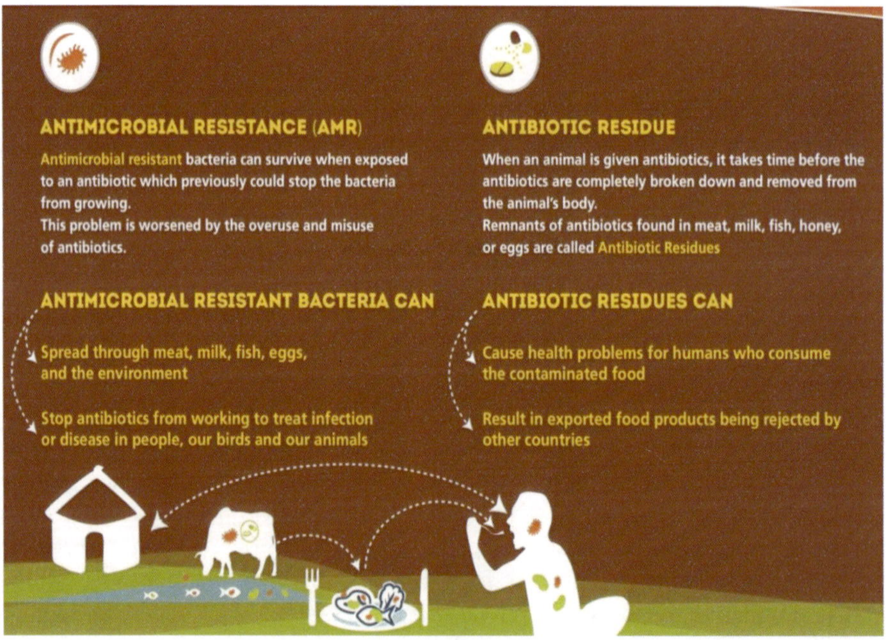

Fig 1. AMR and Antibiotic Residue description according to FAO.

Antimicrobial resistance (AMR) is a global health and development threat. It requires urgent multisectoral action in order to achieve the Sustainable Development Goals (SDGs). WHO has declared that AMR is one of the top 10 global public health threats facing humanity. Antimicrobials – including antibiotics, antivirals, antifungals and anti-parasitic – are medicines used to prevent and treat infections in humans, animals and plants. According to WHO by 2030, India is set to be among the top five nations with the highest proportion of global antimicrobial usage (Van B.T.P. et.al 2015).

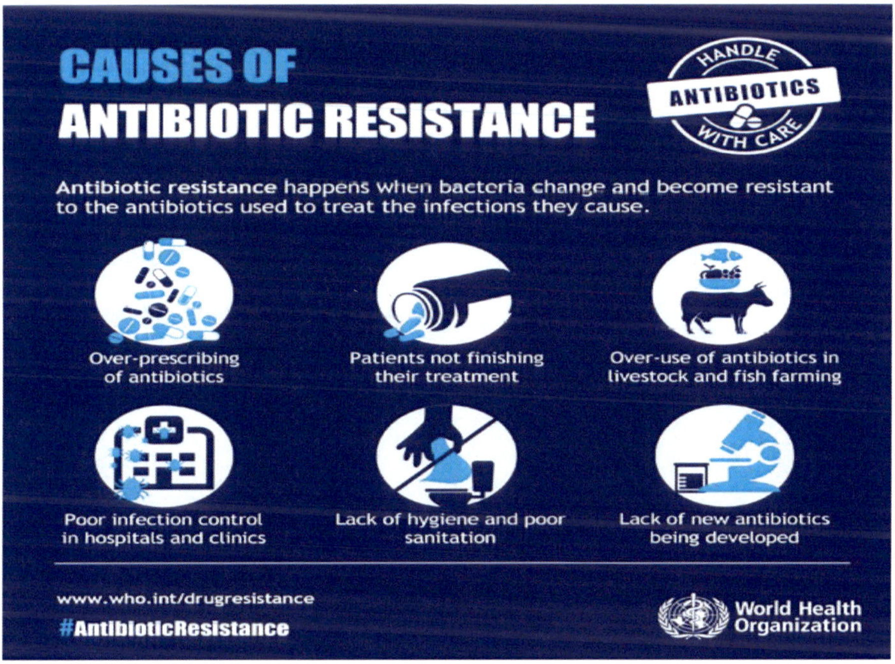
CAUSES OF
ANTIBIOTIC RESISTANCE
HANDLE ANTIBIOTICS WITH CARE
Antibiotic resistance happens when bacteria change and become resistant to the antibiotics used to treat the infections they cause.
Over-prescribing of antibiotics
Patients not finishing their treatment
Over-use of antibiotics in livestock and fish farming
Poor infection control in hospitals and clinics
Lack of hygiene and poor sanitation
Lack of new antibiotics being developed
www.who.int/drugresistance
#AntibioticResistance
World Health Organization

Fig 2. Causes of Antibiotic Resistance as described by WHO

The Role of Livestock Farming Communities

Farming communities are critical stakeholders in addressing antibiotic resistance. Livestock producers, in particular, rely heavily on antibiotics to maintain animal health and productivity. However, the misuse and overuse of antibiotics in livestock can contribute significantly to the development of antibiotic-resistant bacteria. Animals do get diseased occasionally and for managing animal health we need veterinary medicine & antibiotics. For more than 85 years, antibiotics have been used in animals, humans, and agriculture. (Gilchrist M.J. et.al, 2007).

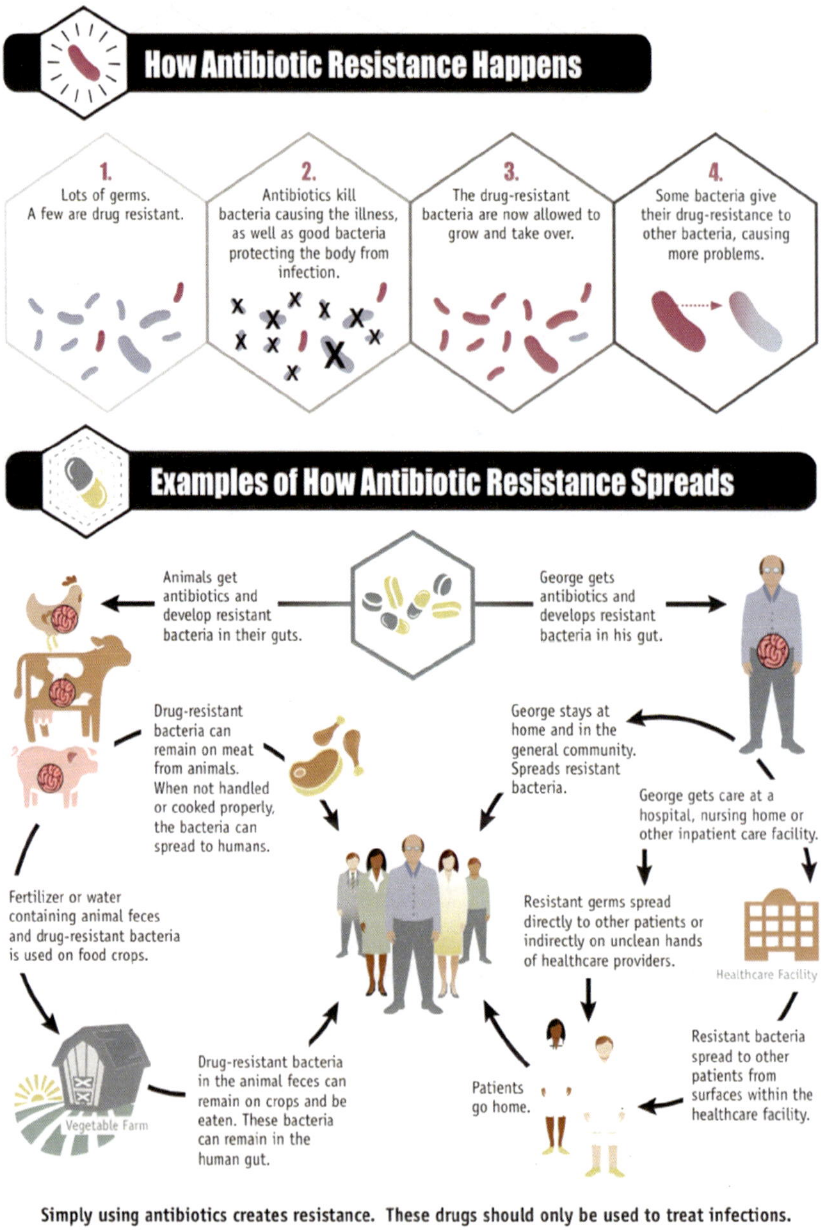

Fig 3. Antibiotic resistance infographic. Photo by CDC/Wikimedia Commons

Causes of AMR

Antibiotics during illness are to be used on prescription of veterinarian. Antibiotic resistance has been linked to an extensive "over-the-counter" drug supply available to farmers and improper dispensing by para-veterinarians. (Sharma A. et.al,2022). Antibiotics cannot be used routinely nor to compensate for poor hygiene, inadequate husbandry, or poor farm management. The overuse and misuse of antibiotics have been identified as significant drivers of AMR. Irregular usage of antibiotics may make it more likely for microorganisms to evolve resistance. AMR cannot be stopped, but it may be controlled and manage (Ferdous J. et.al, 2019). The use of growth-promoters is largely a problem of intensive farming methods and the problems caused by their use are largely those of developed rather than developing countries. The result of the use of growth promoters is an improvement in daily growth rates between 1 and 10 percent resulting in meat of a better quality, with less fat and increased protein content. There is controversy surrounding the use of growth promoters for animals destined for meat production, as overuse of any antibiotic over a period of time may lead to the local bacterial populations becoming resistant to the antibiotic. The cattle industry depends on growth promoters as cattle have high energy requirements that cannot be met easily without the use of growth promoters. High energy rations increase muscle growth and fat deposition in beef cattle, and help to improve milk productivity in dairy cattle. Such rations are associated with side-effects, such as bloat and lactic acidosis, which can be debilitating or even fatal.

Development of Antibiotic Stewardship and Its Concept in Livestock Sector

In 1996, John McGowan and Dale Gerding first applied the term antimicrobial stewardship, where they suggested a causal association between antimicrobial agent use and resistance.

Stewardship: defined as "the careful and responsible management of something entrusted to one's care".

Antimicrobial stewardship (AMS): AMS is a coherent set of actions which promote the responsible use of antimicrobials. This definition can be applied to actions at the individual level as well as the national and global level, and across human health, animal health and the environment (Dyar et.al, 2017). Thus, Antimicrobial Stewardship (AMS) refers to the optimal selection, dosing, and duration of antimicrobial treatment resulting in the best clinical outcome with minimal side effects to the patients and minimal impact on subsequent resistance (Jt Comm J Qual Improv. 2001). Responsible stewardship practices include actions that preserve the effectiveness of antibiotics while maintaining animal health. Only using antibiotics when necessary to manage illness in animals. Establishing best management practices, like use of vaccines, and disease prevention plans to reduce the overall need for antibiotics. Livestock owners and veterinarians working together to make decisions that improve animal health and welfare in long-term.

Antimicrobial Stewardship for a Sustainable Tomorrow

AMS is a mindset: It is all about setting a general action plan, with the ultimate goal being to preserve human and animal health and the effectiveness of antimicrobial medications.

To foster a culture of continuous improvement, experts have recommended the 5 R approach to AMS:

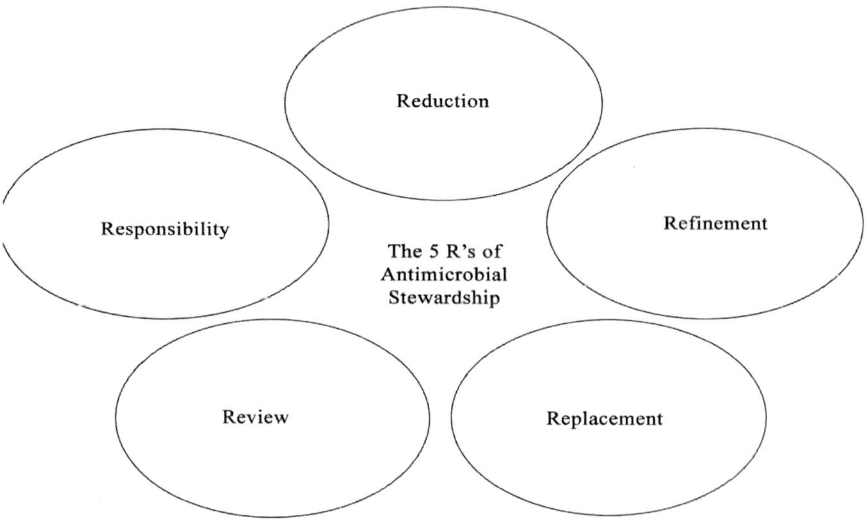

Fig 4: Five R's of Antimicrobial Stewardship

- **Responsibility:** Everyone who uses antimicrobials acknowledges that use can cause harm beyond the animal being treated. Any time we use these drugs, the reward should outweigh the risk. When we do use an antimicrobial, we should take actions that reduce the risk for future animals and the public's health
- **Reduction:** Whenever we can, we need to look for ways to reduce our reliance on antimicrobials
- **Refinement:** When we use antimicrobials, we should ensure that we are using the right drug, at the right dose, at the right time, treating the right bug, for the correct length of time

- **Replacement:** Consider non-antimicrobial products that could be used to promote good health and prevent disease
- **Review:** Everyone on the farm management team (owners, herdspeople, nutritionists, veterinarians, other advisors) needs to sit down and look at farm records on a regular basis. When we do this, we should be critical of every instance that an antimicrobial was used and decide on a specific strategy for making further improvements and reductions in use

It is important to realize that these distinctions are not mutually exclusive — they are all intimately interconnected. Efforts to replace antimicrobials with other products should naturally lead to a reduction in antimicrobial use without compromising animal health or welfare.

Extension Approach to Promote Antibiotic Stewardship

Extension services can play a crucial role in promoting antibiotic stewardship in farming communities. An extension approach can facilitate the adoption of responsible antibiotic use practices by providing farmers with the necessary knowledge, skills, and support. Farming communities can play a vital role in promoting antibiotic stewardship by adopting responsible antibiotic use practices. This includes using +antibiotics only when necessary, following proper dosing and administration guidelines, and implementing alternative disease prevention and management strategies

The following components can be included in an extension approach to promote antibiotic stewardship:

- Awareness and Education: Organize workshops, training programs, and demonstrations to educate farmers on the risks associated with antibiotic misuse and the importance of responsible antibiotic use.
- Technical Assistance: Provide farmers with technical guidance on alternative disease prevention and management strategies, such as vaccination, biosecurity, and sanitation.
- Demonstration and Training: Establish demonstration plots and provide hands-on training to farmers on integrated disease management practices, including the use of antibiotics.
- Farmer-to-Farmer Education: Encourage experienced farmers to share their knowledge and best practices with peers, promoting a culture of responsible antibiotic use.
- Collaboration with Veterinarians: Work with veterinarians to provide farmers with expert advice on antibiotic use and disease management.

Implementation Strategy

To implement the extension approach, the following steps can be taken:

- Conduct a Needs Assessment: Identify the knowledge gaps and training needs of farmers in the target area.

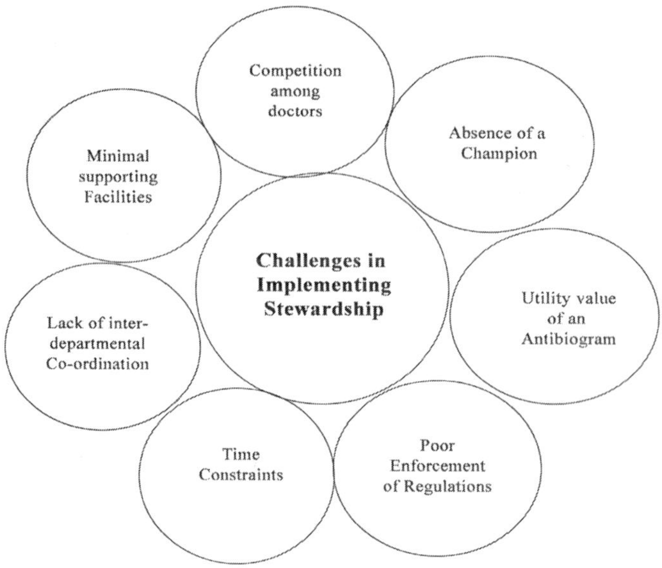

Extension Model for Antibiotics Stewardship

- Direct education through workshops, seminars, demonstrations etc.
- Media outreach (Radio, TV , Social Media).
- Peer to peer education and farmer groups.
- Collaboration with farmers for better herd health management.

Key Strategies for Promoting AMS

- Educating farmers on proper dosage, timing, and alternatives.
- Educating farmers on the risks of misuse of antibiotics.
- Encouraging record keeping and monitoring of antibiotic use.
- Educating farmers on the human health risk due to presence of antibiotic residue in food chain.
- Training programs for farmers for promoting AMS.

- Training programs for the professionals including veterinarian, extension workers, and other stakeholders.
- Collaboration required between essential stakeholders eg: between farmers, veterinarians, policy makers, extension agents.
- Collaboration for Stewardship between government, NGOs etc.
- NGOs like BAIF and collaboration with Pfizer has helped to increase awareness against AMR.

Project Parivartan: The flagship programme under this umbrella is Project Parivartan that focuses on addressing the current infection prevention and control (IPC) challenges in healthcare facilities. This is a multi-year project that Pfizer supports to develop a model for institutional capacity building and deliver facility-based IPC and antimicrobial stewardship (AMS) training in small and mid-size hospitals across India. The goal is to demonstrate that a tangible impact on infection prevention can be made through antimicrobial stewardship activities to improve key outcome indicators in hospitals, such as a reduction in hospital acquired infections.

National Action Plan on Antimicrobial Resistance (NAP-AMR)

In 2015, understanding the gravity of the problem of antimicrobial resistance (AMR), the World Health Assembly (WHA) has adopted the Global Action Plan on AMR (GAP-AMR) in collaboration with the World Health Organization (WHO), Food & Agricultural Organization (FAO) & World Organization for Animal Health (WOAH).

Six Strategic Priorities in National Action Plan for Antimicrobial Resistance in India

1. Improve awareness and understanding of AMR through effective comunication, education training	1. Strengthen knowledge and evidence through surveillance	3. Reduce the encidence of infection through effective infection prevention and control
4. Oprimize the use of antimicrobial agents in health, animal and food	5. Promote investments for AMR activities, research and innovations	6. Strengthen India's leadership on AMR

(NMC Module for prescribers, 2024)

Kerala Antimicrobial Resistance Strategic Action Plan (KARSAP)

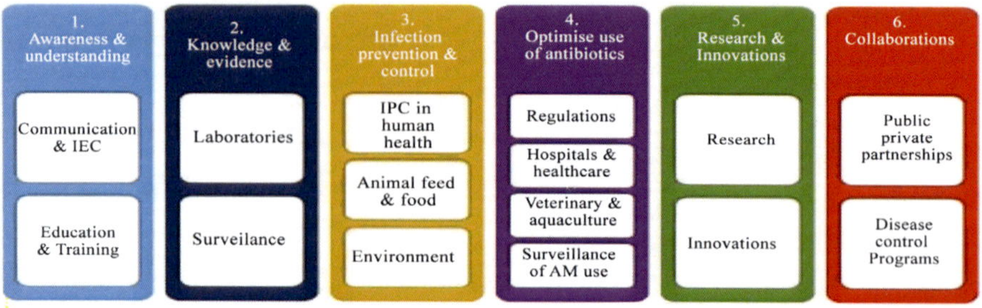

(Government of Kerala October, 2018)

Role of Ethno Veterinary Medicine (EVM) in AMS for Livestock Management Practices

Ethno-veterinary practices concern to animal healthcare comprised of belief, knowledge, practices and skills pertaining to healthcare and management of livestock acquired through practical experience and has traditionally been passed down orally from generation to generation. The plant based traditional medicine systems continue to play an essential role in health care, with about 80% of the world's farmers, shepherds and animal growers relying mainly on traditional medicines for treating routine remedies for their livestock (Lulekal et al., 2008 and Devi et al., 2009). EVM is not restricted to treatment of animal diseases alone, but also involves a myriad of disciplines with all aspects of people's knowledge and practices in animal healthcare, productivity and performance that include their diagnostic and ethological understandings; preventive, primitive and therapeutic skills and treatment; and a wide range of health-related management techniques (Lans et al., 2007). Ethno-veterinary medicine plays important role in livestock development especially in the developing countries. It is viewed as a potential tool to overcome the side-effects of modern drugs and promote organic farming in both developing and developed nations. They are often cheap, safe, time tested and based on local resources and strengths. These can provide useful alternatives to conventional animal health care (Kumar et al, 2002).

EVM is recognized as a potential resource that can play pivotal role in grassroots development and poverty alleviation, empowering people by enhancing the use of their own knowledge and resources in the developing countries (Iqbal et al, 2005).

Recommendations

- Integrate Antibiotic Stewardship into Extension Programs: Incorporate antibiotic stewardship into existing extension programs, ensuring that farmers receive comprehensive guidance on responsible antibiotic use.

- Develop Context-Specific Training Programs: Design training programs that address the specific needs and knowledge gaps of farmers in different regions and production systems.
- Foster Collaboration between Farmers, Veterinarians, and Extension Agents: Encourage collaboration between farmers, veterinarians, and extension agents to promote a culture of responsible antibiotic use and provide comprehensive support to farmers.
- Monitor and Evaluate Extension Programs: Regularly monitor and evaluate extension programs to assess their impact on antibiotic use practices and identify areas for improvement.

Conclusion

Fostering antibiotic stewardship in farming communities is critical to addressing the global threat of antibiotic resistance. An extension approach can play a vital role in promoting responsible antibiotic use practices among farmers. By providing farmers with the necessary knowledge, skills, and support, extension services can help reduce the misuse and overuse of antibiotics in agriculture, ultimately contributing to a safer and more sustainable food system.

- Antibiotic Stewardship is crucial for sustainable agriculture and public health.
- Extension services and Veterinarian play vital role in promoting responsible antibiotic use
- Raising farmers understanding in the use and misuse of antibiotics is the core to resist the resistance.
- Control of AMR should be taken as a GLOBAL PRIORITY before it becomes too grim.

Suggested reading

Basic Animal Husbandry Statistics. (2024). Department of Animal Husbandry and Dairying, Government of India.

Devi, K. R., Singh, T. K., & Devi, L. (2009). Traditional Veterinary Practices in Manipur, India. Indian Journal of Traditional Knowledge, 8(2), 245-249.

Ferdous, J., Islam, M. R., & Alam, M. S. (2019). Antimicrobial Resistance in Livestock and Its Impact on Human Health. Journal of Environmental Science and Health, Part B, 54, 257-265.

Food and Agriculture Organization of the United Nations. (n.d.). Antimicrobial Resistance in Animal Production. Retrieved from <(link unavailable)>

Gilchrist, M. J., Greko, C., Wallinga, D. B., Beran, G. W., Riley, D. G., & Thorne, P. S. (2007). The potential role of concentrated animal feeding operations in infectious disease epidemics and antibiotic resistance. Environmental Health Perspectives, 115(2), 313-316.

Government of Kerala. (2018). Kerala Antimicrobial Resistance Strategic Action Plan (KARSAP).

https://commons.wikimedia.org/wiki/File:CDCinfographicANTIBIORESISTANCE.png

https://openknowledge.fao.org/bitstreams/69b24b62-08ff-4d08-b727-a1ebe216bfb5/download

https://www.amstewardship.ca/faast-reviews/antimicrobial-stewardship/the-5-rs-of-antimicrobial-stewardship/

https://www.pfizer.co.in/our-community-efforts/csr-initiatives/resisting-the-resistance-together

https://www.who.int/europe/multi-media/item/causes-of-antibiotic-resistance

Iqbal, Z., Lateef, M., Khan, M. N., & Jabbar, A. (2005). Ethnoveterinary Medicine: A Review. Journal of Ethnopharmacology, 96(1-2), 1-13.

Kumar, A., Kumar, S., & Kumar, R. (2002). Ethnoveterinary Medicine in India: A Review. Indian Journal of Traditional Knowledge, 1(2), 141-148.

Lans, C., Turner, N., Khan, T., & Bauer, G. (2007). Ethnoveterinary Medicine: A Review of the Literature. Journal of Ethnobiology and Ethnomedicine, 3, 15.

Lulekal, E., Kelbessa, E., Bekele, T., & Feleke, A. (2008). An Ethnobotanical Study of Medicinal Plants in Mana Angetu District, South-Eastern Ethiopia. Journal of Ethnopharmacology, 117(1), 10-22.

National Medical Commission. (2024). Module for Prescribers on Antimicrobial Resistance.

Pfizer India. (n.d.). Resisting the Resistance Together. Retrieved from <(link unavailable)>

Press Information Bureau, Government of India. (2024). Livestock Sector in India.

Sharma, A., Sharma, S., & Kumar, A. (2022). Antimicrobial Resistance in Livestock: A Review. Journal of Veterinary Pharmacology and Toxicology, 21(1), 1-9.

Van Boeckel, T. P., Brower, C., Gilbert, M., Grenfell, B. T., Levin, S. A., Robinson, T. P., Teillant, A., & Laxminarayan, R. (2015). Global trends in antimicrobial use in food animals. Proceedings of the National Academy of Sciences, 112(18), 5649-5654.

World Health Organization. (n.d.). Antimicrobial Resistance. Retrieved from <(link unavailable)

27

Smart Animal Health: Transforming Animal Welfare Through Digital and AI Powered Technologies

Pranav Kumar, Anna Singh[2] and S.R. Upadhyay[3]

[1]Division of Veterinary & A.H. Extension Education, Faculty of Veterinary Sciences & Animal Husbandry (VAHEE), SKUAST-Jammu, Jammu & Kashmir
[2]Division of VAHEE, Faculty of Veterinary Sciences & Animal Husbandry SKUAST-Jammu, Jammu & Kashmir
Veterinary and Animal Husbandry Extension Education, Faculty of Veterinary Sciences & Animal Husbandry, SKUAST-Jammu, Jammu & Kashmir

By 2050, the global population is projected to reach approximately 9.8 billion, requiring a 70% increase in food production to meet the growing dietary demands. The livestock sector will play a crucial role in addressing this rising need through sustainable animal production, contributing to food security, poverty alleviation, public health, and food safety. To tackle the challenges posed by population growth and to achieve the United Nations Sustainable Development Goals (SDGs), technological advancements and innovations will be essential in transforming the food and agriculture sectors.

In light of these challenges, Veterinary Services are more critical than ever. They are essential for enhancing livestock health and productivity, ensuring high-quality food that meets safety standards, and mitigating risks associated with animal diseases and public health. Additionally, Veterinary Services must contribute to global efforts in addressing issues such as food security, antimicrobial resistance, climate change, and the depletion of natural resources.

Over the past century, scientific and technological advancements have driven significant changes in livestock farming and animal health. The integration of innovative breeding techniques, automated feeding and milking systems, and modern housing solutions has led to the intensification of farming systems, enabling increased food production for the growing global population. Furthermore, developments in animal health biotechnologies—such as vaccines, antimicrobials, and diagnostic tools—have been fundamental in reducing disease burdens, improving animal welfare, and enhancing product quality, all of which have contributed to the expansion of the livestock sector.

Currently, rapid technological progress—including cutting-edge biotechnologies, nutritional innovations, and digital solutions—is reshaping the industry. Among these, digital technology has emerged as one of the fastest-growing fields, significantly influencing modern life and gaining prominence in recent years as part of the Fourth Industrial Revolution (Industry 4.0). This revolution is driving disruptive innovations that are transforming multiple sectors, including food and agriculture. Key technologies facilitating this transformation include mobile applications, the Internet of Things (IoT), cloud computing, big data analytics, artificial intelligence, blockchain, and other advanced digital tools.

The integration of these digital technologies in agriculture is opening new pathways for improved livestock policies and management practices, fostering more sustainable and resilient food systems. As a key component of agriculture, animal health plays a vital role in this shift. Veterinary Services must actively participate in this digital transformation by reassessing their organizational structures and ensuring the effective adoption of these technologies for policymaking, decision-making, and strategic planning. In alignment with its vision to strengthen global animal health governance and enhance Veterinary Services' resilience, the World Organisation for Animal Health (OIE) conducted a survey to identify external factors that could impact the sector over the next decade. Among the 17 key factors identified by experts and stakeholders, the increasing reliance on big data analytics and other advanced technologies was highlighted, underscoring the need for Veterinary Services to adapt to these evolving trends.

Digital Health Technologies in Veterinary Care

Big Data and Analytics

Big data is playing a crucial role in veterinary sciences by enabling predictive analytics, disease modeling, and epidemiological studies. By aggregating large datasets from electronic medical records (EMRs), wearable devices, and farm management systems, veterinarians can make more informed decisions regarding disease outbreaks, herd health, and treatment efficacy.

Big Data and analytics are revolutionizing the veterinary and animal husbandry sectors by enabling more precise decision-making, improving animal health, enhancing production efficiency, and fostering sustainability. In the realm of animal health, data-driven insights are proving invaluable for early disease detection and prevention. By analyzing large volumes of health-related data from farm records, sensor data, and environmental factors, veterinarians can detect disease outbreaks early and take proactive measures to prevent their spread. Personalized treatment plans are also made possible by analyzing individual animal health data, which can lead to better recovery rates and more targeted medical interventions, reducing the need for unnecessary treatments.

In breeding and genetics, Big Data is playing a significant role in accelerating the improvement of livestock breeds. Through the analysis of genetic data, breeders can identify desirable traits such as disease resistance, higher milk yield, and better growth rates. This enables more informed breeding decisions, leading to livestock that are more productive and resilient. Additionally, big data analytics helps optimize reproductive management, ensuring that breeding schedules are more efficient and that animals are in optimal health for reproduction, which in turn reduces time to market for livestock.

In terms of supply chain management, Big Data enables more efficient planning and resource allocation. Predictive analytics tools help farmers predict the best times for slaughter, transportation, and sales based on various data inputs. This reduces waste and increases the efficiency of the entire supply chain. Furthermore, the integration of blockchain with Big Data allows for enhanced traceability and transparency, ensuring that consumers can track the origins of their food products. This not only ensures food safety but also builds consumer trust in the integrity of the supply chain.

The use of Big Data in disease surveillance and control is another critical area. Real-time data from farms, veterinary clinics, and diagnostic labs is analyzed to track the spread of infectious diseases. This allows authorities to act quickly and implement containment measures, minimizing the impact of outbreaks. Additionally, livestock movements are monitored, ensuring compliance with health protocols and reducing the risk of cross-border disease transmission.

Big Data also supports sustainability in animal husbandry by providing analytics on environmental impacts. By tracking data on water usage, feed consumption, and greenhouse gas emissions, farmers can make informed decisions to reduce their environmental footprint. Data analytics also helps farmers adapt to the challenges posed by climate change, such as extreme weather patterns that can affect livestock productivity. This is particularly valuable in developing strategies for climate-resilient farming practices.

Finally, decision support systems, powered by Big Data, are becoming essential tools for farmers. Mobile apps and digital platforms, which integrate real-time data analytics, allow farmers to receive actionable insights regarding animal health, breeding cycles, and production management. These tools make it easier for farmers, even in remote areas, to make informed decisions that enhance productivity, improve animal welfare, and contribute to more sustainable farming practices.

Telemedicine and Remote Monitoring

Telemedicine has emerged as a transformative solution in veterinary care, enabling veterinarians to deliver remote consultations, monitor pet health, and provide guidance to pet owners from a distance. This approach offers convenience and accessibility, allowing real-time connections between veterinarians and pet owners, regardless of geographical barriers. Through telemedicine platforms and mobile applications, veterinarians can conduct remote consultations, assess health conditions, and offer preliminary diagnoses, thereby reducing the need for physical travel and enhancing overall pet care.

Digital platforms enable real-time monitoring and remote consultation for animals, reducing the need for frequent veterinary visits. Wearable sensors and IoT devices continuously collect data on an animal's vital signs, movement, and behavior, allowing early disease detection and intervention.

Advancements in telemedicine technologies have further enhanced veterinary practice by facilitating remote diagnosis and treatment modalities. Tools such as teleconsultations, tele triage, and telemonitoring enable veterinarians to evaluate health conditions, provide timely interventions, and monitor patient progress without the necessity for in-person visits. This not only improves access to veterinary expertise but also maintains high standards of care, especially in regions with limited access to veterinary services.

In equine care, telemedicine has revolutionized the approach to remote consultations, enhancing accessibility, efficiency, and quality of service. Studies have shown that telemedicine can significantly improve access to veterinary expertise, reduce travel-related stress for horses, and maintain high standards of care. However, challenges such as technological barriers and the need for physical examinations in certain cases must be addressed to fully realize the benefits of telemedicine in equine practice.

Blockchain for Veterinary Records and Supply Chain Transparency

Blockchain technology is enhancing the security and traceability of veterinary records and the animal health product supply chain. It ensures tamper-proof data storage for vaccinations, medical history, and treatment protocols, improving trust among stakeholders, including veterinarians, farmers, and pet owners.

Blockchain technology is increasingly being utilized to enhance veterinary records and supply chain transparency in the animal husbandry sector. By leveraging blockchain's decentralized, tamper-proof nature, veterinary professionals can securely store and share animal health records across different stakeholders, such as veterinarians, farmers, and animal care specialists. This ensures that medical histories, vaccinations, treatments, and other important data remain accurate, accessible, and resistant to tampering. Blockchain also facilitates real-time sharing of information, enabling faster decision-making and improving the efficiency of veterinary care.

In terms of supply chain transparency, blockchain is proving to be a game changer. Traditionally, the supply chain for veterinary products like medications, vaccines, and medical equipment has been opaque, leading to inefficiencies, delays, and even the risk of counterfeit products entering the market. Blockchain's ability to track each step of a product's journey—starting from production through to distribution—helps mitigate these risks by providing a transparent and immutable record of every transaction. This ensures that stakeholders have access to accurate, up-to-date information, which reduces the chances of fraud, improves accountability, and boosts confidence in the products being used.

Moreover, blockchain's integration with other technologies, such as the Internet of Things (IoT), further enhances supply chain management by enabling real-time monitoring of the condition and location of veterinary products. This allows for proactive management of inventory, reduces waste, and ensures that critical supplies are maintained at the right quality standards. Additionally, blockchain can be used to improve food traceability by recording every step of the animal product's journey, from farm to consumer, ensuring that any issues—such as contamination—can be traced back to their source quickly.

Overall, the integration of blockchain in veterinary records and supply chains is transforming the way animal health is managed and how veterinary products are tracked. It enhances data security, streamlines communication among stakeholders, and offers transparency and accountability throughout the process, all of which lead to improved efficiency, reduced fraud, and better outcomes in veterinary care and animal husbandry practices.

Artificial Intelligence in Veterinary Medicine

AI-Driven Diagnostics and Imaging

AI-powered tools are transforming veterinary diagnostics through advanced imaging techniques, automated radiograph analysis, and deep-learning algorithms for disease detection. AI applications in pathology, for instance, can analyze histopathological slides with higher accuracy and efficiency than traditional methods, aiding in the early detection of cancers and infectious diseases. Artificial intelligence (AI) is revolutionizing veterinary diagnostics and imaging, enhancing the accuracy and efficiency of disease detection and treatment planning. AI algorithms are now capable of analyzing complex imaging data—such as radiographs, MRIs, CT scans, and ultrasounds with remarkable speed and precision. This advancement enables veterinarians to identify abnormalities and diseases more effectively, leading to improved patient outcomes.

A recent study highlighted the integration of AI in veterinary diagnostic imaging, noting that machine learning techniques allow computer programs to analyze large imaging datasets and perform tasks relevant to veterinary diagnostics. The review emphasized the potential of AI to assist in workflow optimization, quality control, and image interpretation, thereby supporting both general practitioners and radiologists in delivering high-quality care.

Furthermore, AI is being utilized to automate tasks traditionally performed by veterinary professionals, such as counting mitotic figures in histopathology slides. The development of AI systems like OncoPetNet demonstrates the capability of deep learning models to perform real-time, expert-level analysis of histopathology images, thereby enhancing diagnostic accuracy and efficiency in veterinary practices.

Precision Livestock Farming (PLF)

PLF leverages AI, IoT, and machine learning to monitor animal health, behavior, and productivity. Smart sensors installed in barns and pastures continuously assess environmental conditions, feed intake, and movement patterns, allowing for real-time intervention in case of abnormalities. AI algorithms process this data to optimize nutrition, enhance reproductive performance, and reduce disease outbreaks. It integrates advanced technologies to monitor and manage livestock health, welfare, and productivity. A recent study conducted a global scientometric review of PLF research, revealing a significant increase in publications over recent years. The research primarily focuses on animal science, veterinary science, computer science, agricultural engineering, and environmental science.

Precision farming has also benefited greatly from Big Data. By collecting and analyzing data on feed, livestock health, and environmental conditions, farmers can optimize the nutrition and care provided to animals. For example, data analytics can help formulate the ideal diet for different animal breeds and ages, improving productivity and reducing feed costs. Environmental sensors also play a role in monitoring temperature, humidity, and air quality in barns and pastures, ensuring that livestock are kept in conditions conducive to their health and growth.

PLF technologies encompass a range of tools, including cameras, microphones, and sensors, to monitor individual animals or entire herds. These tools collect data on various parameters such as feed intake, weight gain, and health indicators. The data is then analyzed to inform management decisions, aiming to enhance productivity and animal welfare. For instance, automated weight detection cameras can calculate a pig's weight without the need for manual scales, offering a non-invasive method to monitor growth. Despite the advancements, the implementation of PLF faces challenges. A study identified twelve potential threats grouped into four categories: direct harm, indirect harm via the end-user, changes to housing and management, and ethical concerns. These challenges highlight the need for careful consideration of animal welfare and ethical implications when integrating PLF technologies into farming practices.

AI for Disease Prediction and Biosecurity

AI-based predictive models analyze vast datasets from global disease surveillance systems to forecast potential outbreaks of zoonotic diseases. Such predictive analytics help policymakers and veterinarians take proactive measures, thereby preventing large-scale animal health crises and ensuring food security.

Artificial Intelligence (AI) is revolutionizing veterinary medicine by enhancing disease prediction and bolstering biosecurity measures. AI algorithms analyze extensive datasets—including medical records, laboratory results, and imaging—to identify patterns indicative of diseases such as Addison's disease in dogs. For instance, researchers at the University of California, Davis, developed an AI-powered algorithm that detects complex patterns in routine blood tests, enabling early and accurate diagnosis of Addison's disease.

Beyond diagnostics, AI plays a pivotal role in biosecurity by predicting and preventing disease outbreaks. By continuously monitoring and analyzing data, AI systems can alert veterinarians to potential health issues, enabling prompt interventions. This proactive approach is crucial in managing infectious diseases and ensuring the health of both animals and humans.

Furthermore, AI aids in predictive modeling, assisting pathologists in anticipating disease progression based on patient history, lab results, and imaging. This capability enhances decision-making and treatment planning, leading to better outcomes for animals.

Challenges

Despite its transformative potential, the integration of digital health and AI in veterinary medicine faces several challenges:

Data Privacy and Security: The adoption of digital health tools and AI systems involves the collection and storage of vast amounts of sensitive data, including veterinary health records, farm management information, and animal welfare data. Ensuring the privacy and security of this data is crucial, as breaches could expose personal or confidential information about farmers, animals, and veterinary practices. For example, unauthorized access to a farm's livestock health records could lead to misuse or exploitation of the data There is a need for robust cybersecurity measures, encryption protocols, and compliance with data protection laws (e.g., GDPR) to safeguard this sensitive data. Additionally, rural farmers may lack the resources to implement such advanced security measures.

Cost and Accessibility: The cost of adopting AI and digital health solutions can be prohibitive, especially for small-scale farmers who may not have the financial capacity to invest in these technologies. For instance, installing automated diagnostic systems or AI-based monitoring tools can require substantial upfront investments in infrastructure and training. This could widen the gap between large-scale commercial operations, which can afford these technologies, and smaller, resource-limited farms, leading to disparities in access to advanced veterinary care and management tools. Ensuring that AI and digital health solutions are affordable and accessible to all farmers is a significant challenge.

Ethical Concerns: As AI systems become more involved in decision-making, there are concerns about over-reliance on technology, potentially at the expense of animal welfare. For example, AI might make decisions based purely on data patterns without considering the nuanced, holistic needs of individual animals. There's also the issue of reducing human involvement in critical care decisions, which can affect the quality of veterinary practice. The ethical dilemma arises from balancing the efficiency of AI systems with the compassion and judgment required in animal care. Ethical considerations also include whether animals might suffer from impersonal decision-making or whether technology might be used in ways that prioritize efficiency over animal well-being.

Technological Adoption: The introduction of digital tools and AI technologies into veterinary medicine requires veterinarians and farmers to learn new skills and adopt unfamiliar systems. This poses a challenge, particularly in rural or less tech-savvy areas where there may be resistance to adopting new technologies. Veterinarians may require specialized training to interpret AI outputs correctly and integrate digital health records into their practices. Similarly, farmers need to be trained on using devices for monitoring animal health or managing farm data. Overcoming this technological gap is vital to ensure that digital tools enhance veterinary practice rather than hinder it. Additionally, technical support and ongoing training are needed to ensure sustained adoption and effective use.

Each of these challenges requires careful consideration to ensure that the integration of AI and digital health in veterinary medicine is ethical, accessible, and beneficial for both animals and farmers.

Future of Animal Welfare in a Digital World

The future of animal welfare will be increasingly tied to digital health technologies and AI. By ensuring that these technologies are developed and implemented with both the welfare of animals and the needs of the farmers in mind, there is potential to achieve a more sustainable, efficient, and ethical system of animal care. As these technologies advance, they will complement the growing understanding of animal behavior and welfare needs. Additionally, the evolution of these technologies will pave the way for enhanced regulatory frameworks that ensure both animal health and welfare are continuously prioritized while navigating the complexities of digital innovation. AI systems could also be used to enforce regulations and ensure that ethical standards are being met across the industry.

References

Ali W., Ali M., Ahmad M., Dilawar S., Firdous A., Afzal A. (2020). – Application of modern techniques in animal production sector for human and animal welfare. Turk. J. Agric. Food Sci. Technol., 8 (2), 457–463. doi:10.24925/turjaf.v8i2.457-463.3159.

American Veterinary Medical Association (AVMA). (2021). The Use of Technology and AI in Veterinary Practice.

Brittany L. K. Miller, T. L. Lawrence, and R. R. Selvaraj. (2022). Advances in Veterinary Medicine and Animal Welfare. CRC Press.

Chesney, J., et al. (2020). "The future of animal welfare in a digital age: Ethical concerns and regulatory frameworks." Animal Welfare Journal, 29(4), 459-467.

Clark, M. P., and Zhang, X. (2019). "AI for animal welfare: Applications and future directions." Computers in Biology and Medicine, 117, 103551

Food and Agriculture Organization (FAO). (2020). The Role of AI in Livestock Health Management.

Food and Agriculture Organization of the United Nations (FAO) (2009). – How to Feed the World in 2050 [background document for the How to Feed the World High-level Expert Forum, 12-13 October 2009]. FAO, Rome, Italy, 35 pp. Available at: www.fao.org/fileadmin/templates/wsfs/docs/expert_paper/How_to_Feed_the_World_in_2050.pdf (accessed on 29 January 2025).

Food and Agriculture Organization of the United Nations (FAO) (2009). –The State of Food and Agriculture: Livestock in the balance. FAO, Rome, Italy, 180 pp. Available at: www.fao.org/3/i0680e/i0680e.pdf (accessed on 29 January 2025).

Food and Agriculture Organization of the United Nations (FAO) (2015). – The Second Report on the State of the World's Genetic Resources for Food and Agriculture (B.D. Shearf & D. Pilling, eds). FAO Commission on Genetic Resources for Food and Agriculture Assessment. FAO, Rome, Italy. Available at: www.fao.org/3/i4787e/i4787e00.pdf (accessed on 29 January 2025).

Grace D., Caminiti A., Torres G., Messori S., Bett B.K., Lee H.S., Roesel K. & Smith J. (2019). – How external factors (e.g. climate change, conflicts, socio-economics, trading patterns) will impact Veterinary Services and the adaptations required [technical item]. In 87th General Session of the World Organisation for Animal Health (OIE), Paris, France, 26–31 May 2019. OIE, Paris, France, 28 pp.

Göncü S. & Güngör C. (2018). – The Innovative Techniques in Animal Husbandry. In Animal Husbandry and Nutrition (B. Yucel, ed.). IntechOpen, London, United Kingdom. doi:10.5772/intechopen.72501.

International Veterinary Emergency and Critical Care Symposium (IVECCS). (2022). AI in Veterinary Medicine: Current Trends and Future Prospects.

Jiang B, Tang W, Cui L, Deng X. Precision Livestock Farming Research: A Global Scientometric Review. Animals (Basel). 2023 Jun 24;13(13):2096. doi: 10.3390/ani13132096. PMID: 37443894; PMCID: PMC10340063. Advancements in Telemedicine for Veterinary Care – Hilaris Publisher

M. S. N. R. A. Bandaranayake and S. P. S. P. L. Anthonypillai. (2021). Artificial Intelligence in Veterinary Science. Springer.

Organisation for Economic Cooperation and Development (OECD) (2019). – Digital technologies for better agricultural policies. OECD Publishing, Paris, France, 234 pp.

Santos, A. L., et al. (2021). "Artificial intelligence in veterinary medicine: Opportunities and challenges." Journal of Veterinary Science, 22(2), 101-109

Smith, T., and Kowalski, K. (2020). "Precision medicine for animals: Leveraging AI and genomics for individualized care." Veterinary Research Communications, 44(3), 273-283

Tedeschi L.O., Muir J.P., Riley D.G. & Fox. D.G. (2015). – The role of ruminant animals in sustainable livestock intensification programs. Int. J. Sustainable Dev. World Ecol., 22 (5), 452–465. doi:10.1080/13504509.2015.1075441.

The Rising Threat of Deadly Diseases Jumping from Animals to Humans- Financial Times

The Veterinarians Preventing the Next Pandemic-The New Yorker

Trendov N.M., Varas S. & Zeng M. (2019). – Digital technologies in agriculture and rural areas – Status report. Food and Agriculture Organization of the United Nations, Rome, Italy, 152 pp. Available at: www.fao.org/3/ca4985en/ca4985en.pdf (accessed on 29 January 2025).

United Nations Department of Economic and Social Affairs (UNDESA) Population Division (2017). – World population prospects: the 2017 revision, key findings and advance tables. Working Paper No. ESA/P/WP/248. UNDESA, New York, United States of America, 53 pp. Available at: https://population.un.org/wpp/Publications/Files/WPP2017_KeyFindings.pdf

Veterinarians Use Artificial Intelligence to Aid Diagnosis of Addison's Disease – University of California, Davis

What Is the Role of AI in Veterinary Pathology? Pathology News

World Animal Health Organization (OIE). (2020). Digital Tools in Veterinary Medicine: Advancements and Challenges.

World Economic Forum (2016). – The Future of Jobs: Employment, Skills and Workforce Strategy for the Fourth Industrial Revolution. Global Challenge Insight Report. World Economic Forum, Geneva, Switzerland, 167 pp. Available at: www3.weforum.org/docs/WEF_Future_of_Jobs.pdf (accessed on 29 January 2025).

World Health Organization (WHO). (2021). Digital Health Technologies: Enhancing Animal Health and Welfare.

Index